YOUR
PERIOD

NICOLE JARDIM

FIX YOUR PERIOD

Six Weeks to Life-Long

Hormone Balance

Vermilion
LONDON

1 3 5 7 9 10 8 6 4 2

Vermilion, an imprint of Ebury Publishing,
20 Vauxhall Bridge Road,
London SW1V 2SA

Vermilion is part of the Penguin Random House group of companies
whose addresses can be found at global.penguinrandomhouse.com

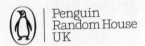

Penguin
Random House
UK

First published in the United Kingdom in 2020 by Vermilion
First published in the United States in 2020 by Harper Wave,
an imprint of HarperCollins Publishers LLC

www.penguin.co.uk

A CIP catalogue record for this book is available from the British Library

ISBN 9781785042560

Printed and bound in Great Britain by Clays Ltd, Elcograf S.p.A.

Penguin Random House is committed to a sustainable future for
our business, our readers and our planet. This book is made
from Forest Stewardship Council® certified paper.

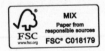

The information in this book has been compiled by way of general guidance in relation
to the specific subjects addressed. It is not a substitute and not to be relied on for medical,
healthcare, pharmaceutical or other professional advice on specific circumstances and
in specific locations. Please consult your GP before changing, stopping or starting
any medical treatment. So far as the author is aware the information given is correct
and up to date as at April 2020. Practice, laws and regulations all change, and the
reader should obtain up to date professional advice on any such issues. The author and
publishers disclaim, as far as the law allows, any liability arising directly or indirectly
from the use, or misuse, of the information contained in this book.

For Marguerite, Chantal, Albertine,
my grandmothers, and great-grandmothers

CONTENTS

PART III: LIVING LIKE A MENSTRUATION MAVEN

FOREWORD

Have you ever been told it's not polite to talk about your period? Or that you can talk about it, but only in your doctor's office? And heaven forbid you share your personal experience in your social circle, let alone on social media. Society's insidious message that the menstrual cycle is taboo for everyday conversation has left many women struggling, confused, and worried about whether what they're experiencing is normal.

Enter a new generation of women, who have started a movement of period positivity, normalising the conversation about women's health and reclaiming their periods with pride. Despite messaging that tells women they should feel ashamed and embarrassed about their monthly bleed, they've forged ahead. And indeed, their frankness in the face of stigma, shame, and social media censorship led *Newsweek* to proclaim 2015 "the Year of the Period."

This was quite a change from what we'd been seeing in the media, which painted a different picture of women's experiences with their cycles. Indeed, ads for menstrual care products have traditionally re-inforced this damaging anti-period rhetoric, portraying "that time of the month" as a shameful malady to be concealed and its symptoms as something to medicate away. Contrast this with the programming we're treated to in between the ads: one minute, you're watching a movie in which someone is being disemboweled, blood spraying everywhere; the next minute, the network cuts to a commercial where blood is considered taboo and a natural biological process is portrayed with images of blue liquid being poured onto pads to demonstrate their absorbency. (For the record, I've never seen any evidence that bright blue fluid is normal discharge from the female body, let alone the human body.)

Not anymore. Today, women throughout the world are redefining the social norms surrounding the menstrual cycle and demanding more open dialogue about what is inarguably one of the most important biological processes in the female body. Rather than feeling ashamed of their periods or their bodies, women are embracing this biological difference as a strength.

This new generation of women is picking up the torch that generations of women before them fought so hard to keep lit, even in the darkest days of medicine. After decades of doctors diagnosing us as hysterical and even telling us our periods didn't matter, this new generation of women has held up the torch to show us another way. Nicole Jardim, one of the many women lighting that path, says, "A woman's body isn't broken, and symptoms aren't its way of betraying you."

Despite what you've been told, problematic periods, mood swings, acne, premenstrual syndrome, and low libido are not "just a part of being female." While these experiences might be common, they are certainly *not* normal. They are your body's way of communicating with you, and given that you're reading this book, I suspect you're ready to listen.

In the pages that follow, you'll learn what those symptoms mean, what your body is trying to convey to you, and how to collect the data that will help you get the answers you need from your next visit to your GP. Let me be clear: this book is not asking you to go it alone, ditch your medications, abandon lab testing, or reject the advances of modern medicine. Instead, it is an invitation to get intimately acquainted with the body you live in, take ownership of your health, and understand how to work with your hormones. It is also designed to help you educate yourself so that you have more productive conversations with your healthcare provider and create an integrative approach to your cycle that serves your unique needs.

Like many people who find their calling in holistic health, Nicole's journey began with a desire to address her own health issues, which ranged from period problems to an autoimmune scare. In her early twenties, she took her issues to doctors, who suspected rheumatoid arthritis and other chronic conditions. Having been told there was no nutrition or lifestyle intervention that could help and that the best they could offer her was "watch and wait," she decided to take her healing into her own hands.

Within months, her symptoms began to disappear and her curiosity grew as she began working with her hormones, honouring how her body responded to different practices, and piecing together her period puzzle from her research. Upon healing herself, she made it her mission to help other women do the same. Nicole has spent years studying under the best women's health practitioners and mentoring with the top evidence-based functional medicine clinicians and countless hours learning and expanding her knowledge. It's been an unconventional path, yet one that has served thousands of women around the globe.

Nicole embraces what science has shown in recent years to be true: that bioindividuality is key to the healing journey. No two women's bodies are the same, and traditional medicine's one-size-fits-all approach has left many women feeling dissatisfied and struggling to make sense of why certain treatments don't help or why they are told their test results are "normal" when they feel anything but.

At the foundation of Nicole's message is the belief that we all experience our periods differently and that no one knows what's best for our bodies more than we do. Her mission is to give women the tools to become their own health advocates so they are no longer excluded from the discussion about their own bodies. She is truly a torchbearer for women's hormonal health, and by reading this book, you can now enjoy the light of that flame. Carry it with you and pass it along; you're now part of the menstrual movement!

In a world that gave public recognition to the period only in 2015, we have a long way to go. You can pay for parking with an app. You can use a credit card at a vending machine. Yet if you want to buy a tampon in a public loo, then you'd better have the right change. Yes, we are far from done in our work to end period shame and ensure that everyone who bleeds cyclically has access to the necessary information and products so they can menstruate with dignity. That work begins with knowing your body, understanding your cycle, and taking ownership of your health. With this book, Nicole will help you do just that.

I encourage you to speak your truth unapologetically. Your story has value. Sharing our stories helps us heal. And you'll never know who will be healed by hearing your story.

The way forward is together, and I'm so honoured to be on this journey with you!

—Dr Jolene Brighten, author of *Beyond the Pill* and
Healing Your Body Naturally After Childbirth

WHAT'S UP WITH YOUR PERIOD?

The Curse. Monthly Menace. Shark Week. On the Rag. Not very endearing euphemisms, are they? But I see why periods have received a bad rap. Bloating, pain, acne, moodiness, messiness—periods can and do suck. Most of us sacrifice a week or more out of every month to dealing with or anticipating our periods. And often they're not just an inconvenience, but a colossal disruption. Maybe you miss work, school, appointments, or dates because you're doubled over in pain and can't do much more than mainline paracetamol and clutch a hot-water bottle to your abdomen. You find yourself snapping at co-workers, partners, and friends; jeopardising relationships because of mood swings. You discover a constellation of acne on your face when you thought you'd left all that behind in secondary school. Your sex drive is AWOL, and as far as feeling sexy is concerned, you may as well keep the period underpants on permanent rotation and leave the lacy lingerie buried in the drawer. You're tired during the day and try to energise yourself with copious amounts of caffeine and sugar—oh, the cravings!—and then you're plagued with insomnia. Or maybe you have a period that is so irregular or totally absent, and you can't predict when it will appear again.

"Something's gotta change," you say to yourself each month, but when you do seek the help of a doctor for relief from these hideous symptoms, you're told that going on the Pill is the only solution. This magic drug will even out your hormonal imbalance, and everything will be right as rain. Fake hormones will fix what's happening with your real hormones, right? *Wrong!*

If all this sounds familiar, I want you to know you're not alone, that you don't need to struggle with the physical and emotional symptoms of your period every month, and that synthetic hormones are definitely not always the answer.

When it comes to all things menstrual cycle-related, medical professionals often tell us that our symptoms (e.g. moodiness, brain fog, fatigue, fertility struggles, and low libido) are normal, or are a natural response to getting older. Nothing to worry about.

With all due respect to those medical professionals, that's bullshit.

Suffering related to your menstrual cycle is unnecessary and most definitely *not* normal. It's *statistically* normal perhaps—for instance, between 45 and 95 per cent of women have painful periods, and 10 to 25 per cent require medication and time off from daily activities[1]—but I promise you that's not the way your body was designed, and it's not the way it has to be. You are not supposed to be doubled over in pain every month or go through multiple tampons or pads before you can even get out the door for work. You're not supposed to constantly wonder when your next period will arrive or live in a perpetual state of fear that every month you'll fall apart the week before your period.

One of the biggest myths perpetuated on women today is that our menstrual issues are not fixable. They are. Still, we don't need a great deal of medical intervention to be healthy, and we certainly don't need to medicate our cycles with various forms of hormonal birth control and other drugs. What we do need is a more comprehensive understanding of how our bodies function so we can discern what they're telling us and know how to give them what they need.

The reality is that you can naturally improve how you experience your period every month. While we've been told forever that periods suck, I've dedicated my career to showing women that they don't have to. Through my private and group coaching programmes, e-courses, my blog, and top-rated podcast, *The Period Party*, I've helped tens of thousands of women around the world cultivate deeper respect for and understanding of their menstrual cycles and the role their hormones play in their health.

HORMONES ARE THE KEY

When it comes to period problems, it's important to know three things:

1. Your body and your menstrual cycle are not as complicated as you have been led to believe.
2. Hormones, your body's chemical messengers, interact with one another all day long and are responsible for almost everything that happens in your body.
3. Your menstrual cycle is governed by a few key hormones (oestrogen, progesterone, and testosterone), and the symptoms you're experiencing right now are probably linked to an imbalance among them.

The thing is, hormones don't just kick in when you're going through puberty or menopause. In addition to menstruation, they play a role in almost every bodily function, which is why we tend to feel pretty terrible physically and emotionally when they're imbalanced.

Hormones have received a bad rap when it comes to periods:

"Oh, she's so hormonal!"

"It must be that time of the month!"

"Puberty sucks!"

"Why can't I stop crying?"

"Ugh, I'm being so bitchy!"

"Menopause is a nightmare!"

I could go on, but you get the gist. Hormones' reputation as disrupters of our moods and health may be deserved, but the real deal is that it is often hormone *imbalance* that is the root cause of painful periods, amenorrhoea, polycystic ovary syndrome (PCOS), premenstrual syndrome (PMS), endometriosis, and other woes. Women who struggle with issues related to their periods don't always connect their problems with hormones or hormone imbalance, but they should. The fact is if we get those hormones under control, we can lessen and, in some cases, even resolve our pesky period problems and other related symptoms.

Poor diet, irregular sleep habits, chronic stress, and overexposure to environmental toxins all have a significant impact on hormonal health. Our reproductive organs are usually the first to let us know that there is something wrong, but rather than medicate away these symptoms, it is important to identify and treat the underlying causes of the hormone imbalance. By investigating your health holistically and making simple lifestyle adjustments, you can rebalance your hormones, and those unwanted symptoms will abate naturally, both as a sign and as a side effect of your getting healthier.

A NEW WAY TO THINK ABOUT YOUR PERIOD

Each month, your body tries to tell you something about your health. PMS, a heavy period, no period—whatever you're experiencing isn't the result of your body randomly rebelling against you. Rather, these issues are your body's way of communicating with you. Just as a fever is a sign of infection, your period problems are a sign of your body needing attention. Your body is always working for you, not against you. As with a fever or a sore throat, your period symptoms are your body's way of telling you what's happening inside—only, it's speaking a language many of us have never learned.

I first heard the term *body literacy* from renowned writer and women's health critic Laura Wershler. She came up with the concept after reading a novel that got her thinking about how illiteracy and a lack of education disempowers women and girls all over this planet. She was struck by the fact that women in the West struggle with another kind of illiteracy: We are not taught to "read" our own bodies. In fact, we are taught to distrust and even fear them. How many times have you ignored your symptoms because you were told they were a normal part of being a woman? That's especially true of our periods. According to Wershler, body literacy "is acquired by learning to observe, chart, and interpret our menstrual cycle events" so that we're able to understand how our total health and wellness are connected to our cycles.

Inspired by Wershler, I decided to make "period literacy" the first thing I spoke about with clients in my own practice. As a certified women's health coach with a speciality in hormonal and menstrual health—heck, I'm known online as "the Period Girl"!—I knew that if my clients were not aware of how their bodies worked, or were scared of how they worked, they would not be able to make the best decisions for their own unique period challenges. And now, with this book, I want to help you recognise the various signs and symptoms linked to your menstrual cycle and be better able to interpret what they're telling you about what's going on "under the hood": what's working well and what needs some attention. When it comes to our overall health, our periods hold a lot of answers. Unlock those answers, and you unlock your power. When you become period literate, you'll know *why*, for example, you're experiencing an irregular, long, or heavy period and will be able to make informed decisions about how to address that issue.

Becoming period literate changed my life. At fourteen, I found that my periods were getting heavier and heavier—a situation that culminated in one of those mortifying accidents at school. I was wearing a tampon, a pad, and shorts under my school uniform, and I still sprung a leak! It went all the way through my dress. I distinctly remember pretty much wanting to leave the planet. Another time,

I was visiting friends in New York City when I experienced what is known as flooding: I was changing tampons and pads every thirty minutes. I mean, when you miss your train because you're bleeding through all your clothes in the loo in Grand Central Station, you know you have a problem.

Not only was my period ridiculously heavy each month, but it was also incredibly painful, the kind of pain that made me see stars. And the pain became more and more excruciating as time went on. Each month, I'd miss a day or two of school; and when I had to attend for an obligatory event or test, I'd take a handful of ibuprofen and power through. It was awful.

Then my period started to show up days or weeks late. Eventually, it was coming every two or three months. At first this seemed like an improvement—except that when it finally made an appearance, it arrived with a vengeance. All my friends seemed to have similar period problems, and because this was normal for my mum during her teen years, too, I just assumed it was also my normal.

Because no one sounded the alarm, it went on like this for about three years, until I finally saw a gynaecologist. Hope and potential relief at last! I sat down across from her and explained all my symptoms in great detail. She didn't give me an explanation, but instead pulled out her pad and wrote a prescription for the birth control pill to "fix" my period problems.

Finally! I was thrilled to be joining the ranks of my super cool pill-popping friends. I knew from them that this magic pill would give me my life back. No more missing school, parties, and dates because I was too incapacitated to get out of bed. And indeed, during my next period, I didn't have many of the symptoms I'd been experiencing for so many years: my pain was considerably reduced, my flow was significantly lighter, and I wasn't about to pass out from exhaustion. I was overjoyed. I'd found my period panacea.

Fast-forward a few years. While I was no longer having any issues with my period—I was bleeding for a grand total of only one day each month—new symptoms started cropping up, ranging from thinning hair and excruciating joint pain to chronic yeast infections.

I was twenty years old and a hot mess express. None of the dozens of specialists I visited could figure out what was wrong with me, even after extensive (and expensive) tests. Much like my gynaecologist, all they did was jot down a prescription for pain pills, antibiotics, and other treatments that never really worked. It wasn't until a fortuitous visit to my friend's acupuncturist that I got some answers and learned that my not-so-healthy diet and lifestyle habits combined with my years on the Pill were messing up my hormones and wrecking my health.

I had seen so many different doctors for all my seemingly unrelated ailments, and not one of them had ever said that the birth control pill could be linked to, much less cause, any of them. But my acupuncturist nailed it: to get well, I had to fix my hormones. With his help, I tried resolving my symptoms by ditching the Pill and overhauling my diet, exercise, sleep habits, and stress management. And you know what? After some trial and error, this approach worked. And when my period came back after coming off the Pill, it was totally manageable.

My period panacea was not the Pill after all. Rather, it was a holistic, whole-body approach. Yes, it required a great deal of patience, self-compassion, and experimentation, but I got my life back—and you can, too.

My experience inspired me to show others how to approach their health in this same way. You can absolutely fix your period problems without the use of the Pill. If you're struggling with painful or heavy periods, PMS or PMDD (premenstrual dysphoric disorder), or irregular or missing periods, the programme in this book will help you balance your hormones and correct these common period problems. If you're trying to get pregnant or are interested in optimising your fertility for when you may want to get pregnant later on, you'll benefit from this programme, too. Most of the clients I work with are cisgender women—however, I recognise that not all women menstruate and not everyone who has a uterus and menstruates identifies as a woman. This programme is designed for *anyone* with a menstrual cycle in their twenties, thirties, or early forties who wants to address the root causes of their issues in a natural way. They're tired of using synthetic hormones that they feel inadequately address their symptoms and, in many cases, mess up their natural hormones even more. By the time they come to me, many have stopped using hormonal birth control such as the Pill, patch, vaginal ring, shot, injection, implant, or hormonal IUD.

Getting off hormonal birth control is really the first step in balancing your hormones naturally. (For more on why this is so, see "So, I *Can't* Take a Pill for That?" below) If you stay on the Pill or another form of hormonal birth control while following this programme, you will feel better—for example, you'll probably have better digestion and better moods—but you won't be able to balance your hormones. It's simply not possible to balance your hormones while taking synthetic hormones designed to create imbalance. Yes, I know: it can be scary to change your birth control, but you have several excellent natural options (see Chapter 12), and I encourage you to consider them.

SO, I *CAN'T* TAKE A PILL FOR THAT?

Like me, you may have been prescribed the birth control pill to "fix" your period problems. You're not alone: 58 per cent of American women who are on the Pill take it for reasons other than preventing pregnancy.[2] That's right. Every month more than half of the women who take the Pill do so because they have menstrual cycle-related symptoms that are so disruptive that they need a powerful synthetic hormonal cocktail to address them. Why? In the mid-1980s, when direct-to-consumer marketing of prescription medication became legal in the US, pharmaceutical companies started promoting their contraceptives as more than birth control. They became so-called lifestyle drugs, marketed to improve a person's quality of life by treating conditions that were not as serious as preventing pregnancy.[3] Typically, these conditions included acne, PMS or PMDD, missing periods, heavy periods, and painful periods. In addition, something I hear a lot is that the Pill can be used for "period regulation." This drives me crazy. The Pill most definitely does not regulate a period. And this goes for other forms of hormonal contraceptives, too (the patch, IUD, vaginal ring, implant, and the contraceptive injection (in the UK, for instance, this could be Depo Provera or Noristerat)).

Here's what the Pill and these other forms of hormonal birth control *actually* do: they stop you from ovulating.[4] No ovulation, no natural hormone changes, no more period problems. But there's a catch: because your body is no longer going through its natural monthly cycle of hormone production, you are no longer producing sufficient amounts of sex hormones, which support your mood, libido, vaginal lubrication, and bone health. As you can see, these natural hormones control many of our body's major systems; no wonder the side effects of hormonal birth control are so wide-ranging: from migraines, acne, and mood swings to irregular bleeding, weight gain, low libido, and depression.[5]

And I've got news for you: that bleeding you experience during the days you take the placebo (sugar) pills is not a real period because you never ovulated. It's what's known as a "withdrawal bleed" or "pill bleed," and it occurs only because your hormone levels drop enough to cause your uterine lining to shed. Again: no ovulation, no period.

The straight truth is that the Pill and other hormonal birth control methods override your body's natural processes and merely mask any underlying hormonal imbalance. While on the Pill, no woman's body is capable of functioning at its optimal level. This is why the Pill will never be an actual fix for your period problems, but rather, a temporary sticking plaster that will hide what's actually going on under the surface.

So, if you're using any kind of hormonal birth control for your period problems, I encourage you to consider whether it is the right choice for you. I know going off the Pill is a big decision. You may be afraid your symptoms will come back. Or perhaps you're worried about being able to find an effective alternative form of birth control. These are important things to consider, and the decision should not be made lightly. Only you can decide the best way to support your health, and I hope the information I share in this book will help you make that decision.

YOU ARE IN CONTROL

If you want any of your period-related discomfort to change, you must first make a decision. You must decide that you have what it takes to attain a normal, healthy—and dare I say happy?—period. Trust me. You do.

Unfortunately, our current healthcare model is designed in such a way that the woman suffering from menstruation-related symptoms is often taken out of the equation of her own healing. When she is diagnosed (usually based on a set of generic guidelines) and provided with a treatment plan, her unique biology and lifestyle are hardly ever taken into consideration. This approach to women's health is obviously a huge problem and has resulted in the one-size-fits-all course of treatment. But just as no two women are alike, no two menstrual cycles are alike, and what is normal for one woman is not likely normal for the next.

Anyway, outsourcing your healthcare hardly ever works. You know what is best for your body, not anyone else. You don't have to give your power away to doctors; you can be your own health advocate. Yes, health professionals can help—I'm one!—but no one else can give you your health back. Your well-being is a gift you must give yourself. But in order to be empowered on your health journey, you have to educate yourself. And making yourself familiar with your period health will make you a key player in solving your period-related issues. I passionately believe that *all* women can (and should) be active participants in supporting, improving, and maintaining their health, and I'm dedicated to showing you how to put yourself in the driver's seat, starting today.

HOW TO USE THIS BOOK TO FIX YOUR PERIOD

While I can't do the work for you, I can give you the right set of tools and information to empower you to take a closer look at your diet, stress levels, gut health, sleep patterns, and genetics to find the source of your period problems. This book will give you access to the most up-to-date, research-backed information and provide lots of practical steps you can take to put yourself back in the driver's seat and put your period problems in the rearview mirror.

A note about the language used in this book. While I often make references to "women" or "females" throughout the text, I recognise that not everyone who menstruates identifies as a woman—trans men and non-binary folks get periods, too, and can benefit from the recommendations in this book. Ultimately, I want anyone who menstruates to be included in the conversation and in the decisions involving their own healthcare.

Like a grown-up version of "the talk," the first part, "Mapping the Menstrual Cycle: How It All Works," is a road map that leads you through your menstrual cycle from start to finish, so you are no longer guessing or mystified by how your hormones impact your health. But this is more than just a book about the mechanics of menstruation.

Part 2, "Six Weeks to Fix Your Period," guides you through the Fix Your Period programme to address the root causes of your menstruation-related symptoms, rather than just spot-treating them. It will not only give you information on the importance of your period but also transform you into a full-fledged menstruation maven by providing you with natural, healthy solutions to your period problems.

Each week of the programme covers a key contributor to hormonal balance, digs into the role it plays in your period problems, and tells you everything you need to know for your body to run optimally. The protocol for each week includes specific diet and lifestyle changes you can make right now to start moving the needle on your health in a big way.

By the end of week six, as good habits are carried forwards week by week, you'll have a revamped lifestyle optimised for hormonal balance and the opportunity to experience a pain-free, regular period accompanied by fewer mood swings and more energy.

You may be tempted to skip straight to the week that speaks to you the most or to dig through the book looking for a to-do list for your particular situation. Here's the thing: no matter what your symptoms or condition, you will benefit the most by completing the programme in the way I've presented it. Your brain and endocrine glands talk to each other via hormones, and this programme is designed to reopen those channels of communication and keep the conversation flowing. And favouring one voice, one hormone, over another won't yield the long-term results I know you're looking for.

Part 3 is the final piece of the period puzzle, syncing everything into hormonal harmony and showing you how to live in accordance with your cycle. You'll be working smarter, sleeping better, feeling more amazing than ever before, and living a more audacious life.

Make sure to head to fixyourperiod.com to download the accompanying workbook to use in conjunction with the programme. In the appendices, you'll find additional resources, including quick and easy recipes to follow during the six-week programme and beyond; information on hormone testing; and lists of books, websites, and products to support you on your hormone-healing journey. And be sure to check out appendix C for the supplement brands I recommend.

When you follow the advice in this book, you'll have better periods and, perhaps most important, you will have reclaimed an essential part of yourself: the ability to navigate your hormonal landscape and your cycle in a way that you may never have thought possible or didn't even know existed. You *can* be healthy and rewrite your period story.

PART I

MAPPING THE MENSTRUAL CYCLE: HOW IT ALL WORKS

PERIODS 101

GET TO KNOW YOUR FLOW

In those medical dramas on TV, the doctors and nurses say things like "We have to monitor the patient's vitals." What they mean is they have to make sure the patient's heart rate, respiratory rate, blood pressure, and body temperature (the four established vital signs) are within the healthy range for him or her to stay alive. Well, your period is a vital sign, too, of your overall health.

Back in 2005, the Society for Menstrual Cycle Research—yes, this research body exists—co-sponsored a scientific forum called "The Menstrual Cycle Is a Vital Sign." Ten years later, in 2015, the American College of Obstetricians and Gynaecologists released a report on girls and adolescents which acknowledged that menstruation should be recognised as a vital sign.[1] But despite this progress, period-related issues are still often dismissed as the unfortunate consequence of being a woman—as if high blood pressure was the unfortunate consequence of having a heart. There are positive signs that this is changing, but until it does, it's imperative that women take back ownership of their health with the understanding that their menstrual cycle is a barometer of their health. Congratulations for being one of these women!

Ovulation—or, more important, *regular* ovulation—is a sign of health and fertility.[2] (Believe it or not, your body's ultimate goal each month is pregnancy.) Ovulation that occurs on a consistent basis is the driver for sufficient levels of oestradiol (the body's most potent form of oestrogen) and progesterone, the two key female sex hormones. While these two hormones are known mostly for their role in the menstrual cycle and childbearing, they play significant roles in other bodily functions, too. In fact, oestrogen makes sure your heart and blood vessels are working well,[3] progesterone can protect your breasts and uterus from cancer,[4] and both are essential to keeping your bones strong[5] and your brain working optimally. (No brain fog or mood swings here!)[6]

As you can see, a number of body systems are impacted by the same hormones that control our menstrual cycle. So, if the menstrual cycle is not functioning within what are considered "normal" parameters, our overall health is at risk. That's right. Your period is a marker for general well-being, underlying medical conditions, and even chronic disease states.[7] Think of it as your body's early-warning system: it will sound the alarm if your body needs attention.

For instance, irregular periods (i.e. periods that don't arrive consistently every 25 to 35 days) could indicate that your body is under too much stress or there is a nutrient deficiency.[8] Painful periods, especially the ones that leave you in the foetal position on the bathroom floor, could be a sign of system-wide inflammation, pelvic floor dysfunction, or even endometriosis.[9] Heavy periods could be linked to fibroids, adenomyosis (tissue similar to that of the uterine lining that grows into the muscular wall of the uterus, causing it to thicken), or even low thyroid function.[10] Missing periods mean you're not ovulating, and thus not making the sex hormones you need each month to build your endometrium (the lining of the uterus) and subsequently shed it.[11] These period problems should never be ignored or dismissed as "normal." That said, the early-warning system won't help you if you don't know how to interpret its signals, so it's crucial that you understand how a period should work.

There is no perfect period, and periods are not the same for everyone. Your period is a reflection of your genetics, lifestyle, and overall health, which means there is a lot of variation out there. I want you to know how *your* cycle is intended to work, why it works that way, and what can influence it. By getting comfortable with your cycle, you'll have a better idea of what's going on in your body and what your symptoms are telling you. So, let's take it from the top. Don't worry. This is going to be a lot more interesting than the cringe-worthy sex talk you had with your mum when you were a pre-teen.

THE FOUR PHASES OF YOUR MENSTRUAL CYCLE

Female bodies are cyclical by nature, producing varying quantities of hormones at different points in our monthly menstrual cycle— namely, oestrogen, progesterone, and testosterone. (See Figure 1, page 6.) Other hormones, such as follicle-stimulating hormone (FSH), luteinising hormone (LH), anti-Müllerian hormone (AMH), prolactin, oxytocin, and cortisol; and neurotransmitters such as serotonin, epinephrine, and dopamine, also fluctuate. And the whole point? To get you pregnant.

We'll get into the nitty-gritty of these hormones in a minute, but for now it's enough to know that they are responsible for four distinct phases of the menstrual cycle. As in the natural world, our bodies are constantly ebbing and flowing, and each phase of the monthly cycle brings about significant physical and emotional changes; for women who are getting their period every 25 to 35 days, this occurs on an almost weekly basis.

Mastering your internal rhythms is the key to feeling more connected to your body and the first step to solving a lot of the physical and emotional complaints associated with your cycle. This knowledge will help prepare you for your own natural ebbs and flows and will provide important clues about whether your hormones are functioning the way they are supposed to in the various phases.

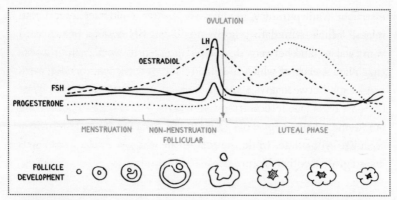

Figure 1: The four phrases of the menstrual cycle, the main hormones involved, and the stages of follicle development

Phase 1: The Bleeding Phase (Menstruation)

You may have been taught that your menstrual cycle ends with your period, but actually, day 1 of your menstrual cycle is the first day of bleeding. On average, the bleeding phase lasts for 3 to 7 days. Right before your period, your progesterone level plunges, causing the breakdown and shedding of your uterine lining. As menstruation gets under way, your key female sex hormones, oestrogen and progesterone, are at the lowest they will be in your entire cycle, with progesterone staying low until after ovulation.

When menstruation starts, the proverbial floodgates open, and you likely feel a sense of release and even relief after the anxiety or feelings of anticipation you felt leading up to it. During this week, you may feel tired, withdrawn, introspective, and emotionally vulnerable.

Your cervix, the cylindrical-shaped tissue that connects the vagina and uterus, changes position throughout your cycle. In this first phase, it is firm to the touch, sort of like the tip of your nose; in a low position; and slightly open to allow menstrual blood to pass through.

The bleeding phase also marks the first half of the follicular phase, during which a region of your brain known as the hypothalamus secretes gonadotropin-releasing hormone (GnRH), which instructs your pituitary gland (the "master endocrine gland") to release follicle-stimulating hormone. This FSH communicates with your ovaries, and between days 1 and 4, it recruits a handful of ovarian follicles, each of which is a little balloon-like sac that contains a single egg. Between days 5 and 7, just as menstruation is wrapping up for most of us, one follicle from the selected group is chosen. It's kind of like the *Hunger Games* of egg selection, because only one follicle is recruited to ovulate, while the rest of the follicles in the group will disintegrate. Mother Nature doesn't play around!

Phase 2: The Follicular Phase

Next, we move into the non-menstruation half of the follicular phase, which is the time in the menstrual cycle when the ovaries continue preparing for the big *O*—ovulation, that is, not orgasm, but let's hope you're having orgasms during that time, too!

The maturing follicles produce oestradiol in increasing amounts. Around day 8 of the menstrual cycle, or halfway through the follicular phase, that chosen follicle from the group starts to flex its muscles and dominate—thanks to the inhibitory effect of anti-Müllerian hormone on the others.[12] As oestradiol continues its ascent, it signals the brain to slow down FSH production and crank up luteinising hormone production by the pituitary gland. Rising LH stimulates production of androstenedione and testosterone (male sex hormones), which play a supporting role in the act of ovulation.

As ovulation approaches, oestrogen also prepares the uterus for pregnancy, thickening the blood vessels of the uterine lining. The cervix gradually moves higher in the vaginal canal and opens. Cervical fluid is pretty non-existent the first few days after menstruation. Then, as oestrogen builds and stimulates the cervix, cervical fluid begins to take on a wetter consistency, often looking pasty, creamy, or like lotion. You are most fertile in the second half of the follicular phase leading up to ovulation, and a barrier method of birth control should be used then if you are not planning to get pregnant.

Phase 3: The Ovulatory Phase

Contrary to popular belief, ovulation, not menstruation, is the star of the menstrual cycle show. As Dr Lara Briden, author of *Period Repair Manual*, says, "Ovulation is how we make hormones." The ovulatory phase is the shortest phase, but it's the one that packs the biggest hormonal punch. It is the culmination of all the hard work your body has been doing throughout the follicular phase.

During this phase, oestradiol levels rise in parallel to the size of the maturing dominant follicle.[13] Increasingly high levels of oestradiol tell the hypothalamus to trigger the mid-cycle LH surge that is needed to initiate ovulation. Then, right before the LH surge, the oestradiol level falls, which is often the cause of mid-cycle/ovulatory spotting. LH and progesterone increase levels of prostaglandins and proteolytic enzymes, which are responsible for weakening the walls of the follicle, so the egg can more easily get out.[14]

In a remarkably short period of time—the ovulatory process is only twenty-four to forty-eight hours long—this complicated dance of LH, FSH, oestradiol, and progesterone results in an egg bursting out of the follicle on the ovarian surface and into the peritoneal cavity, where it is ushered into a fallopian tube by the fimbriae (finger-like projections on the tubes) and pushed along towards the uterus. Once an egg is released, it survives for twelve to twenty-four hours. (Within that window, another egg could be released. That second egg will also survive for twelve to twenty-four hours. If both are fertilised, this can result in fraternal twins.) The egg will either be fertilised on its journey through the fallopian tube by a sperm cell or it will disintegrate.[15] The remainder of the follicle then becomes a temporary endocrine gland called the corpus luteum, which is an important player in the next and final phase.

Fun fact: ovulation occurs randomly from either ovary on any given cycle, but some studies have indicated that ovulation occurs more frequently from the right ovary and that ovulation on the right side has a higher potential for pregnancy.[16]

At this point, your cervix becomes soft, moves up higher in the vaginal canal, and opens. This positioning helps your released egg get the best (strongest, healthiest) sperm, as those sperm will have to swim further to get to the cervix, where they take a pitstop and then move on in their quest to reach the released egg.

In preparation for the sperm, your cervical fluid transforms into what is known as fertile-quality cervical fluid, becoming clear (translucent) and viscous (think raw egg white) and highly elastic or very wet and watery. When looked at under a microscope, the fluid will contain channels that help sperm swim up through the cervix. Fertile-quality cervical fluid nourishes the sperm, protects them from the vagina's natural acidity, and guides them towards the egg.[17]

Phase 4: The Luteal Phase

This phase typically ranges from 11 to 17 days but is about 12 to 14 days in most women.[18] The length of the luteal phase is based entirely on how long the corpus luteum (the follicle that released the egg) maintains its progesterone production.

After ovulation, FSH and LH levels decline, with LH remaining low for the rest of the cycle and FSH rising slightly before menstruation to get the next round of follicles ready.[19] Oestrogen continues its sharp decline, while progesterone continues its climb thanks to the corpus luteum's progesterone output.[20] Progesterone will stay high throughout the luteal phase.

Progesterone is a thermogenic, or heat-inducing, hormone: it raises your basal body temperature for the remainder of the luteal phase. This rise in temperature is an important indicator of whether you've ovulated.[21] Progesterone also further prepares the endometrium for a possible pregnancy. It transforms cervical fluid from stretchy and wet to opaque and sticky, or less fluid-like. If examined under a microscope, it would appear to have a basket-weave texture, which serves as your vagina's very own sperm barrier. This is why it is referred to as infertile cervical fluid, as it's particularly hard for sperm to swim through it at this stage.

During the second week of the luteal phase, oestrogen makes one more appearance, in a last-ditch effort to further prep your body for pregnancy. Due to the higher oestrogen, you may notice an increase in cervical fluid resembling that seen in the lead-up to ovulation. (Don't worry, this is not fertile-quality cervical fluid, so you can't get pregnant.) You might also find you've got increased energy, and a sex drive might blow in from nowhere. This is very exciting for those of us who struggle with PMS symptoms, as sex is often the last thing on our minds during this time!

If the egg is fertilised, it starts producing human chorionic gonadotrophin (hCG) hormone and continues to make its way down the fallopian tube to the uterus. The hCG will signal the corpus luteum to keep making progesterone as well as oestrogen, to support a pregnancy in its early stages.

If there is no pregnancy, the corpus luteum function begins to decline at about 9 to 11 days after ovulation.[22] The drop in oestrogen and progesterone that follows will tell the uterine lining it's time to go.

Whew! Isn't your body remarkable? I mean, no juggler in the world could keep so many balls in the air at one time. It's easy to see how the slightest miscue could lead to a collapse of the system and the rise of period problems. But just because our cycles are intricate does not mean nurturing them is complicated. You don't need to learn to juggle to have a healthy menstrual cycle; you just need to give it the support it needs and then kick back and watch the show. If your symptoms are a real slog, you might not be as excited about this hormonal juggling act as I am, but keep reading, because everything is about to change for you.

WHAT IS MY PERIOD SUPPOSED TO BE LIKE?

Now that you know what's going on inside your body throughout your menstrual cycle, you probably want to get clued in to what a period should look like. Over the years, I have received a bazillion questions from women about the nature of their periods, ranging from "How long should my period be?" and "Is it normal to spot before or after my period?" to "What should my period blood look like?" and "Are clots just a part of having a period?"

Remember the days of Sex Ed? Or, more important, remember what you learned in those classes? Yeah, I don't, either! I went to a Catholic secondary school, so my Sex Ed class was called Christian Family Life Education. CFLE class consisted of discussions on why we shouldn't have sex. It was, for obvious reasons, of little use to me or my classmates. I certainly wasn't getting the answers to any of my burning questions, and I'm willing to bet you didn't either.

That's probably why I've been asked these questions and variations on them *a lot* over the years. So, I'm going to walk you through an ideal cycle. Knowing what one looks like will help you establish your menstrual baseline and get a sense of the type of cycle you should be working towards.

What Is a Period, Anyway?

Women are often confused by the terms *period* and *menstrual cycle*. Your menstrual cycle is the entire cycle, from day 1 of bleeding to the last day before your next bleed. The term *period* is used to describe vaginal bleeding that lasts roughly 3 to 5 days and occurs approximately every 28 days. But the thing is, unless ovulation has occurred prior to the bleed, you're not having an actual period.

Whoa, what?

Yup. A true period is always preceded by ovulation. This is important, so let me say it again: a true period is *always* preceded by ovulation. If you're not ovulating, then you're experiencing what is known as an anovulatory cycle. In this case, none of the steps I describe in the previous section occur, and instead, you experience a kind of ongoing follicular phase without the rise of progesterone that normally follows ovulation. Some of us may skip a period because of this, while others will have a bleed. If you experience a bleed, the only way you'll know you had an anovulatory cycle is if you've been tracking your cervical fluid patterns and basal body temperature, which are signs of fertility.

Do I Need to Have a Period?

So, all this raises the question "Why do so many doctors maintain that we don't need to have a period?" Yup, you've probably heard that having a period is not necessary. I'll never forget seeing those ads back in the day for Seasonique (in the US), an extended-cycle birth control pill that gives you four periods a year, and thinking there was something wrong with that picture. I don't know about you, but no matter how far we've come in the field of medicine, I just can't wrap my head around the idea that artificially suppressing your period for months at a time is a good idea.

So many times I've heard "But, Nicole, my doctor says it's fine, and I've read articles written by other doctors that tell me it's totally okay, too."[23] It's true. Many doctors and healthcare practitioners don't believe a period is physically necessary. Well, I disagree. Having a healthy menstrual cycle is necessary, and a regular period is part of the deal.

How Long Should My Menstrual Cycle Be?

The length of your cycle is the number of days between periods, including the first day of your period until the day before your next period starts. The average length of a cycle is 29 days.[24] This is determined by the length of your follicular phase and the day you ovulate. Let's say you ovulate on day 15 of your cycle. Then your period would be expected to come anywhere from 11 to 17 days after that, depending on the health of your corpus luteum.[25]

There is a persistent belief that each and every menstrual cycle should be 28 days long, with ovulation occurring on day 14. A quick Google search for "How long should my menstrual cycle be?" will bring up dozens of results reinforcing this idea.

This is possibly due to the notion that before artificial light took over our world many women ovulated with the full moon and menstruated on the new moon (the moon cycle is 29.5 days long). Well, things have changed a fair bit since then. Nowadays, very few women have a consistent 28-day cycle.

And, if you think about it, the rhythm method—a calendar-based method of birth control developed in the early 1900s, which asserts that menstrual cycles are 28 days long with ovulation occurring about 14 days before the next period—has contributed to this misconception (pardon the pun). Additionally, the widespread use of the birth control pill since the 1960s, with its monthly dose of 28 neatly packaged pills to give you that "perfect" 28-day cycle and 5 to 7 days of bleeding, is likely skewing the data. Whatever the reason, the myth of a 28-day cycle with ovulation occurring precisely on day 14 is just that, a myth.

Practitioners differ regarding what constitutes a normal menstrual cycle length, with studies showing that a healthy cycle can fall within the range of 21 to 35 days.[26] However, in my professional experience, a 25- to 35-day cycle is ideal for optimal hormone health and fertility. Women I've worked with over the years with cycles shorter than 24 days tend to have lower progesterone or excess oestrogen and too-short luteal phases, which can impair their ability to get pregnant. So, while these shorter cycles might technically be considered "healthy," remember that fertility and menstrual health are intricately tied together. While pregnancy might not be *your* endgame, it is your *body's*, and a truly healthy cycle is one that gives your body a chance to reach this goal. In my experience, this is achieved with a 25- to 35-day cycle.

Regarding ovulation, contrary to the myth of the perfect day-14 egg release, ovulation actually changes from cycle to cycle. This fluctuation depends on a variety of factors, which we'll get to, but I like to see ovulation occur between days 12 and 21 in my clients' cycles.

Cycles that regularly fall outside the 25-to-35-day range are usually indicative of deeper hormonal issues. Often, longer cycles indicate polycystic ovary syndrome (PCOS) or something else that might be causing oestrogen not to reach its threshold, which delays ovulation; while shorter cycles could mean a luteal phase defect (a luteal phase that is too short), ovulation that is occurring too early, or anovulatory cycles.[27]

More important than the length of any individual cycle, though, is the consistency of your cycle. In other words, there shouldn't be a lot of fluctuation from month to month. For instance, one month you've got a 25-day cycle, then the next month it's 35 days, and the third month it's 26 days. True, each of these cycles is within the "ideal" length, but the fluctuation is itself a sign that ovulation is not happening consistently, as it should for you to be at your healthiest. The goal is to have cycles that fluctuate by only 2 to 3 days. For instance, my cycle ranges from 27 days to 31 days but is almost always 28 to 30 days long, minus one to two atypical cycles each year that are 26 or 32 days long.

When there is a lot of ovulation day fluctuation from cycle to cycle, it's important to look at what's happening in your life. Have you experienced an extremely stressful situation that could have disrupted ovulation? Maybe you had a lot of air travel, were ill, partied too hard, or ate poorly because you were busy with work. All these factors can influence your body's carefully laid plans for when an egg is released each cycle.

If you experience this kind of irregularity, don't freak out and go digging through your calendar to figure out what particular event caused this change. Studies show that up to 46 per cent of women experience cycle length fluctuations of more than 7 days in a year.[28] However, it's important to know that women included in these studies had cycle lengths shorter or longer than the ideal 25 to 35 days, which is why I'd rather see cycle length fluctuations of no more than 2 or 3 days. In short, my goal for you is not statistical normalcy but true health.

How Long Should My Period Be?

Just like the difference in opinion about the normal length of a cycle, there is also a lot of debate about how long our periods should last. In my experience, a normal period should range between 3 and 7 days, with 4 to 5 days being ideal for most women (and 5 days being the statistical average).[29] This signifies that you had adequate levels of oestrogen to sufficiently build up the uterine lining in the first half of your cycle prior to ovulation.

At the point when I finally went off the Pill in my early twenties, my period had gone from 5 medium/heavy days to 1 very light day. While on the Pill, my diminishing period seemed like the best thing ever, but the health consequences of a practically non-existent period and very low levels of oestrogen soon became glaringly obvious. Think chronic urinary tract infections, headaches, joint pain, a practically non-existent sex drive, painful sex, and melasma (brown patches) on my face, to name a few.

I had no idea what was going on in my body, but in a nutshell, my sex hormone production had been shunted (thanks to no ovulation), and with every month I spent on the Pill, I was operating on a growing deficit of oestrogen, progesterone, and testosterone. Add to that a high-stress college environment, two internships, and a job search, and I was a disaster.

The full-body negative impact of a sex hormone deficit is why I like to see periods in my clients that last 3 or more days. Two days or fewer often signifies insufficient oestrogen to maintain all the other functions in the body that are dependent on this critical hormone. Low-oestrogen symptoms include vaginal dryness, painful sex, low libido, joint pain, an inability to focus, crankiness, anxiety, sleep disruption, and night sweats.[30] Take it from someone who experienced it!

Keep in mind, if you have always had a 2-day period and you're rockin' life without any symptoms, then you're probably just fine and a 2-day period is likely the norm for your particular body and hormonal makeup. Again, consistency is key. However, if your period has always been 5 days long and has gradually or suddenly dropped to 1 or 2 days, this could indicate that your oestrogen production is compromised.

On the other end of the spectrum, if your period lasts 8 days or longer, this is often a sign of oestrogen dominance (when oestrogen is too high in relation to progesterone) and/or low thyroid function.[31]

How Much Blood Loss Is Considered Normal?

Normal periods consist of an average blood loss of 60 ml or less with an average range of 35 to 50 ml, although the range women experience is much wider.[32] Not sure what that looks like? I encourage you to pour 35 ml and 50 ml of water into a measuring cup to get an idea.

Each soaked regular pad or tampon holds roughly 5 ml (or 1 teaspoon) of blood, so it's considered normal to soak about six to ten pads and/or tampons during each period.[33] Most of us don't wait until our pad or tampon is fully soaked and different brands have varying absorbencies, so if this number seems low to you, it may be because of the brand you use or because you change your pads or tampons more often.

Measuring menstrual blood loss is tricky and has limitations. This is because, in addition to blood, you're also expelling tissue, uterine lining, clots, and other fluids, so in terms of menstrual fluid volume, according to the scientific research, you're potentially losing more than I've described. This is why it comes down to the individual. Only you can know what's normal for your unique body, but if you're consistently experiencing any of the signs of a heavier-than-average period (see "How Much Am I Bleeding?"), it's time to speak to your GP or gynaecologist.

HOW MUCH AM I BLEEDING?

One fully soaked regular tampon or pad holds approximately 5 ml, or 1 teaspoon, of blood, and a fully soaked super tampon holds 10 ml. A half-soaked regular pad or tampon equals 2.5 ml, and a half-soaked super tampon equals 5 ml.[34]

Make a note in your period-tracking app or in the Notes app on your phone every time you change your pad or tampon, period underwear, or menstrual cup—note how full it is—each day of your period to determine if you have a heavy period. If the number of fully soaked regular pads or tampons is higher than sixteen; or if you've fully soaked "regular flow" period underwear four or more times a day on at least 3 days of your period; or if you've changed a half-full 30 ml menstrual cup more than six times during your period, then you likely have a heavier-than-normal flow.

If you're losing more than 80 ml of blood per cycle or you're soaking more than sixteen regular tampons or pads per cycle, then this is a sign of menorrhagia, or an excessively heavy flow.[35] Other signs are periods that last longer than 8 days, flooding (when you're literally bleeding through pads/tampons every thirty to sixty minutes), and clots that are 2.5 cm (one inch) long or bigger.

Although not as talked about as heavy periods, excessively light periods are problematic, too. Just as short periods can indicate a lack of adequate oestrogen, so can a light or scanty period. In my personal experience and throughout my work with clients, if bleeding lasts for just 1 to 2 days each cycle and blood loss is such that only a total of five pads or tampons (25 ml, or roughly 5 teaspoons or less) are used during your entire period, this is a sign that oestrogen is not where it's supposed to be to build a substantial-enough uterine lining.

As always, it's important to determine what is normal for *you*. These statistics provide helpful benchmarks but may not necessarily represent your body's norm.

What Should My Period Look Like?

I once mentioned my preference for period underpants on social media, and someone asked, "Do period underpants work for those bulky smashed blood clots?" I'll get to that question later, but the point I want to get across here is that this is not how a period should look. If your period looks like this regularly, then you're reading the right book.

Menstrual fluid consists of sloughed-off endometrial tissue, red blood cells, and other fluids. Your period should ideally start with a saturated red colour. A relatively wide range of reds can be used to describe healthy menstrual blood. These include ruby, berry, cherry, currant, crimson, scarlet, and rose, so don't worry if your blood isn't fire-engine red.

If the blood is brown or very dark, that's a sign of slower-moving blood at the beginning or end of your cycle. Slow-moving blood is exposed to more oxygen, and oxidised blood is darker. According to Barbara Loomis, a specialist in abdominal therapies and Visceral

Manipulation, "When the uterus is in a flexed or severely tipped position it may slow down the flow of menstrual blood leaving the body. The blood then becomes brown in colour due to the oxidation process. Additionally, this malposition makes it harder for the uterus to expel all the blood, so you may see brown blood flow or spotting from a previous cycle." This may be accompanied by pelvic pain, menstrual cramps, constipation, and low-back pain during your period. I recommend working with someone trained in Visceral Manipulation, a pelvic physical therapist or a certified Arvigo therapist if you suspect your uterus is malpositioned.

In the years I've worked with clients, I've also observed many see a shift from brown blood to a more vibrant red colour after following my programme, so pay attention to whether that happens for you after the six-week programme.

The blood should have a consistency like high-quality maple syrup—that is, it should flow easily. Period blood that is clotted; clumpy; that looks like blueberry, raspberry, or blackberry jam; or that is pasty like mud could be indicative of oestrogen dominance and progesterone deficiency. Period blood that is thinned out, too little, lighter in colour, and pink rather than red (i.e. like watermelon juice or watered-down cranberry juice) could mean there is an oestrogen deficiency.

Is It Okay If I'm Spotting Before or After My Period?

Spotting causes a great deal of distress, so it's important to know that there are different types of spotting—some are okay, some are not so great.

For many of us, our periods begin with spotting. (Please note that spotting is not considered your period, and if you're tracking your cycle, spotting should not be counted as the beginning of menstruation.) Premenstrual spotting for 1 to 2 days before your period begins is no big deal; this blood is often darker red or brown because it's slow moving or is leftover blood from the previous cycle, which is common with a flexed or tipped uterus. However, spotting for more than 3 days leading up to your period is not considered normal. In fact, it is often a sign that your progesterone is dropping too quickly and could also indicate a condition such as endometriosis, uterine fibroids, or hypothyroidism.

On the flip side, when your period ends, you should experience bleeding that tapers off over a day or two rather than spotting that lingers for 3 or more days. The latter could also be indicative of those same conditions I just mentioned.

Spotting around ovulation is also quite common, and in most cases it is considered normal. Ovulation spotting usually lasts for around 1 to 3 days and shows up in your fertile-quality cervical fluid as bright red, light red, or pink. This spotting occurs as oestrogen levels drop right before ovulation, causing a slight partial shedding of the uterine lining.

Cervical inflammation can also cause spotting; this blood usually looks bright red in colour. This inflammation can be caused by an infection such as chlamydia, gonorrhoea, or bacterial vaginosis and should be checked out by a doctor. This kind of spotting will usually show up after sex if the cervix was bumped.

What's the Typical Pattern of Bleeding?

The first day of your period is the first day of your typical flow, when you experience significant bleeding and need a pad, tampon, period underwear, a menstrual cup, or some other form of period protection. A period typically starts out heavier and then moves to medium and then light before ending. But because each of us is unique, some women experience periods that start out lighter, become heavier, and then become lighter again. In others, the flow is consistent every day of the period and then abruptly ends or tapers off with some spotting. Each of these scenarios is considered healthy and nothing to worry about.

When it comes to the pattern of bleeding, start-and-stop periods are probably the biggest concern for most women. Their periods are like evening traffic on the motorway: starting and then suddenly coming to a screeching halt around day 3 or 4 and then starting up again twenty-four hours later. There are a number of possible reasons for this, including too-high oestrogen, progesterone not dropping uniformly once your period begins, the position of the uterus, and how the uterine muscles are contracting.

Ultimately, you want to examine every aspect of your period and menstrual cycle when trying to determine if it's normal for you. Your typical period may not be the same as your BFF's typical period. Remember that your period will be affected by diet, stress, and other lifestyle factors throughout the previous month, so keep all this in mind when evaluating your period from month to month.

STAGES OF THE MENSTRUAL LIFE CYCLE

My friends in their thirties are always asking me about changes they've noticed in their periods from when they were in their twenties. This is definitely a thing, ladies. Your period evolves (sometimes significantly) between your teens and your late thirties. Many of these changes are due to major events such as pregnancy, the postpartum period, times of extreme stress, and use of hormonal birth control. All these aside, your period shouldn't really change too significantly until you hit your forties. If you notice something out of the ordinary that lasts for more than three months, it's time to do some digging.

Periods in Your Teens

Hello, erratic! During puberty and the teenage years, a girl goes from a completely anovulatory state to a state of regular ovulation and periods—a challenging transition. And her periods reflect that transition by being a little all over the place.

In the first five to seven years after a girl's initial period, as her reproductive system adjusts to its new role, she will likely experience occasional anovulatory cycles, slower follicle development, and a smaller dominant follicle than adult women.[36] Anovulatory cycles and inadequate follicle development may result in skipped periods, irregular cycles, or more frequent or heavier bleeding because of the lack of progesterone both to hold the uterine lining in place and to slow oestrogen's growth of the uterine lining.

Unfortunately, girls are often put on the Pill or some other form of hormonal birth control (IUD and implant) to "treat" these symptoms when, really, they might just be indicative of their ovulation process getting its bearings. Trust me, I get it. I went on the Pill as a teenager because of my excruciatingly heavy and painful periods, too. But by not letting the body grow into itself, we ultimately inhibit its development and potential. As humans, we must first learn to crawl, then walk, then run. We don't get upset at newborns when they fail to qualify for the Olympics, and our endocrine and reproductive systems need the same patience and nurturing.

I've also seen many instances of teenage girls being given a diagnosis of polycystic ovary syndrome (the number one cause of ovulatory infertility in the United States) based on their irregular cycles, and as a result of this diagnosis they were falsely told they will have trouble conceiving later in life. This is hugely detrimental to a girl's psyche, and I've met lots of women who still hold that belief into their twenties and thirties. This is why period literacy is necessary from the very start. Teenage periods are just as susceptible to the effects of food and lifestyle, and girls need to pay attention to these aspects of their health, too.

There are several signs that there could be deeper issues happening with a teenage period. If any of the following symptoms is present, it's important to see your doctor:

- A missing period or lack of ovulation;
- Heavy bleeding or periods that consistently last more than 8 days;
- Extreme period pain that disrupts daily activities and school attendance; and

- Consistently having two periods in one month or very irregular bleeding patterns.

Periods often start to regulate and normalise as a girl approaches her late teens. Keep this in mind before going on (or putting a daughter on) a form of hormonal birth control to fix teenage period problems. All the suggestions in this book apply to teenage girls as well as adult women, so for teens experiencing any of these symptoms for more than three months, I highly recommend you start here.

Periods in Your Twenties and Thirties

Now that you've left your tumultuous teenage years behind you, it's time to really own your menstrual cycle. This phase of a woman's menstrual cycle involves a lot of life changes such as college, graduation, getting a first job or starting a business, moving into your own place, getting married, and having kids.

While this is an exciting time, full of new life adventures, it's also straight-up stressful, which will affect your hormones. I've found that most women in their twenties who are not on hormonal birth control notice one of three things: they experience a continuation of their issues from puberty, their periods start to regulate and normalise, or they start developing period problems they didn't experience as teenagers. This is why paying attention to the foundations of health—diet, stress management, and proper supplementation—is critically important. You have youth on your side, so you'll find you feel better within a short period of time. Kind of like everything in your twenties (colds, hangovers, and boyfriends), you'll bounce back fast from period problems if you implement a few key practices.

Pregnancy and the postpartum time are considered phases within this phase of the menstrual life cycle because your period is affected by both these events. In fact, what I have observed with a significant number of clients is that their pregnancy completely reset their hormonal equilibrium and that their periods changed significantly postpartum. I continually hear from women that their periods became heavier and more painful after they gave birth, while others have said their periods were lighter and less painful. There is also greater variability in menstrual cycle length in the first few cycles after ovulation returns in the postpartum stage.[37]

One of the biggest concerns is a shift in menstrual cycles in the early thirties. Most women tell me they start to notice their cycles getting shorter and their periods getting heavier during this time. For others, their periods shorten and get lighter. I chalk this up to the dietary, stress, and environmental burdens that often increase in our thirties, and the fact that our guts and livers are not as resilient to these stressors as they were when we were in our twenties. Supporting your gut and liver health during my six-week programme will be extra beneficial.

While perimenopause, the transition period between our regular cycling years and the onset of menopause, officially begins at age thirty-five, you don't just suddenly start experiencing symptoms. What most women notice as they approach forty is a few anovulatory cycles each year, which lead to diminished levels of progesterone. Lower progesterone causes an increase in sleep issues, such as difficulty sleeping through the night, along with worsening moods, especially in the late luteal phase. Otherwise, it should be business as usual for women in their mid- to late thirties who are ovulating and menstruating on a regular basis.

Periods in Your Forties and Beyond

Your forties are gonna be a different story! Just like the time after your first period, the decade leading up to your ovaries shutting their doors for good and your very last period can be rather turbulent. However, please know that contrary to popular belief, perimenopause doesn't have to be terrible, and suffering during this transition time is optional.

As perimenopause gets under way, women tend to experience earlier ovulation and shorter menstrual cycles, along with increased anovulatory cycles and decreased progesterone, which leads to heavy periods, or flooding.[38] This decrease in progesterone relative to oestrogen (also known as oestrogen dominance or oestrogen excess) can go on for a number of years. Some women experience an irregular pattern of bleeding, with some months being heavy and long while others are short and light. There may be spotting (at different times in the cycle), and most women will start to skip periods here or there during this phase of perimenopause.

As menopause gets closer, things begin to shift. Oestrogen starts to drop, along with progesterone, which leads to longer and longer menstrual cycles and fewer periods each year. Menopause officially starts once you've ceased to have a period for twelve months.

TRACKING YOUR CYCLE

Now that you know all about your period, let's get to tracking it! Cycle tracking is the first step in getting acquainted with your menstrual cycle and attaining period literacy. Quantifying things such as the length of your menstrual cycle, how many days you bleed, and your period-related symptoms will empower you to make more educated decisions about your health and wellness. While this may seem strange or off-putting at first, I promise you'll get used to it quickly.

If you don't already, I recommend that you start tracking your cycle using an app. There are literally dozens of available apps, so I recommend you find one that works for you. Or feel free to track using a paper chart—but let's face it, tracking your menstrual cycle on your smartphone is much easier and more convenient for most people. Reviewing trends in your cycle-tracking data over months or years is easier when you use an app, and you can share your charts with a partner or your health practitioner via email.

If you have never tracked your cycle, follow the instructions in the "Basic Cycle Tracking" section. If you have tracked your cycle before or are currently tracking the basic symptoms, then check out the "Advanced Cycle Tracking" section to start charting your basal body temperature and cervical fluid patterns so you can determine if and when you are ovulating in your cycle.

> **PRO TIP:** When choosing an app, always check its privacy policy. Yes, some app companies might actually sell your intimate data!

Basic Cycle Tracking

No matter what app you choose, or even if you go old school and keep track of your cycle via paper charts, I suggest you track just the basics first to get into the habit of tracking and avoid overwhelm. Even if this basic tracking is all you do, you'll still learn a lot about your menstrual health. As part of basic cycle tracking, you should track:

- the first day and the last day of bleeding;
- a few key details such as how heavy or light your flow was on each day—pay particular attention to heavy bleeding days (and if they feel unusually heavy for you);
- any spotting you experience either before or after your period, or at other times in your cycle; and
- any physical and emotional symptoms you experience during your period and throughout the entire month. Make a quick note in your app or chart of your most bothersome symptoms, such as pain that keeps you from doing what you want or need to do, cravings, energy levels, sleep, bowel movements, significant mood swings, breakouts, fatigue, brain fog, or anything else that feels distressing to you.

Just so you know, once you've entered multiple cycles, many apps will make predictions about ovulation and when your period will arrive, which can be helpful for planning your life.

It can be overwhelming to try to keep track of all of this at once. So, start simple, and then work through this section as many times as you need to help you fully optimise your menstrual health. Owning your health is a journey. You'll get the best results when you're patient and make small changes over time.

Advanced Cycle Tracking

Now, for those of you who are real nerds (like me!) about this cycle-tracking stuff, you can get even more granular about your data collection. The more data that you have, the more you can learn about and improve your cycle.

With more advanced tracking, you're really tracking three things: cervical fluid, body temperature, and cervical position.[39] Considered together, these three things will tell you if and when in your cycle you're ovulating, which will give you a picture of your unique menstrual cycle patterns and fertility.

This kind of data will be invaluable to you on this journey and in the long term. It puts your cycle in context, meaning that you will know the nuances of your unique menstrual cycle and be able to pinpoint when there are abnormalities long before something serious develops. Imagine being able to compare your current data to data in the coming months once you've done the six-week programme to see how your menstrual cycle parameters have improved. This is bio-hacking at its finest!

Record your temperatures and cervical fluid in an app or a paper fertility chart. (See "Workbooks" under "Fertility Awareness Method (FAM) Further Education and Resources" in appendix C).

STEP 1: TRACKING YOUR CERVICAL FLUID

When we know our unique cervical fluid patterns, we are able to determine when we are fertile and when we are not. After your period, you may notice little to no cervical fluid and a "dry" vaginal sensation: when you touch your vulva it feels only slightly moist, and when you wipe yourself it feels dry. As oestrogen begins its ascent, your cervical fluid will take on a "wetter" consistency, often becoming creamy (like lotion) or milky, and white in colour.

As you enter your fertile window, you may notice it becoming slippery, viscous, stretchy (like egg white), or watery. This is known as fertile-quality cervical fluid. You will also experience a wet or slippery vaginal sensation, meaning that when you touch your vulva, it feels very wet, or the toilet paper will feel slick when you wipe. After ovulation, with the rise of progesterone, the fluid becomes thicker, with a sticky, tacky, or pasty texture, or it may dry up completely.

For the remainder of the luteal phase, you will likely notice little to no cervical fluid and a dry vaginal sensation similar to what you experienced right after your period. You may notice the wetter-quality fluid again around the middle of your luteal phase (about 5 to 7 days before your period). This happens because of a rise in oestrogen during that time and is *not* a sign of ovulation.

I suggest checking for cervical fluid each time you use the toilet to get into the habit. It's a good idea to wear black or dark-coloured underwear so it's easy to see the cervical fluid when you use the loo throughout the day. Then make sure to note the consistency and amount of cervical fluid you see each day in your app or on your paper chart.

If you're not seeing any on your underwear, which is quite common after coming off hormonal birth control, use a finger to check internally. Be patient with your body as she begins to readjust to having ovulatory cycles again.

If you have not been on hormonal birth control and you don't produce a lot of cervical fluid in the 5 to 7 days before ovulation, don't worry; it doesn't necessarily mean there is something wrong. There is a range for cervical fluid production, fluid production declines with age, and everyone is different. If you notice 2 days or less of cervical fluid in your fertile window, and this doesn't increase after implementing the Fix Your Period programme—give it three months—you should work with a trained fertility awareness practitioner and a functional medicine or naturopathic doctor to dig deeper and determine the contributing factors.

The dry-wet-dry cycle is a typical pattern, but there can be deviations from this. If you continue to experience the wet cervical fluid after ovulation occurs, or if you generally notice cervical fluid throughout your cycle, this often indicates endocrine disruption. Keep in mind that your cervical fluid is produced in response to rising oestrogen. If you have PCOS or your oestrogen is dominant over your progesterone for another reason, such as a thyroid condition, then this could be the cause.

A yeast infection, bacterial vaginosis, or a sexually transmitted infection can also throw your cervical fluid for a loop. If you have a thick white discharge that smells like yeast and is accompanied by itching or irritation, you may have a yeast infection. A fishy-smelling, grayish discharge could be bacterial vaginosis. If you experience any of these symptoms, see your doctor for testing immediately.

How to Tell If You've Ovulated by Observing Cervical Fluid

The first step in determining if you have ovulated is to identify your peak day. Your "peak" day is not necessarily the day of the greatest quantity of cervical fluid or the most wetness, but rather, the last day that you observe fertile-quality cervical fluid or have a wet vaginal sensation in any given cycle.

The peak day usually occurs a day or two before you ovulate, but it can also occur on the day of ovulation. You will be able to determine your peak day only in retrospect: it's the day before your cervical fluid starts to become sticky or tacky or dry up, and the wet vaginal sensation has dissipated. Knowing your peak day will help you determine the end of your fertile window: if you observe that your cervical fluid has changed consistency or been dry for 3 days after your peak day, then it's one sign you've ovulated.

STEP 2: CHARTING YOUR BASAL BODY TEMPERATURE

A basal body temperature is a person's temperature first thing upon awakening. Before ovulation, your waking temperature will be on the lower side, often anywhere from 36.11 to 36.50 degrees Celsius (97.0 to 97.7 degrees Fahrenheit). A day or two after ovulation, your temperature will typically rise at least two-tenths of a degree and stay elevated until right before your next period. Post-ovulatory temperatures usually rise to 36.55 degrees Celsius (97.8 degrees Fahrenheit) or higher. This is caused by the production of the heat-inducing hormone progesterone.

How to Chart Your Basal Body Temperature

To get an accurate reading, you need to take your temperature first thing upon awakening after at least three consecutive hours of sleep and before any other activity such as using the toilet, brushing your teeth, or texting. Your temperature tends to rise about two-tenths of a degree per hour, so aim to take it at roughly the same time every day.

Record your temperature in an app or, if you're using a paper fertility chart, use a pencil to circle your daily temperature. Each day you can then draw a line connecting your daily temperature to the previous temperature (see "Workbooks" in "Fertility Awareness Method (FAM) Further Education and Resources" in appendix C). You should also note any events such as illness, air travel (especially across time zones), alcohol consumption, or periods of excessive stress, and any temperatures taken earlier or later than usual. You should take all these factors into consideration when interpreting your temperature pattern.

The reason you chart your temperature in conjunction with observing cervical fluid is to determine if and when you have ovulated in any given cycle (see Figure 2 on page 30). Pay attention to when your temperature rises more than two-tenths of a degree above the previous six temperatures, and stays elevated for at least 3 days. This is the first step in determining that you've ovulated. And once you have combined this temperature shift with the change in your cervical fluid from wet to dry, you can confirm ovulation has occurred.

For many women, it takes three to four months to see a pattern in their temperature readings, so don't freak out if your basal body temperature appears to be all over the map when you're just starting out. If you're ovulating, there should be a pretty distinct difference in the temperatures between the first and second halves of

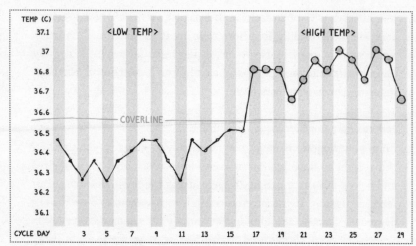

Figure 2: Temperature chart depicting ovulation

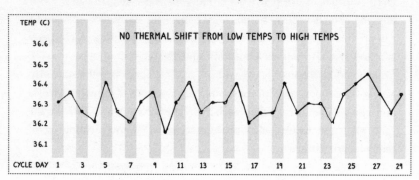

Figure 3: Anovulatory (no ovulation) temperature chart

your cycle. If there isn't, it may be a sign that you are not ovulating (see Figure 3 above), or you may have low progesterone, a thyroid imbalance, or a stealth issue that you should address with a practitioner.

STEP 3: MONITORING YOUR CERVICAL POSITION
Your cervical position is the third sign of fertility that you would pay attention to during your cycle. This is not a necessary step, as it merely confirms what your cervical fluid and temperature have told

you, but if you want to feel for your cervix, you damn well should! Your cervix is usually firm and remains low and closed throughout most of your cycle. However, as oestrogen increases during the lead-up to ovulation, it causes the cervix to become soft, move up higher in the vaginal canal, open up, and produce the characteristic fertile-quality fluid. The cervix position can be felt by checking internally using your middle (or longest) finger. Please make sure to wash your hands before feeling for your cervix.

Tracking Irregular or Missing Periods

Regular cycles are great, but let's face it, all women experience times in their life when their cycles are irregular or stop altogether. These times most commonly include when your period begins (puberty), after coming off hormonal birth control, during travel or weight change, postpartum or after a miscarriage, during breastfeeding, and in perimenopause. The great thing about tracking your period is that it can be a tool during all these phases, not just when your cycles are regular.

If your cycles are irregular, keep tracking as normal. Take your temperature at the same time and track your cervical fluid daily. You'll be able to glean lots of information by tracking, such as if and when you're ovulating, when your period is coming, and when you're potentially fertile.

If you are not ovulating but are having a bleed, your charts won't show a biphasic temperature pattern (the shift from low pre-ovulatory temperatures to high post-ovulatory temperatures) or a clear cervical fluid pattern. Rather, your temperature will bounce up and down (refer back to Figure 3 on page 30), and your cervical fluid will display a basic infertile pattern, rather than going from dry to wet to dry again. When ovulation does return, your chart will alert you to this as well. Seeing a functional medicine or naturopathic doctor is recommended if you have not been ovulating for six months or more (and you're not pregnant or breastfeeding).

Charting while making these changes will help you to identify emerging patterns so you can support your hormones as they move towards balance. Continue charting this way until a period returns.

And you thought it was just a period! Now you are aware, in a way you probably never have been before, of all that is happening in your body each month. This knowledge provides you the opportunity to be engaged with your menstrual cycle in a whole new way. And look, we're just getting started. Hormones are involved in every aspect of your menstrual cycle. Let's dig a little deeper into these major players in the next chapter.

2

THE HORMONAL HIERARCHY

When I created my Fix Your Period programme, I polled a lot of women, asking them what came to mind when they heard the word *hormones*. Most of their responses were along the lines of:

"I think of menopause, complete with hot flashes and night sweats."

"Hormones make me think of puberty or pregnancy."

"What comes to mind is terrible PMS, raging periods, and bad moods."

No one said they thought of hormones in a positive way, as the essential chemical messengers they are. In fact, until I started studying hormones, I'd never heard of their being referenced in a positive way, as helpful to women. They were always talked about as if they were the bane of every woman's existence.

Hormones have a really bad rap, and it's high time they got a reputational makeover. After all, they are responsible for almost every process in your body. They are the stars of the show, not some understudy, and frankly, they should be revered.

From the time we're born (long before PMS problems and menopause), our hormones are in charge of a plethora of bodily functions not related to our menstrual cycle, such as our appetite, sleep patterns, how we respond to stress, our digestion, whether we're happy

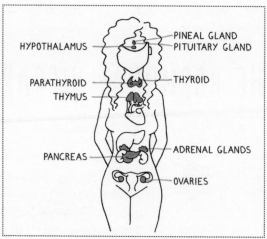

Figure 4: Endocrine glands

or anxious, and everything in between. This is why it's so important for women of every age to have a basic grasp of the endocrine system, the collection of glands that produce hormones, and how those hormones work. Otherwise, they'll be simply feeling around in the dark for decades, trying to piece together an understanding of what the heck is going on in their bodies.

There are several major glands in the endocrine system, such as the hypothalamus, pineal, thyroid, adrenals, ovaries, pancreas, and, most important, the pituitary gland—also known as the master gland because it tells other endocrine glands what to do (see Figure 4 above).

Collectively, they produce *a lot* of hormones, more than fifty, in fact. The hormones and the glands in your endocrine system work like a symphony; each of them has to play in tune for you to be in a state of vibrant health. And just as when one player in an orchestra is off-key, when one hormone veers off course, the others follow suit and disharmony ensues.

You've probably been in a need-to-know relationship with your hormones, ignoring them only until they start to malfunction, so I want to give you the lowdown on nine of the most important of these chemical messengers: cortisol and insulin; pregnenolone and DHEA;

and oestrogen, progesterone, testosterone, thyroid hormones, and melatonin.

HORMONE TIERS

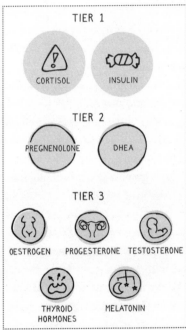

Figure 5: The hormonal hierarchy

Let's think of these hormones as being in a tiered system—a hormonal hierarchy, if you will (see Figure 5). I consider the tier 1 hormones, cortisol and insulin, the queen bees of the endocrine system. If they become imbalanced, they disrupt the tier 2 hormones, pregnenolone and DHEA. Subsequently, if *those* hormones go on the fritz, they impact the tier 3 hormones: oestrogen, progesterone, testosterone, the thyroid hormones, and melatonin. But the tier 1 hormones can also directly disrupt the tier 3 hormones. See how important they are?

Tier I: Cortisol and Insulin

Cortisol and insulin are at the top of the hormonal hierarchy because they're "life and death" hormones. When you are in a dangerous or threatening situation, cortisol is the hormone that will prompt the release of glucose in your body, and insulin will efficiently move that glucose into your cells so you can fight for your life or run like hell.

These tier 1 hormones are heavy duty, and they'll go out of their way to prove they mean business. And when they rise to unsustainable levels, they can wreak havoc on *all* the other major hormones: pregnenolone, DHEA, oestrogen, progesterone, testosterone, the thyroid hormones, and melatonin.

When thinking about **CORTISOL**, I want you to visualise yourself twenty thousand years ago as part of a hunter-gatherer tribe. You're out one day foraging for berries when out of the corner of your eye you spot a lion stalking you from the tall grass. The moment your brain registers this formidable threat, it instructs your adrenal glands to start pumping cortisol into your bloodstream. In a split second, that hormone turns you from a calm, relaxed, daydreaming forager into an efficient, focused fighting machine. Cortisol acts like a rocket booster, giving you the strength and mental focus to either fight or flee. It also prioritises your body's functions, taking offline those that are least important in this situation, such as your digestive and reproductive systems. (I mean, when you're face-to-face with a lion, digesting your lunch and getting pregnant are not high on your to-do list, right?)

In this situation, cortisol has just saved your life—or, at least, it gave you a better chance of survival. Pretty cool, huh? So why does this badass hormone get so much bad press? The problem is that, these days, lions have been replaced with traffic jams, tax returns, work deadlines, and financial woes. While most of these stressors are not life threatening, our bodies react to them as though they were. And while twenty thousand years ago we might have encountered a lion once or twice a year, these modern-day stressors are there every day, all day long, all year long, triggering the adrenal glands to release cortisol into our bloodstreams almost constantly.

Over time, this elevated level of cortisol (and of other "survival" stress hormones) starts to have an effect on the "subordinate" endocrine glands, namely, the thyroid and the ovaries. Essentially, cortisol tells your ovaries to slow their roll because your body has perceived this external stress as potentially dangerous—and therefore, this is not a good time to be ovulating or getting pregnant. So, ovulation is delayed, or it may even stop for some time due to the amount of psychological stress you're under. Cortisol also tells your thyroid to take it easy on its responsibilities, so you can conserve your energy for the "threat" you're facing.

And . . . BAM! You start experiencing irregular periods or your period disappears completely. Your PMS takes on a life of its own, and your periods become heavier or more painful. Your sex drive withers, and you start feeling like you'd rather be gardening than getting it on with your partner. Or, maybe you start gaining weight for no apparent reason, your hair starts falling out, or you develop what feels like unmanageable fatigue.

It's easy to demonise this hormone. Chronic stress and constantly elevated levels of cortisol have become an epidemic in our caffeine-fueled, overstimulated, high-stress, fast-paced society. We're constantly told, and rightly so, to reduce our stress levels and keep our cortisol down at all costs. But when kept in check, cortisol, far from being our enemy, is actually one of our body's dearest friends.

INSULIN also has a say in how all the other hormones in the body behave. Like cortisol, it affects our sex hormones to such a degree that if it is out of whack, attempts to get those hormones in balance will be minimally effective at best. Insulin's main job is to help keep blood sugar levels stable. When food enters the body and is converted to glucose, the pancreas releases insulin to help move that glucose from the bloodstream into your cells so you can use it as energy.

The problem arises when you eat too many carbohydrates—and unfortunately, this happens on a daily basis for pretty much everyone. Glucose levels in the body are tightly regulated, so when we dig into, say, two scoops of vanilla ice cream (which has about 28 grams of sugar), our pancreas has to step up production of insulin big-time.[1] Too much glucose in our blood can be toxic, so our body is quite aggressive in getting any excess out of there. And just to be on the safe side, it usually errs on the side of removing more glucose than is necessary. This swift reduction in glucose in the blood leads to what's known as a blood sugar crash. What happens when your blood sugar drops so quickly? You feel faint and lethargic and you get "hangry." How many times a week do you feel this way?

You know what else raises insulin levels? Stress. Stress raises cortisol levels, and cortisol raises your blood sugar. As your blood sugar goes up, your insulin levels rise, too. High blood sugar and insulin levels are directly and indirectly linked to PMS, PCOS, endometriosis, fibroids, heavy and painful periods, migraines, depression, anxiety, acne . . . and the list goes on. Just about every cell in your body is affected by too much insulin. The link between insulin hyperproduction and your sex hormones is why hormonal imbalances always—yes, *always*—improve when you eat to stabilise your blood sugar.[2]

Tier 2: Pregnenolone and DHEA

I consider pregnenolone and DHEA, both produced in the adrenal glands, the "parent hormones." In addition to having their own specific roles in the body, they also give birth to a number of more well-known downstream hormones.

PREGNENOLONE is often referred to as the "mother hormone" because it is converted from cholesterol to produce many other hormones. It's the precursor to A-list celebrities such as progesterone and cortisol, neither of which could exist without it. Yet most people know next to nothing about this unsung hero.

Pregnenolone protects neurons from damage and is also known for enhancing memory, motivation, and mood.[3] In fact, pregnenolone supplements are often used to relieve the symptoms of many neuropsychiatric disorders, including anxiety and depression.[4] Other benefits of pregnenolone include better-quality sleep, a reduction in PMS and menopausal symptoms, an improvement in immunity, and repair of the myelin sheath (the protective fatty tissue covering nerve cells). Like many of the sex hormones, pregnenolone levels naturally peak when we are younger, and then decline with age.

DHEA is a precursor to star players such as oestrogen and testosterone, but it is still derived from pregnenolone, so I consider it to be a bonus parent. In addition to its parental role, it's also known as the "fountain of youth" hormone because it's been shown to help reduce inflammation, improve insulin sensitivity, reduce belly fat, boost libido, and improve depression.[5] DHEA levels hit their peak during our mid-twenties and then steadily decline as we get older.[6]

Oh, those glorious twenties! For those of you still in your DHEA prime, don't take those days for granted. For those of you who have passed your DHEA peak, you might be asking, "Why don't we just pump our bodies full of this 'fountain of youth' hormone?"

Well, like all things in life, more isn't always better. DHEA is an androgen, or male hormone, so women who supplement with DHEA can experience symptoms such as aggression, adult acne, and unwanted hair growth. Trust me, you don't want to go popping DHEA pills. As with all hormones, DHEA supplementation should be done under the guidance of a trained and experienced practitioner.

Tier 3: Oestrogen, Progesterone, Testosterone, Thyroid Hormones, and Melatonin

These hormones fall into the third tier because they are most influenced by the hormones just described. They're at the bottom of the hierarchy, and when they become imbalanced, it shows up as those symptoms you most recognise: problems with sleep and energy, period-related issues, and mood swings.

We usually think of **OESTROGEN** as a single hormone, but oestrogens are actually a family of hormones that plays an important role in women's sexual and reproductive health. Oestrogen is made mostly in the ovaries, although the adrenal glands, fat cells, and brain also make small amounts of it.

More than fifteen forms of oestrogen have been identified, but there's no need to memorise them. We'll just focus on the three main oestrogens: oestrone, oestradiol, and oestriol. Each of these has specific functions.

1. **OESTRONE**, or O1, takes over from oestradiol as the dominant oestrogen in postmenopausal women and is sometimes elevated when younger women experience what is known as primary ovarian insufficiency (formerly, premature ovarian failure), which, put simply, is early-onset menopause.

2. **OESTRADIOL**, also known as O2, is the predominant form of oestrogen in females of reproductive age who are not currently pregnant. O2 aids in the cyclic release of eggs from the ovaries during ovulation. Elevated oestradiol in relation to progesterone is often linked to heavy periods and PMS.

3. **OESTRIOL**, or O3, is the weakest of the three oestrogens and the one that's released in large amounts from the placenta during pregnancy.

Oestrogen (oestradiol, in particular) is the "feminine hormone" because it is responsible for the physical features that we associate with being female. It is also a proliferative hormone: as it begins to rise in young girls, it triggers the onset of puberty and the physical changes that come with it (commencement of the menstrual cycle; the formation of thighs, hips, and breasts; and the growth of pubic and underarm hair). In adult women, oestradiol is responsible for most of what happens with your menstrual cycle—in particular, kicking off ovulation and the stimulation and growth (i.e. proliferation) of the uterine lining.

Oestrogen has had a bit of a raw deal, and is often demonised in the world of women's health. For example, many birth control pills are touted as having the lowest dose of oestrogen possible, as if oestrogen were some kind of evil villain and even the slightest bit in our bodies could be catastrophic. (FYI: The Pill doesn't even contain oestrogen. It contains ethinyloestradiol, a potent synthetic form of oestrogen.) Then there is a lot of talk about "oestrogen dominance," or "oestrogen excess," and its connection to *all* the terrible things, such as breast and uterine cancer and conditions such as endometriosis and fibroids. But it's important to understand that oestrogen dominance occurs only when oestrogen hangs out unopposed in our bodies for too long, meaning that there is not enough progesterone in the body to keep oestrogen's proliferation tendencies in check. (We'll get to that in a second.)

According to Dr Felice Gersh, "Oestrogen is the unsung hero of female well-being." That's right, the oestrogen made in your body is all that and a bag of chips. Though primarily known for its role in the menstrual cycle and pregnancy, oestrogen has so many other roles—regulating brain function, for example, and supporting the health of your urinary tract, heart and blood vessels, GI tract, immune system, bones, breasts, skin, hair, mucous membranes, and pelvic muscles. Oestrogen is *life*.

How does oestrogen have such far-reaching effects? Oestrogen receptors (kind of like ports where hormones pull up and "dock" to drop off their instructions to the cell) are located throughout the body,[7] which is why women in oestrogen-deficient states—think missing periods or, in many cases, being on hormonal birth control—often feel so universally crappy.

PROGESTERONE is the other primary female ovarian sex hormone. I call it the "Keep Calm and Carry On" hormone, because of its ability to soothe our nervous systems during those often less-than-dignified PMS days. Progesterone is best known for its role in preparing the endometrium, the lining of the uterus, for the potential of pregnancy after ovulation. Think of oestrogen as the hormone that builds the house and progesterone as the hormone that furnishes and decorates it.

Where does progesterone come from? Well, once an egg is released, the egg's follicle transforms into the corpus luteum, a 2-to-5 cm transient endocrine gland produced in the ovary during the second half of the menstrual cycle,[8] which starts pumping out progesterone. (Yes, ladies, each month, your body is capable of making a mini endocrine gland in under twenty-four hours!)

If you were to get pregnant, the progesterone produced by the corpus luteum would support the embryo for the first three months, before the placenta took over. If there is no pregnancy, the corpus luteum breaks down and turns into scar tissue known as the corpus albicans.

Like oestrogen, progesterone has some other pretty fundamental roles in the body. These include supporting the health of our breasts, heart, thyroid, and nervous system. But maybe most important, progesterone helps to maintain healthy brain function and mood regulation. This eases anxiety and promotes healthy sleep in the second half of your cycle.

Progesterone circulating in the bloodstream has direct access to the brain and nerves. In fact, one of progesterone's main jobs is to protect the brain from damage and help repair it after injury. It does this by promoting the growth and repair of the myelin sheath, the layer of fatty tissue protecting nerve fibres that aids in communication between neurons.[9] From an evolutionary perspective, progesterone chills us out to help facilitate the development of an embryo if we were to be pregnant. (Remember, your body is *always* preparing for pregnancy.)

Oestrogen and progesterone work together like dance partners. When one is out of sync, the dance is disrupted. For example, if progesterone levels are low, there isn't enough available to counter the effects of oestrogen, and symptoms of oestrogen dominance (e.g. heavy periods, sore breasts, and migraines) appear.

Ah, **TESTOSTERONE**, the hormonal driver of big muscles, competitive sports, and pub fights. It's typically considered a hormone only men should care about, but this is a myth. If you've been told that testosterone is totally irrelevant to women, then you'll want to pay extra attention here.

While it is true that testosterone is responsible for many physical and emotional characteristics in men, from facial and body hair to assertiveness and aggression, adequate levels of testosterone in women help build muscles, keep skin supple, boost our moods, help us handle stress and uncertainty like a boss, and get us in the mood for sex. Roar! This is why I refer to it as the "strong, sexy, confident" hormone. Testosterone is what gives us women a sense of power, motivation, and assertiveness.

Produced by the ovaries and in the adrenal glands, testosterone in women peaks right before ovulation, which is hardly surprising given that it drives libido, which is your body's way of trying to entice you to have sex and get knocked up.

THYROID HORMONES. The thyroid gland produces two main hormones: triiodothyronine, or T_3; and thyroxine, or T_4. I like to refer to the thyroid hormones collectively as the "go go go" hormones because they are responsible for helping us feel energetic and upbeat.

(You might be asking, "What about thyroid-stimulating hormone, or TSH?" This is produced by the pituitary gland, not the thyroid.)

T_3 is the active form of T_4. While the body does make a little bit of T_3 on its own, approximately 80 per cent of the active thyroid hormone is converted from T_4. T_3 plays an incredibly important role in regulating the body's metabolism, heart function, digestion, muscle control, brain development, bone maintenance, and your menstrual cycle. In other words, T_3 helps your body maintain a normal weight, prevents brain fog, and keeps you feeling happy.

Most women don't realise that the health of their thyroid is connected to their periods. In fact, women with hypothyroidism, or low thyroid function, have reduced levels of T_3, which can actually lower progesterone production, which itself further impacts the thyroid, reducing its T_3 output even more.[10] This is just one of the ways your thyroid can affect your period, and it's also an amazing example of the interconnectedness of the glands in our endocrine system and the numerous feedback loops in our bodies.

MELATONIN is produced mostly in your gut and also by the pineal gland at night. This hormone is responsible for regulating your circadian rhythm, also known as the sleep/wake cycle. Basically, it helps you fall asleep and stay asleep. Your sleep/wake cycle is governed by light exposure (sunlight, moonlight, and artificial light). Unfortunately, overexposure to crazy amounts of blue light from computers, smartphones, and TVs reduces your body's capacity to produce melatonin, which can seriously mess with your ability to sleep properly. (If you bring your smartphone to bed with you, I'm looking at you.)

Here's the kicker: not only does low melatonin disrupt sleep, but it is also linked to a lack of ovulation, infertility, and even chronic pelvic pain in endometriosis.[11] Yes, your sleep/wake cycle is intricately connected to your menstrual cycle. Who knew?

Melatonin supplements have become super popular in recent times due to our fast-paced, hectic, artificial light-flooded lives. However, giving yourself a large dose of melatonin isn't the same as having a healthy circadian rhythm and naturally regulated melatonin levels. Large amounts of melatonin (sometimes way above what your body would make naturally) can actually delay or even stop ovulation. This can potentially change the timing of your menstrual cycle or stop it altogether.[12] Now you know: too little or too much melatonin via supplementation can do a number on your cycle, so prioritising sleep so you can produce your own melatonin is uber important.

Now that you have been schooled in the basics of your menstrual cycle and the key hormones that influence it, let's take a look at some of the most common period problems and the symptoms you may be experiencing, and start to uncover what your hormones are telling you. Remember, symptoms are your body's way of alerting you that something needs your attention. Knowing where your hormones are going wrong will point you towards the best way to tame them and resolve those symptoms.

3

DECODING YOUR PERIOD

WHAT YOUR PERIOD PROBLEMS ARE TRYING TO TELL YOU

So, what's a hormonally imbalanced girl to do? First, it's important to always remember the interconnectedness of your hormones and the endocrine system as a whole. While you might be experiencing multiple, seemingly disparate symptoms, many times these can all be traced back to one or two underlying imbalances in key hormones. Remember the hormonal hierarchy and its tiered system? (See Figure 5 on page 35.)

As we learned in the previous chapter, any imbalance in tier 1 hormones cascades down to tier 2 and tier 3 hormones. Have you ever heard the line "When a butterfly flaps its wings in one corner of the globe, it triggers a storm halfway across the world"? This is the butterfly effect, a concept used by mathematicians to study the effects of changes in interconnected systems. The endocrine system is one of these interconnected systems. When a small change occurs in the tier 1 hormones, it can result in a large change in the lower-tier hormones. This interdependence is why we can't spot-treat our period problems: the symptoms you experience are really just manifestations of other, underlying issues. So, to understand the symptoms you're experiencing, you must search for the butterfly and not get lost in the storm.

The good news is that resolving the smaller initial issues that have led to larger problems is usually a whole lot easier than trying to treat every symptom you're dealing with. So, no matter how overwhelming this all sounds, it's really not that complicated to fix your period.

We'll get into the specifics of what you can do to ignite hormone balance in Part 2, but first, let's look at what causes the common period problems.

YOU ARE NOT BROKEN

Women struggling with period problems often tell me that they feel their bodies have betrayed them. Usually a doctor made them feel this way during an appointment at which they were told they had "XYZ condition" and that they were likely doomed to a future of excruciating pain, trouble getting pregnant, an unmanageably heavy flow, or some other insert-worst-case-scenario-here. Or, they were told that what they were experiencing was "normal" and just a natural part of being a woman.

I've said it before, but it bears repeating: suffering related to your period is not normal. If you've ever found yourself thinking that your body is broken, or that maybe you should just suck it up and deal, I want to help you flip the script. The truth is that no matter what period problem or hormonal imbalance you're experiencing, your body is *not* damaged or defective. Your body is amazing and beautiful, and these symptoms are just her way of communicating—okay, sure, sometimes screaming—that something needs your attention.

Your period problems aren't just telling you that you need to buy more tampons or stock up on paracetemol. They're alerting you to a potential system-wide malfunction. That's right, menstrual issues are our proverbial canary in a coal mine. By recognising your period symptoms and the signs of hormonal imbalance, you'll be able to take action and personalise a plan that's right for you, ending your period problems and improving your overall health.

WHAT'S YOUR BODY TELLING YOU? COMMON PERIOD PROBLEMS

Your period problems are an indicator of the hormonal conversation gone awry. They're not in your head. They don't just come with the territory of being someone who menstruates. They're not something you can ignore. And they're not something you can just forget about if your healthcare provider shrugs them off. They are trying to tell you something, and you have to listen.

You may know something's up because you're experiencing a constellation of symptoms. Take a moment now to list them. Note their frequency and severity. Good. Now I'm going to lay it all out here so you can make a direct link between what you're experiencing and the common conditions indicated by your symptoms. I promise this isn't as confusing or as overwhelming as you've been made to believe.

Let's take a look at some of the most common period problems and how to connect the dots to the hormones involved. First, the problems:

- PMS and PMDD (you're saying and doing unreasonable things, but you can't stop);
- Period pain (truly, you have my utmost sympathy);
- Mid-cycle, or ovulatory, pain (ouch!);
- Heavy periods (enough, already!);
- Light or short periods (like, was that even a period?);
- Short cycles, or too-frequent periods (bleeding more often than should be legal);
- Infrequent, or irregular, periods (you have no idea when she's making an appearance);
- Missing periods (you haven't seen a trace in months);
- Spotting or bleeding in between periods (can't stop, won't stop bleeding);
- Vaginal infections (itchy much?);
- PCOS (more symptoms than you can count); and
- Endometriosis (this much pain should be illegal).

PMS and PMDD

Premenstrual syndrome (PMS), or premenstrual tension (PMT), refers to a collection of physical and psychological symptoms that arise in a cyclical pattern, and coincide with the second half of the menstrual cycle (the luteal phase).[1] The symptoms often show up around 2 to 10 days before your period begins, and usually resolve when menstruation starts.

Approximately half of all women worldwide experience PMS symptoms,[2] and a number of studies have shown that roughly 91 per cent of women experience at least one PMS symptom each month.[3] Yet many women are surprised that PMS is even considered a legitimate condition. In our culture, it's just another "normal" negative part of the experience of being a woman, lame jokes and all. If ever there was a condition that needed a societal makeover, this would be it.

PMS's bigger, badder sister, premenstrual dysphoric disorder (PMDD), is considered a severe mood disorder and is characterised by significant emotional and physical symptoms that occur in the luteal phase.[4] It is estimated that PMDD affects about 2 per cent of women worldwide,[5] but some estimates suggest that 3 to 8 per cent of women are impacted.[6] For these women, it's not just a matter of feeling a little bitchy each month; it is more comparable to experiencing debilitating and sometimes traumatic symptoms that negatively impact relationships, careers, and mental well-being.

PMS and PMDD symptoms can range in severity because they are highly influenced by nutrient deficiencies, excess psychological stress, genetic factors, gut health issues, and blood sugar abnormalities[7] that drive oestrogen to become dominant over progesterone (your "Keep Calm and Carry On" hormone). These two hormones also heavily influence chemicals in the brain, including serotonin, dopamine, and oxytocin, which all affect mood and even gastrointestinal health. This is also why there is such an assortment of PMS and PMDD symptoms.

While the symptoms women experience are indeed legitimate, I prefer to think of them as a message from your body that something is awry. Declaring these symptoms as a syndrome or disorder tends to set us up to feel like we are doomed to a life of monthly PMS or PMDD purgatory, when the truth is that even if you have been diagnosed with either of these conditions, the correct diet and lifestyle changes can drastically improve your experience in the days leading up to your period.

I mean, when you think about it, how can half the entire female population on the planet have a syndrome that affects them every month? Your body was not created in such a way that you would be miserable for one to two weeks each cycle. Most definitely not. Your menstrual cycle is a marvel of nature, not a design flaw. At this time in your cycle, your body is just giving you a heads-up that good ol' Aunt Flo will be making an appearance soon. Depending on how well you're taking care of yourself, you might barely notice these symptoms—or your life might turn into a cliché montage of you thinking and saying (gasp!) unreasonable things at the slightest provocation, receiving knowing looks from the supermarket cashier as she scans your box of tampons and your two tubs of Ben & Jerry's, and not being able to zip up your favourite jeans because you're so bloated. (Oh, and, hell, let's throw in the teenage acne and the overreacting to everything.)

Again, feeling like your body and your life are completely out of control before your period is a sign it's time to address what's going on below the surface. You don't need to be a slave to PMS or PMDD.

MOST COMMON PMS AND PMDD SYMPTOMS

Women who experience PMS or have been diagnosed with PMDD may have one or more of a range of physical, mental, or emotional symptoms. Brace yourself: this is not a short list. While there is conflicting evidence on the number of symptoms associated with these two conditions, the most common include:

- bloating and fluid retention;
- cramping;

- lower-back pain;
- acne;
- change in appetite, especially a big increase in hunger or food binges and increased cravings for salt or sugar (hello, crisps and chocolate!);
- stomach upset, nausea, or vomiting;
- sleep problems (usually insomnia) and often excessive fatigue;
- headaches and menstrual migraines;
- breast tenderness or pain;
- lowered libido (sex or ice cream? Hmm, let me think about that);
- anxiety (can this period just show up already?);
- irritability, anger, or rage (your partner never knows if happy you or angry you will walk in the door);
- feeling down and not like yourself; and
- brain fog or forgetfulness (where did I put my keys again?).

When it comes to PMDD, women often describe experiencing (on top of the symptoms just listed) what feels like a mini-depression every month that includes feelings of sadness, hopelessness, worthlessness, extreme anxiety, and explosive anger. Others report being totally overwhelmed by life and having suicidal thoughts. These complaints should never be dismissed, and if you experience them, it's important to seek help from a trained medical professional.

I want to re-emphasise that because these conditions are driven by lifestyle factors, you have much more control over your PMS or PMDD than you think. Most symptoms can be reduced or eliminated altogether when their underlying causes are addressed. If you regularly suffer from PMS or have been diagnosed with PMDD, you'll want to pay special attention to stabilising your blood sugar, improving the state of your gut health, and supporting your liver's detoxification ability, as all these play a role in your levels of inflammation and the amount of oestrogen circulating in your body. Both of these are heavily connected to PMS and PMDD symptoms, so weeks three, four, and five of the six-week programme are going to be especially important for you.

FEELING PMSY AROUND OVULATION?

You're not crazy! For some women, PMS symptoms are more erratic, often occurring around ovulation, a time when we're supposed to feel great. This is likely a sign of oestrogen dominance and/or the inability to detox oestrogen properly, combined with something known as histamine intolerance, or histamine sensitivity, which we discuss in Chapter 7.

PMDD AND TRADITIONAL MEDICINE

I'm not one to discount anyone's experience, but the diagnosis of PMDD feels a bit like overpathologising women's health and experiences, especially because I've seen so many Fix Your Period programme success stories over the years. PMDD is listed in the *DSM-5* (the *Diagnostic and Statistical Manual of Mental Disorders*), and, in fact, in the early 2000s, the Food and Drug Administration in the US approved four anti-depressants to treat PMDD before the American Psychiatric Association had even designated it a psychiatric condition.[8]

I don't doubt that women suffer these symptoms, but to push severe period-related problems as a mental disorder seems extreme; it also supports the narrative that women "lose their minds" every month. If you suffer extreme symptoms prior to your period, you are not crazy, and you shouldn't be treated as such. At the same time, you should be querying why this is happening to you.

Finally, I believe we should all be questioning the jump from how we treat PMS symptoms (conventionally with the Pill and holistically through lifestyle changes and supplementation) to how we treat PMDD, whose main treatment is a brain-altering drug. Don't get me wrong: if this is what you feel you need to do, then you should make that decision for yourself. But I strongly encourage you to give the six-week programme a chance first.

Period Pain (Dysmenorrhoea)

Period pain, or dysmenorrhoea, is perpetually normalised in our society, but I'm here to tell you that it's not normal and should not be ignored. When we have back pain or migraines, we seek treatment, and doctors often pull out all the stops to help us address them. Why would uterine pain be any different? I know it's hard to unlearn what we've been indoctrinated to believe, but it's time to move away from the idea that women should be "sick and suffering" and to raise the standards for ourselves.

The symptoms here are pretty obvious: pain, and lots of it. In addition to pelvic pain, other symptoms I consider as falling under the period pain umbrella include pain that radiates down your legs, lower-back pain, nausea, vomiting, diarrhoea, sweating, and head-aches. Any number of these can happen just before or during your period, and they may last from a few hours to 2 or 3 days. A full-on period party!

But how much pain qualifies as too much? If you experience anything more than mild cramping, your body is trying to tell you something. Pain that is disrupting your life and/or that requires medication (more than one dose a day of 200 mg to 400 mg of ibu-profen, for instance) or time off from work, school, or your day-to-day routine could very well be a sign of unaddressed inflammation or an underlying condition like endometriosis.

If this is you, you're not alone. Dysmenorrhoea is the most common gynaecological condition experienced by women on the planet. Studies have found that between 45 and 95 per cent of women have painful periods, and 10 to 25 per cent require medi-cation and time off from daily activities.[9] In fact, period pain is one of the top reasons women miss work—second only to missing work to look after sick children. Ugh. Why do we put up with this? It's just not right.

WHAT CAUSES DYSMENORRHOEA?

Primary Dysmenorrhoea

There are two types of dysmenorrhoea. Primary dysmenorrhoea re-fers to cramping pain related solely to your period. When you feel this pain, it's just your uterine muscles doing their monthly thing, working to push menstrual blood out. Primary dysmenorrhoea is considered a natural part of your cycle, meaning there is an absence of pelvic disorders such as endometriosis, uterine fibroids, or cysts,[10] and it usually starts soon after your first period or during your teen years. If you have primary dysmenorrhoea, you'll notice pain beginning just before or right after your period starts, and lasting anywhere from a few hours to 3 days.[11]

One cause of primary dysmenorrhoea includes high levels of prostaglandins, hormone-like substances that cause the uterus to contract. Prostaglandins exist in all human tissue, and different types of prostaglandins do different things. For example, prostaglandin E_2 and F_2 stimulate inflammation, contract uterine muscles, and constrict blood flow to the damaged area to prevent blood loss. When you begin to shed your endometrial lining, a large amount of prostaglandins is released. This constricts blood vessels in the uterus and causes it to contract. Higher levels of prostaglandins will cause more severe uterine contractions, which can lead to the painful cramps that are familiar to many of us.

So, you'd think the answer would be to inhibit prostaglandins, and, in fact, that is the go-to recommendation by doctors for period pain. Prostaglandin-inhibiting medications include nonsteroidal anti-inflammatory drugs (NSAIDs) such as aspirin, ibuprofen (Nurofen is one brand name), naproxen (brand names: Feminax Ultra, Period Pain Reliever, and Boots Period Pain Relief), and medications used to treat osteoarthritis and rheumatoid arthritis.[12]

But there's a potential problem. Prostaglandins also trigger the egg's release from the ovary, so prostaglandin-inhibiting medications may prevent the follicle from rupturing and releasing an egg. While it is controversial in humans, there is some evidence linking NSAIDS to delayed ovulation or anovulatory cycles, and I've seen this in some clients who were taking pain medication on a daily basis.[13] Pretty crazy, right? Don't stress, though. If these medications are the cause of your ovulatory problems, once you stop taking them, ovulation should normalise. More than anything, I want you to be querying why you might need pain medication regularly, and pay attention to whether your pain is reduced once you do the six-week programme.

Women with a "tilted uterus" (also known as a retroverted or retroflexed uterus) also commonly experience primary dysmenorrhoea.

Possible factors that contribute to a tipped/tilted uterus include pelvic misalignment (e.g. from habitually wearing high heels), regularly sitting improperly on the sacrum (the large triangular bone at the base of your spine), and falls that directly impact the sacrum.

In addition to period pain, if you have a tipped/tilted uterus you might also experience painful sex and mild to severe lower-back pain before and during your period. If your doctor has said you have a tilted uterus, work with a trained pelvic physical therapist, a certified Arvigo therapist, and/or someone trained in Viceral Manipulation in addition to following this six-week programme.

Secondary Dysmenorrhoea

Secondary dysmenorrhoea is due to a medical condition, the most common cause being endometriosis.[14] Pain from secondary dysmenorrhoea usually begins earlier in the cycle, sometimes one to two weeks before menstruation even starts, and lasts longer (sometimes throughout your entire period) than the menstrual cramps associated with primary dysmenorrhoea. As if the pain weren't bad enough, secondary dysmenorrhoea is often accompanied by heavy periods and irregular menstrual bleeding or spotting outside your period or during sex.[15] The conditions that cause secondary dysmenorrhoea include:

ENDOMETRIOSIS: an inflammatory disease in which tissue that is similar to the kind that lines the uterus grows outside the uterus. No matter where it is in the body, this tissue builds up and attempts to shed with each menstrual cycle, often causing excruciating pain and other symptoms. Endometriosis is believed to affect at least one in ten premenopausal women worldwide.[16] (For more on endometriosis, see page 77).

UTERINE FIBROIDS: the most frequent benign tumours found in the female pelvis. Occurring in up to 70 per cent of women before menopause,[17] fibroids can lead to heavy and prolonged bleeding and sometimes severe menstrual cramps.

ADENOMYOSIS: a condition in which endometrial tissue grows into the muscular wall of the uterus, causing the uterine walls to thicken and become enlarged.[18] Think of it like a thick sponge lining the uterine cavity. Similar to endometriosis, adenomyosis causes the affected tissue to thicken and shed in accordance with hormone fluctuations, which leads to extremely heavy bleeding and cramping. Adenomyosis occurs in about 20 per cent of women with endometriosis.[19]

PELVIC INFLAMMATORY DISEASE (PID), CHLAMYDIA, OR GONORRHOEA: PID doesn't necessarily cause painful periods, but rather, ongoing pelvic pain. One of the symptoms of both chlamydia and gonorrhoea is lower-abdominal pain. If left untreated, both these STIs can cause PID.[20]

OVARIAN CYSTS: cavities filled with fluid that grow on the ovaries. In most cases, these cysts are the follicles on your ovaries that grow each month as part of the ovulation cycle. They are known as functional ovarian cysts and are quite common during your childbearing years. Most ovarian cysts are harmless and resolve on their own, but some can become dangerously large, leading them to potentially rupture and damage the ovary. Increasing mid-cycle pain or ovulation pain could be a sign of a problematic ovarian cyst. If you experience such symptoms, please see your doctor for a diagnosis.

THE COPPER IUD: a birth control device that creates an inflammatory response in the uterus, which stops implantation. It is believed that this localised inflammation is part of the reason why many women experience debilitating cramps for the first three to six cycles after this type of IUD is inserted. Menstrual cramps and pain outside the menstrual window are the number one reason for removal of the Paragard IUD.[21] If your period pain doesn't improve or subside within six months, consider having your IUD removed. This kind of pain may be mitigated through my six-week programme, but ultimately, if the IUD is causing it, it's unlikely to subside completely.

Remember, disruptive period pain might be statistically normal, but it's not biologically normal. It is really important that you see a doctor to determine the cause of your pain, as that will determine how to address it. If a practitioner has downplayed or dismissed your pain, I encourage you to stick to your guns and find a doctor who will take your pain seriously and work with you to figure out its cause. In the meantime, the Fix Your Period programme will be instrumental in addressing the sources of your pain. These can include your diet, blood sugar, gut inflammation, stress response, and thyroid health.

Mid-cycle or Ovulatory Pain

It's completely normal to feel a twinge or even a slight ache or cramp in your lower abdomen when ovulation occurs. The pain is usually one-sided, coming from the ovary releasing the egg, and may be due to a small amount of blood being released when the follicle ruptures through the ovarian wall. I've found that this pain can last from a few minutes up to a few days and may be accompanied by vaginal bleeding lasting from a few hours to a few days. For most women, this pain is bearable, an expected part of their cycle. For others, however, it is debilitating, even requiring a day off from school or work. (If you are in the latter group, please see your doctor for an ultrasound to determine what's going on.)

If you have inflammation or excess prostaglandin production—remember, prostaglandins play a role in the release of the egg from the ovary—you may notice more severe pain at this time. You may also experience this kind of pain if you have ovarian cysts or endometriosis. Because this higher level of pain is linked to inflammation and excess oestrogen the six-week programme will be highly effective in minimising or eliminating it.

Heavy Periods (Menorrhagia)

Menorrhagia. Sounds serious, right? Like, "Whoa, you have menorrhagia?" But *menorrhagia* is just a fancy term for "heavy periods," which aren't exactly life threatening, but can put a real damper on life's activities. From working to dating to going to the beach to exercising—a heavy flow can affect many aspects of a woman's life and feel unmanageable, not to mention be potentially *mortifying*. Women complain to me constantly about leaks, accidents, ruined underwear, and stained outfits; feeling stressed about simply leaving the house or performing normal activities; and experiencing the full-on exhaustion that comes with excessive blood loss.

We covered an excessively heavy flow a bit in Chapter 1. To recap: if you're losing more than 80 ml of blood per cycle or you're soaking more than sixteen regular tampons or pads per cycle, it could be a sign of menorrhagia. You'll know you have a heavy period when:

- your period consistently lasts 8 days or longer;
- you're changing regular tampons, pads, or period underwear more than every two hours each day or a full 30 ml menstrual cup more than twice a day;
- you need both a pad *and* a tampon or a tampon *and* period underwear to control your menstrual flow;
- you have to get up and change your pads, tampons, or period underwear during the night;
- you have a menstrual flow with blood clots 25 mm long or longer; or
- your period generally wipes you out—you experience tiredness and lack energy, you find yourself short of breath, or you've been diagnosed with low iron or iron-deficient anaemia.

WHAT CAUSES HEAVY PERIODS (MENORRHAGIA)?

Heavy bleeding can occur at any age, but it is most common at either end of the reproductive age spectrum, during the teenage years and then again during perimenopause, when oestrogen levels tend to be higher in relation to progesterone. These two times of life are characterised by irregular ovulation, and thus sporadic progesterone production.[22]

Adolescents experience heavier periods likely because of their immature endocrine system—in particular, the immature hypothalamus function. (The hypothalamus talks to the pituitary gland, which talks to the ovaries and tells them when to ovulate. So, if the hypothalamus is still developing, there are likely to be hiccups in the ovulatory process.) These anovulatory cycles increase oestrogen and decrease progesterone, causing heavier periods.

Perimenopausal women experience heavier periods because of waning ovarian function. As the ovary ages, it is less likely to complete the ovulation process. Without consistent ovulation, there will be a lack of adequate progesterone, which is often a cause for heavier periods.[23]

The causes of heavy periods and conditions related to heavy periods are grouped into three main categories:

Hormonal Imbalances

HIGH OESTROGEN. A period that is heavy, clotted, or clumpy or that resembles what crushed-up frozen blueberries look like when they've started to melt is indicative of higher oestrogen levels in relation to progesterone.[24]

HYPOTHYROIDISM, OR LOW THYROID FUNCTION. Thyroid hormone and progesterone are inextricably linked. If your body is not producing adequate thyroid hormone, your progesterone levels may drop, causing oestrogen to become dominant over progesterone.[25]

Uterine Problems

ENDOMETRIOSIS (see page 77).

ADENOMYOSIS (see page 54).

FIBROIDS (see page 54). The two types of fibroids most likely to cause heavy bleeding are intramural fibroids, which grow in the wall of the uterus, and submucosal fibroids, which grow inside the uterine cavity. Fibroids are generally fed by oestrogen excess and progesterone deficiency, which can also thicken the uterine lining and worsen heavy bleeding.[26]

UTERINE POLYPS. When these benign growths protrude into the uterine cavity, they can cause abnormal uterine bleeding, but it is usually not heavy. See "Spotting or Bleeding in Between Periods" (page 70).

MISCARRIAGE, ECTOPIC PREGNANCY, AND THE POSTPARTUM TIME can all cause heavy bleeding. Women often report to me that their periods are much heavier after they give birth. If this has happened to you, it's a good idea to track how much you're bleeding. Read Chapter 9 and get your thyroid tested to rule out postpartum thyroiditis.

Other Illnesses, Disease, or Medication

PROGESTIN-ONLY BIRTH CONTROL OPTIONS. The Depo-Provera injection and the Nexplanon implant are both linked to ongoing, irregular bleeding. These progestin-only birth control options inhibit ovulation in most women using them. According to obstetrician and gynaecologist Dr Shawn Tassone, "Progestins in these forms of birth control work similarly to natural progesterone in that they thin out the uterine lining, but because of the high doses, they potentially thin out the endometrial lining so much that the underlying basal blood vessels are exposed, causing excessive bleeding. This is why many women on the Depo-Provera shot and the Nexplanon implant experience irregular bleeding patterns."[27]

THE PARAGARD (AKA COPPER) IUD. This non-hormonal form of birth control can cause extremely heavy and prolonged periods, irregular bleeding, and spotting. Approximately 70 per cent of users experience these symptoms in the first three to six months of use.[28]

VON WILLEBRAND DISEASE. The most prevalent inherited bleeding disorder in women,[29] von Willebrand disease impairs the way blood clots and is a common cause of heavy menstrual bleeding and excess bleeding during childbirth. If you've had heavy periods for as long as you can remember, ask your doctor to test you for von Willebrand disease. About 13 per cent of women with heavy menstrual bleeding test positive for this disease.[30]

If your flow is on the heavy side, weeks four and six in the Fix Your Period programme will be particularly important for you. The focus of these weeks is liver detoxification and thyroid support, which are both linked to runaway oestrogen levels and heavy periods.

Light or Short Periods

At the opposite end of the spectrum are women who do not bleed heavily during their periods. While this may seem welcome to some—"I want a heavier period," said basically no woman ever—a light or short period can be a problem too.

There is a very wide range of blood loss in menstruating women, but in my experience, I consider a light period to be typically 25 ml or less with only 1 to 2 days of bleeding. In more practical terms, during the span of a light period you might use five regular tampons/pads or fewer. If you use a menstrual cup, depending on which one you use—they range in capacity from around 15 ml to 40 ml—you'll probably fill it only once. You might also notice your blood doesn't really flow consistently and instead seems more erratic, kind of like spotting. In terms of colour, it may be watery and light red or pink or brown, rather than a vibrant red.

WHAT CAUSES LIGHT OR SHORT PERIODS?

Prior to going on the Pill, my client Jamie had extremely heavy periods: she'd go through a pad and a super tampon every two hours for 7 days each month. After being on the Pill for five years, her periods became significantly lighter: she experienced barely 2 days of bleeding and had to change her pad only once or twice a day. I know what you're thinking. What's wrong with that? Well, Jamie wanted to work with me because she was having migraines and at least two weeks of terrible mood swings each cycle.

The Pill's dose of ethinyloestradiol and progestin (aka the synthetic versions of oestrogen and progesterone) had turned off her ovulatory cycle, and thus her body's production of oestrogen and progesterone. Her pill was of the low-dose variety, so she didn't have enough ethinyloestradiol in her system to grow her uterine lining to have a substantial bleed each month. Lower oestrogen (whether it's your own or the type that comes in the Pill) means your uterine lining does not build up as much each month, and this leads to lighter periods and sometimes cessation of bleeding over time.

In addition, the Pill raises the liver's production of a protein called sex hormone-binding globulin (SHBG), which binds to oestrogen and reduces its levels in the body even further.[31] When she came to me after coming off the Pill, Jamie's SHBG was pretty high, and she was barely spotting each month.

We worked on addressing her lack of ovulation by addressing the nutrient deficiencies and gut health problems that developed while she was on the Pill. Within three months she started ovulating again and got a period, albeit a very light one. She was no longer getting migraines, and her chaotic moods had stabilised. Over the next six months on the Fix Your Period programme, she saw her period gradually become a 3-day bleed as ovulation regulated and her oestrogen levels returned to normal.

If you're not on the Pill, a light period can be a sign that you're not ovulating. The first thing to do is establish if you're ovulating by charting your cycle (see "Tracking Your Cycle" in Chapter 1).

- If you're *not* ovulating, you'll need to identify the underlying causes, which often include chronic psychological stress,[32] sudden weight loss, low body weight or body fat, a vegetarian, vegan, or low-carb diet (this is not the case for everyone but I've seen this scenario a lot—don't shoot the messenger!), too much soy,[33] thyroid disease, too few nutrients or malabsorption of nutrients (particularly fat), and conditions such as PCOS[34] or hypothalamic amenorrhoea (see page 68).[35]
- If you *are* ovulating, then your body is producing enough oestrogen to trigger ovulation, but it might not be enough to build up your uterine lining significantly.

Both these scenarios are addressed in Chapters 4 through 9. It's helpful to know that if you've always had periods on the lighter side and you're not experiencing any other period-related symptoms such as lack of ovulation, a short luteal phase, or the problems related to oestrogen deficiency (e.g. low mood, anxiety, vaginal dryness, painful sex, urinary tract infections, and decreased ability to handle stress), then don't panic. You may be just fine.

Short Cycles, or Too-Frequent Periods

A typical cycle triggered by ovulation should ideally fall within the 25-to-35-day range. Within that cycle, your period should last 3 to 7 days. When your period comes less than every 24 days or what feels like more than once a month, it is showing up too often. Technically, bleeding that does not follow ovulation is not considered a true period, but it can certainly resemble one.

At some point, you may have been told that having a short cycle is no big deal. But it is, seriously. Because of the potential for higher exposure to unopposed oestrogen over time, there is an increased risk of breast cancer with short cycles.[36] These insufficient cycles are almost always coupled with heavy or long periods—zero fun, if you ask me.

Bleeding every 24 days or fewer is almost always a sure sign that you are:

- not ovulating or ovulating very sporadically (every few cycles for instance);[37]
- ovulating very early in your cycle and having a short follicular phase (shorter than 10 days);[38] or
- ovulating mid-cycle and having a short luteal phase (shorter than 10 days).[39]

As you now know, ovulation is not a simple operation, so there could be a number of hormonal glitches (e.g. elevated oestrogen, low progesterone, or low thyroid function) along the way that are causing your short cycles. (FYI: shorter cycles are also associated with heavy caffeine and alcohol consumption and cigarette smoking.)[40]

Years ago, when I was in a long-distance relationship, travelling back and forth to Europe every few months while running my business—don't feel too sorry for me—I experienced a very short cycle. I arrived home after a particularly stressful trip through three different countries for the better part of an entire day, and I promptly started spotting. I was only on day 13 of my usual cycle, so I figured it was ovulation spotting; but it wasn't: the spotting got worse and became a light flow that lasted for the remainder of my cycle, until I got my next period on day 24, a little more than three weeks after my last one, much earlier than normal for me.

WHAT CAUSES SHORT CYCLES, OR TOO-FREQUENT PERIODS?

Extreme stress sends your adrenals into overdrive, pushing up production of cortisol and other stress hormones, which do a number on your sex hormone production, particularly progesterone. Because progesterone keeps your endometrial lining from sloughing off until your period, if your body doesn't have enough of it, you may experience a shortened luteal phase, cycles shorter than 24 days, and too-frequent periods.

My own short cycle was a potent reminder to me that female bodies are exquisitely sensitive to stress. The early period was my body's way of straight-up telling me that I was seriously overdoing it. (Hello, cortisol!) I knew that if I didn't want another three-week cycle and weeks of bleeding the following month, I would have to clean up my act. I immediately took the hint and made it a priority to take care of my emotional and physical health through daily meditation and journalling, getting eight to nine hours of sleep each night, and stepping up my food and supplement game to support my hormones and soothe my frazzled nervous system.

Obviously, fixing one's period is not always as simple as relaxing, curtailing travel, or paring down a busy schedule, but that might be all it takes for some of us. Again, as a first step, you have to figure out if and when you're ovulating by tracking your menstrual cycle (see Chapter 1). This will help you determine which issue you're experiencing. You then need to start the Fix Your Period programme and focus on cleaning up your diet and managing your stress. This will go a long way towards addressing the scenarios I've just discussed.

Infrequent, or Irregular, Periods (Oligomenorrhoea)

Some months you get a period, other months you don't. Maybe you get two in a row and then have more months without. This erratic menstruation schedule is officially termed *oligomenorrhoea*. I know what you're thinking: Don't most women rejoice at skipping a period here and there? Why, yes, sure. You get a whole month off from the hassle of not having a tampon when you most need one, from binge-eating chocolate, from rage-drinking wine, and from bursting into tears at . . . well, everything! Sign me up. But skipping a period once a year is very different from missing a period for three months in a row.

Most women develop oligomenorrhoea at some point in their lives, especially during postpartum, during times of acute stress, and after coming off hormonal birth control. And while the symptoms of this condition might be better than, say, severe period pain, they are still a sign of an underlying problem that should not be ignored.

Infrequent, or irregular, periods basically translate to infrequent, or irregular, ovulation. You have to ovulate in order to have a true period, but keep in mind, if you have a cycle in which you don't ovulate, you can still have a bleed. With oestrogen building up your uterine lining during the first half of your cycle, at some point, the lining will begin to fall away, and you'll bleed.

WHAT CAUSES INFREQUENT, OR IRREGULAR, PERIODS (OLIGOMENORRHOEA)?

Now that you know how this whole ovulation thing works, it's time to understand what prevents it from happening consistently every month and why you may have fair-weather periods. Infrequent periods/infrequent ovulation is most commonly linked to low levels of oestrogen and/or progesterone. (Noticing a trend here? These two hormones run the reproductive show!) But in order to have enough oestrogen and progesterone, you must be ovulating regularly.

Think of it this way: anything that your body perceives as a stressor (whether an external or internal source or something you don't realise is causing a heightened stress response in your body) is a potential ovulation disruptor. Here are the main causes:

EXCESSIVE OR ONGOING PSYCHOLOGICAL OR PHYSICAL STRESS. An ongoing illness, job-related stressors, or events such as a death in the family, a marriage, or prolonged travel are all possible culprits.

QUITTING HORMONAL BIRTH CONTROL. It may take some time for your cycle to regulate after you discontinue birth control.

TOO MUCH EXERCISE OR OVERTRAINING. CrossFit five times a week, anyone? Not everybody can handle this kind of intense exercise without going into fight-or-flight mode.

POLYCYSTIC OVARY SYNDROME (PCOS). PCOS is an inflammatory endocrine disorder characterised by high androgens (male hormones such as testosterone) and elevated luteinising hormone, both of which prevent your ovarian follicles from reaching the ovulation stage.

EATING DISORDERS. Anorexia or bulimia, low nutrient intake, low body weight, and inadequate body fat can send a signal to your brain that your body is in starvation mode, causing it to respond by shutting down non-essential operations such as ovulation.

THYROID DYSFUNCTION (See Chapter 9 for the ways in which the thyroid affects the menstrual cycle.)

CERTAIN MEDICATIONS. Medication such as antibiotics and antidepressants, and chemotherapy and radiation treatments for cancer can all bring on oligomenorrhoea.

When following the Fix Your Period programme, your main focus should be on weeks two and five, which involve blood sugar balancing and stress management. These two practices will be most effective in addressing irregular periods.

Missing Periods (Primary and Secondary Amenorrhoea)

Your period is missing. Where and why did it go? When will it come back? And why is this bothering you so much when you've wished countless times for your period to go away? Anyone who has had her period disappear on her knows about the anxiety caused by the sudden absence of our monthly visitor. I mean, how dare she just dip out on you when she has accompanied you (without an invitation) to so many dances, dates, beach weekends, and final exams?

Amenorrhoea is defined as a period that is missing for three months or more if you previously had a regular cycle and six months or more if your periods were irregular. It isn't a disease, curse, or illness, but like all period problems, it is a clue that something else is going on in your body. Finding out exactly what is behind your AWOL periods can sometimes be tricky: the absence of a period can be an indicator of a number of underlying issues, but it certainly isn't impossible to get to the root cause.

Here's the bottom line: if you don't ovulate, you won't get your period. Remember, ovulation is the whole reason the menstrual cycle exists, which is kind of a big deal—think the continuation of humanity—so amenorrhoea is as much associated with lack of ovulation as it is with lack of periods.

As with menorrhagia, there are two types of amenorrhoea. With primary amenorrhoea, you're over age sixteen but have never had a period. Secondary amenorrhoea occurs when you have not had a period for three or more months (if you were cycling regularly before) or for six months if you had irregular cycles before.[41]

WHAT CAUSES MISSING PERIODS
(PRIMARY AND SECONDARY AMENORRHOEA)?

The causes behind missing periods are closely linked to the causes behind irregular periods—because, you know, ovulation. In many cases, an irregular period is a gateway to missing periods. First, a woman will experience a skipped period here or there, then a period that arrives every few months, and then, eventually, her period doesn't turn up at all.

Typically, the hormonal imbalances associated with amenorrhoea include a dysregulation of the brain hormones that talk to the ovaries (FSH and LH), low oestrogen, a combination of low oestrogen and low progesterone, elevated testosterone, and hyperthyroidism (elevated thyroid hormones). These hormones need to play well together in order to kick off ovulation and give us a period. When the whole ovulatory process is halted, your endometrium doesn't adequately thicken and subsequently shed (aka produce a period).

The causes for amenorrhoea are very similar to those for irregular or light periods. The three have a lot in common hormonally, but the difference is that with irregular or light periods, ovulation is still occurring (albeit irregularly); with amenorrhoea, it is not. Amenorrhoea has multiple causes.[42] The most common ones are:

HORMONAL BIRTH CONTROL, ESPECIALLY THE PILL. Many women who have come to me have reported developing amenorrhoea while on oral contraceptives.

QUITTING HORMONAL BIRTH CONTROL. Post-pill amenorrhoea is when your period has not returned three months after you've stopped birth control.[43]

THYROID DYSFUNCTION. Hyperthyroidism in particular can cause amenorrhoea.

MEDICATIONS. Anti-psychotics, anti-depressants, and opiates;[44] and chemotherapy and radiation treatments for cancer can all cause amenorrhoea. The last two can cause permanent loss of periods and fertility.

EARLY-ONSET MENOPAUSE CAUSED BY PRIMARY OVARIAN INSUFFICIENCY. Also known as premature ovarian failure, this is when your ovaries stop working normally before age forty.

HYPERPROLACTINAEMIA, OR HIGH PROLACTIN. This may be caused by a pituitary tumour.

PREGNANCY. (Sorry, but I have to say it.) If your period hasn't arrived on time, take a test to rule out pregnancy.

AUTOIMMUNE DISEASES SUCH AS COELIAC DISEASE. No kidding—this autoimmune disease can manifest as amenorrhoea, among other reproductive problems.[45] (We'll discuss this more fully in Chapter 6.)

POLYCYSTIC OVARY SYNDROME (PCOS). This is often defined by irregular periods, but some women with the condition lose their periods for significant amounts of time. For a more detailed explanation of the condition, see page 74.

STRUCTURAL AND GENETIC ISSUES. These include Asherman's syndrome (uterine scarring or adhesions, which can prevent blood from exiting the uterus); a pituitary tumour (which raises levels of the hormone prolactin, which suppresses ovulation and menstruation); and Mayer-Rokitansky-Küster-Hauser syndrome (underdeveloped or a lack of reproductive organs). Dealing with these issues usually requires more than just food and lifestyle changes. Primary amenorrhoea (you've never had a period and are sixteen years or older) is the biggest indicator of these problems or conditions. If you have primary amenorrhoea, see a doctor as soon as possible for evaluation.

NATURAL REASONS. Our body progresses through natural phases and cycles during which amenorrhoea is completely expected, so no need for alarm. These include pregnancy, breastfeeding, the later stages of perimenopause, and menopause.

Hypothalamic Amenorrhoea

This type of secondary amenorrhoea, also known as functional hypothalamic amenorrhoea, occurs when there is a disconnect in the conversation between the hypothalamus and the ovaries.[46] This disruption is caused by something hijacking the hypothalamic–pituitary–ovarian axis, the hormone highway on which FSH and LH travel to the ovaries and on which oestrogen and progesterone send signals back to the brain. With hypothalamic amenorrhoea, the hypothalamus has gone on holiday and is not making gonadotropin-releasing hormone (GnRH), the hormone that instructs the pituitary to make FSH and LH.

Hypothalamic amenorrhoea is diagnosed when other contributing causes (e.g. thyroid disorders; hyperprolactinaemia, or high prolactin; pregnancy; PCOS; and autoimmune diseases such as coeliac disease) have been ruled out. Remember, when your body perceives danger (whether that is too much exercise or not enough food), it will go into energy-conservation mode so as to safeguard other, more vital processes such as brain and heart function. Ovulation takes a *lot* of energy each month, so it will be the first thing to go as part of this process.

WHAT CAUSES HYPOTHALAMIC AMENORRHOEA?

STRESS. Excessive or ongoing psychological or physical stress (e.g. extreme work stress or an ongoing illness) can play a role.

EXTREME DIETING OR EATING DISORDERS. Anorexia and bulimia and/ or extreme weight loss are all causes of hypothalamic amenorrhoea. **TOO MUCH EXERCISE OR OVERTRAINING.** Female athletes, I'm looking at you in particular, but this can be the case for anyone.

I've so often heard women say something along the lines of "Not having a period is a blessing," or "I don't want kids, so why should I care about whether I have a period?" Regardless of whether you want children, it is imperative to understand that your menstrual health is reflective of your overall health; the two are not mutually exclusive. All women should view having a healthy menstrual cycle the same way they view having good gut health or good eyesight; it is an integral part of your overall health and long-term well-being that is not contingent on baby making. Or, seen another way, your menstrual cycle is a promoter of general good health. I view ovulation as a vital process in a woman's life cycle. Just as suddenly being unable to read a street sign indicates that you have vision problems, no longer having (or never getting) a period indicates that something is up with your reproductive organs.

MEDICATIONS THAT CAN DISRUPT YOUR PERIOD

You know all those scary side effects listed on the container of or in the leaflet accompanying most medications? Well, sometimes those lists include missing your monthly cycle. Here are some medications that commonly cause oligomenorrhoea and amenorrhoea:

- Hormonal birth control[47]
- Anti-depressants, including the SSRIs (selective serotonin re-uptake inhibitors) Prozac, paroxetine, and sertraline[48]
- Chemotherapy[49]
- Anti-psychotics [50]
- Antibiotics[51]

Regarding the last item, while missing periods aren't considered side effects of antibiotic use, I've seen delayed or missing periods anecdotally in hundreds of women after they've taken antibiotics.

If your period is missing, you need to investigate what is going on. Ignoring this symptom is only delaying the inevitable. Also, there is the potential for health issues that include osteopenia (low bone mass), osteoporosis (severe loss of bone mass, putting you at risk for fractures), increased risk of heart disease, mood disorders such as anxiety and depression, sexual dysfunction (low or no sex drive and painful sex), and infertility.[52]

Spotting or Bleeding in Between Periods

The medical term for spotting or bleeding in between periods is *abnormal uterine bleeding*. It sounds extreme, but don't freak out. I just want you to know the medical terminology.

My client Catherine was having what felt like two periods a month. Talk about a huge pain in the you-know-what, right? She knew which one was her real period because it came very consistently every 28 days, lasted about 5 to 7 days, and was accompanied by severe cramps and heavy bleeding. Her so-called mid-month cycle, however, was less predictable. It showed up between days 11 and 14 and lasted for a few days to two weeks. There would be a little bit of cramping, and the flow was a lot lighter, like spotting.

Catherine had been having period problems her whole life, but this "mid-month cycle" started in her early twenties, during a time of significant stress. It then stopped for a couple of years, when she started seeing an acupuncturist, but started again when she ended a long-term relationship (a very traumatic experience). When she came to see me, she reported drinking two to three glasses of wine every night to cope with the breakup and the burden of a highly stressful job she wasn't happy in.

While she wasn't actually having two periods—remember, you have to ovulate in order to have a period, and you can't ovulate twice in one cycle—she was experiencing abnormal uterine bleeding during each menstrual cycle.

You may be experiencing abnormal uterine bleeding if your period comes on a pretty regular basis and you notice:

- spotting for more than 2 days after your period ends;
- spotting or bleeding during or around ovulation time that lasts for more than 2 days (e.g. you had your period two weeks ago, but it feels like it's come again);
- spotting that starts soon after ovulation and lasts until you get your period;
- spotting or bleeding anywhere from 3 to 10 days before your period;
- bleeding or spotting after sex; or
- bleeding all the damn time.

I often see spotting, or irregular bleeding, in my practice. And, ugh, is it ever stressful for the women experiencing it. I've had many frantic texts over the years from women asking me WTF is up with their bleeding after sex or their spotting for days and days before their period is due. Aside from being downright inconvenient, this bleeding doesn't feel normal, and it creates a lot of worry about what it means for the state of their current hormonal health and future fertility.

WHAT CAUSES SPOTTING OR BLEEDING IN BETWEEN PERIODS?

Sometimes, bleeding between your periods is totally normal; ovulation spotting is one such instance. In fact, ovulation spotting can be a sign of fertility—provided it happens *only* at ovulation and not at other times in your cycle as well. If you're spotting at other times in your cycle, it might be a sign of endometriosis, adenomyosis, fibroids, or a polyp. Ovulation spotting will look like fertile-quality cervical fluid with some pink, red, or brownish blood in it. This type of spotting may happen on the day of ovulation, when the follicle ruptures as the egg is released into the fallopian tube. Or it may be triggered by the drop in oestrogen right before ovulation, which causes a bit of the uterine lining to detach and release. Once progesterone kicks in, the spotting stops. If you spot at times in the cycle other than ovulation, it could be the result of:

LOW PROGESTERONE. By far the most common cause of spotting or irregular bleeding I've seen in my work with women, spotting due to low progesterone can happen at any time after ovulation right up to the day before your period. (FYI: this would not be a cause of spotting in the follicular phase, that is, the time after your period ends leading up to ovulation.) Progesterone keeps the uterine lining in place until your period comes.[53] If your progesterone levels aren't high enough, your endometrial lining might start disintegrating soon after ovulation. Or your progesterone levels might drop prematurely a few days before your period and cause pre-period spotting. This often ranges in colour from light red to dark red to brownish (i.e. a rust colour). Extreme stress and a low-functioning thyroid can also reduce your precious progesterone and promote premenstrual spotting.

BACTERIAL, YEAST, OR SEXUALLY TRANSMITTED INFECTIONS. The other reason for spotting before a period that I've seen, and experienced myself, is an infection or bacterial imbalance in the vagina. This type of spotting isn't related to fluctuations in hormones, but is more likely due to inflammation. You may see bright red spotting before your period or in your cervical fluid after your cervix has been irritated, such as during sex or following a cervical smear test. Whatever its cause, if you suspect an infection, see your doctor immediately.

FIBROIDS, ENDOMETRIOSIS, OR ADENOMYOSIS. More serious conditions like these also contribute to spotting and irregular bleeding. Numerous factors play a role in their development, including immune system problems, genetics, nutrient deficiencies, blood sugar and insulin imbalances, an imbalance in the ratio of oestrogen to progesterone, obesity, and gut-related conditions. Some of my clients who experience spotting in their follicular phase (that is, before ovulation) have endometriosis, fibroids, or adenomyosis.

HORMONAL BIRTH CONTROL. A number of hormonal birth control methods can cause spotting and irregular bleeding. The Pill (especially the progestin-only pill), the Depo-Provera injection, and the Nexplanon implant have all been linked to spotting in between periods. (Please check out Chapter 12 for a full discussion on birth control.) Of course, speak to your doctor if you experience spotting while on any of these contraceptives.

ENDOMETRIAL CANCER. This may cause abnormal uterine bleeding in the form of spotting or bleeding in between periods.[54]

BROWN SPOTTING

I've been asked about brown spotting more times than I can count. Brown blood that appears at the beginning or end of your period is usually just older blood that has taken longer to come out of the uterus. When blood is exposed to oxygen, it changes from red to brown. Think of when you get a cut. Initially, the blood is red, but it quickly changes to darker red and then brown. I discussed possible reasons for why you might see brown blood on page 17 in Chapter 1. Once you address the root causes of brown spotting, you'll start to see shades of red blood leaving the uterus.

I don't consider spotting a benign problem, so if you've had this issue for any length of time, there is most definitely something going on beneath the surface. For instance, a client of mine struggled for years to get pregnant when she was in her twenties. She was in an extremely stressful work environment, eating lots of sugar to cope, and not taking care of herself. She was experiencing ongoing spotting every month, sometimes up to 10 days before her period came. It was the one symptom she was having that could have been linked to her failure to get pregnant, but no doctor took her concerns seriously or did any testing to figure out the cause. As you have just learned, she might have had low progesterone due to her stress and diet. After five years of trying to get pregnant naturally, she did a round of in vitro fertilisation (IVF) and was finally able to get pregnant.

What's the lesson here? Your body is always trying to tell you what's up. It's your responsibility to decipher its messages so you can take preventative action and possibly avoid costly procedures down the road.

Vaginal Infections

Oh gawd, vaginal infections. Every woman's favourite topic! While these aren't period problems per se, they are very much linked to the menstrual cycle, and as such, they must be discussed in conjunction with menstrual health. Not only are vaginal infections a nuisance, but your body is not meant to fight infection for any length of time, so you gotta get this taken care of, girl! In addition to a visit with your doctor for diagnosis and treatment, you'll find week three of the programme (on gut health and its connection to your vaginal microbiome) especially helpful in kicking these infections to the curb for good.

The most common types of vaginal infections are yeast infections and bacterial vaginosis. I have *a lot* of experience with these. (I know. The horror! We hate talking about our vaginas, much less vaginal infections, but here I am, letting it all out.) When I was on the Pill, I used to get the worst yeast infections. It was debilitating. My gynaecologist's office was a revolving door, and after each visit I'd walk away with yet another prescription. After years of this, I discovered that I needed to work on my gut microbiome. Who knew? Once I fixed my gut, my vaginal problems and my life were forever changed.

Most women who experience vaginal infections feel like their vaginas are punishing them. The constant itching, the burning, the smell—oh the smell—and the repulsive discharge are a special kind of hell. If you suspect you have a vaginal infection, please see your doctor to find out which infection you have and treat it accordingly.

Polycystic Ovary Syndrome (PCOS)

This inflammatory endocrine disorder prevents the ovarian follicles from reaching the ovulation stage, causing significant delays in ovulation (or even preventing it), which then causes irregular or non-existent periods.[55] It affects over a hundred million women worldwide, making it the most common endocrine disorder in women of reproductive age and the leading cause of ovulatory infertility.[56]

Polycystic ovary syndrome is a bit of a misnomer; it's a collection of symptoms that may have different causes, and might not even include polycystic ovaries. In fact, approximately 20 per cent of women who do *not* have PCOS have cysts on their ovaries, and about 30 per cent of women who *do* have PCOS *do not* have cysts.[57] Even more important, these "cysts" are actually follicles that haven't gone through the maturation process.[58] In addition to "cysts," irregular or absent ovulation and periods, and fertility problems, some of the more common symptoms of PCOS include:

- insulin resistance;
- elevated androgens (male hormones);
- mid-cycle, or ovulatory, pain;
- acne or oily skin;
- hair growth, on the face and other parts of the body, like the chest;
- male-pattern baldness; and
- unwanted weight gain, an inability to lose weight, and obesity.

I could go on—depression, anxiety, sexual dysfunction, sleep apnea—but you get the idea. The variety of its symptoms and the fact that PCOS presents differently in each woman—one woman may have ovarian cysts and acne, while another may not have cysts or acne but may struggle with male-pattern baldness—has made getting a PCOS diagnosis a challenge.

To help sort things out, the European Society of Human Reproduction and Embryology and the American Society for Reproductive Medicine agreed to "the Rotterdam criteria." To be diagnosed with PCOS, a woman must present with two out of the following three conditions:

- Oligo-ovulation (irregular ovulation) or anovulation (absent ovulation);
- Hyperandrogenism (elevated levels of androgens such as testosterone); and/or
- Polycystic ovaries (i.e. enlarged ovaries each containing at least twelve follicles measuring between 2 and 9 mm when shown on an ultrasound).

Given how widely the presentation of symptoms can vary, these criteria aren't a perfect diagnostic tool. In fact, you may deal with PCOS symptoms yet not meet the Rotterdam criteria. Or you may have pill-induced (or post-pill) amenorrhoea, a temporary condition with many of the same symptoms as PCOS. Or perhaps you've been told you have PCOS based on an ultrasound when you may not. PCOS is often a catchall diagnosis for a constellation of period-related problems, especially for teenagers, a period of life when many PCOS-like symptoms show up.

Are you sensing that conventional medicine doesn't quite know how to handle PCOS? Me, too. Indeed, instead of investigating root causes, doctors resort to spot-treating the symptoms—you know how well that works!—with medications such as the birth control pill and metformin (a drug often prescribed to treat diabetes as it helps control high blood sugar and promotes insulin sensitivity). Conventional practitioners also emphasise genetics as the cause of PCOS, a finding that has led to the widespread misconception that it is unpreventable and irreversible—not to mention leaving women with a PCOS diagnosis feeling too hopeless to take control of their own recovery.

Genetics plays a role, but it is not your destiny. Yes, studies show that a woman with PCOS has a 40 per cent likelihood of having a sister with the syndrome and a 35 per cent chance of having a mother with it,[59] suggesting a genetic connection that may be stronger in some women than in others. But having a predisposition to PCOS does not mean you'll get it. Genes are turned on and off by environmental and lifestyle factors, such as diet and exposure to certain toxins like BPA. Eating an unbalanced diet filled with refined sugars, a habit we often pick up from our families, is a larger root cause of PCOS than genetics, and a factor you can control.

PCOS AND INSULIN RESISTANCE

A significant number of women with PCOS have hyperinsulinaemia (elevated levels of insulin), or insulin resistance.[60] Getting to grips with your blood sugar is key no matter what your genetics. If you've been diagnosed with PCOS or have PCOS-related symptoms, week two of the Fix Your Period programme, "Step Off the Blood Sugar Roller Coaster," will be critical for your recovery. Once you treat insulin dysregulation or insulin resistance through diet and lifestyle changes, your PCOS symptoms should diminish significantly or, in some cases, completely disappear.

PCOS AND ANDROGEN LEVELS

According to Dr Fiona McCulloch, a naturopathic doctor author of *8 Steps to Reverse Your PCOS*, "true PCOS is centered on lifelong androgen excess." In fact, 60 to 80 per cent of women with PCOS have excess androgens.[61] High androgen levels are often the result of too much insulin. Excess insulin causes the liver to make less sex hormone-binding globulin (SHBG), the main protein that binds testosterone and keeps it from running amok. This creates more free testosterone, and the potential for PCOS symptoms. High insulin also causes the ovaries to make excess androgens, in particular testosterone.

The takeaway: PCOS is not a life sentence; it is absolutely treatable. Whether you've been officially diagnosed with it or are experiencing PCOS-related symptoms, the six-week programme will help you by targeting the root causes.

Endometriosis

Endometriosis can cause pain, sometimes severe pain. For some women the pain is cyclical, and for others the pain is more constant or between periods.

Endometriosis is a disease where lesions made from tissue that is similar to (though not exactly the same as) the tissue that lines the uterus form outside the uterus.[62] These growths are most commonly found in and around the pelvis such as on the fallopian tubes, on the surface of the uterus, on the ovaries, and on the lining of the pelvic cavity. The lesions are also commonly on or near the intestines or the bladder, and can be found as far away as the lungs or the inside of the nose.

The tissue making up these growths and lesions responds to the hormone fluctuations that govern the menstrual cycle in the same way the tissue lining the uterus would, building up and shedding. But unlike the blood and tissue that make up your uterine lining, which exits the body via the vagina, this tissue has no way to exit the body. This produces inflammation, adhesions, and scar tissue that build up around the endometrial lesions.

Every woman with endometriosis has a unique experience of pain and other symptoms because the severity of the lesions does not directly correlate with the symptoms. If you have any kind of pelvic pain, either cyclically with the menstrual cycle or even between periods, you should work with your healthcare team to rule out endometriosis. Some common symptoms of endometriosis include:

- severe pelvic or period pain that can disrupt your life, forcing you to miss work, school, or social activities for a day or more;
- periods that last longer than 7 days;
- heavy to very heavy menstrual flow;
- bowel dysfunction with IBS-like symptoms, such as constipation, diarrhoea, or both;
- concurrent vaginal or bladder pain with diagnoses including vulvodynia, interstitial cystitis, and pelvic floor dysfunction;[63]
- nausea or vomiting, especially when the pain increases;
- bloating;
- fatigue;
- depression and anxiety;
- pain during sex; and
- infertility.

Endometriosis is estimated to affect approximately one in ten women of reproductive age—that's approximately *176 million women* worldwide.[64] Countless women (20 to 25 per cent of them to be exact) don't even realise they have endometriosis until they are trying to conceive and lesions are found.[65]

Shockingly, studies have shown a delay of between three and eleven years from the onset of endometriosis symptoms to final diagnosis—with an average of *9.28 years* passing before the patient receives a proper diagnosis![66] This is not okay, and it's a pretty glaring example of how often women's health concerns (especially pain) are dismissed or ignored. Often, women suffering from this debilitating condition are prescribed pain medication for their "killer cramps" and antidepressants and sent on their way, which is why it can take an unconscionably long time to get a diagnosis.

And as if that weren't enough, the procedure necessary for a diagnosis of endometriosis is both invasive and expensive. Performing an exploratory laparoscopy surgery to obtain a biopsy of the tissue is currently the only truly accurate method to diagnose endometriosis. (In other words, if a doctor diagnoses you with endometriosis or dismisses the idea that you might have endometriosis based on lab testing or imaging, please find another doctor as soon as possible.)

WHAT CAUSES ENDOMETRIOSIS?

So what causes endometriosis? It's unclear, but there are a number of theories about the contributing factors to endometriosis, including genetics, inflammation, environmental factors (like xenoestrogens), progesterone resistance, and autoimmunity.[67] While endometriosis does have genetic underpinnings, thankfully genetics isn't your destiny, and a number of lifestyle interventions can mitigate this condition. My entire six-week programme is designed to reduce inflammation, and optimising the health of your gut and liver (weeks three and four, respectively) will be especially important because of their role in inflammation and the development of autoimmune disease.

While it's important to continue to seek a clear diagnosis from an expert doctor who specialises in endometriosis, this protocol will help to lower your inflammatory load in the meantime and may significantly reduce your endometriosis-related symptoms, whether or not they are usually worse with your periods.

A little overwhelmed by all the symptoms and symptom overlap? Don't worry, we got this. Fixing your period is not that complicated. The good news is that while hormones are usually the problem, they are also the solution. The food, lifestyle, and supplement adjustments found in the six-week programme in Part 2 will not only help alleviate your most frustrating hormone-related symptoms but could lead to a complete resolution of them. You ready for that? Okay, let's get your hormones working *for you*, and put you back in charge of your period!

SIX WEEKS TO FIX YOUR PERIOD

4

WEEK ONE

ENLIST THE POWER OF FOOD
TO FEED YOUR HORMONES

Welcome to week one of the Fix Your Period programme. Are you ready to completely revitalise your body and hormones and put your symptoms in the rearview mirror? Over the next six weeks, the step-by-step changes you make in how you eat, supplement, and live will transform your experience with your period and your fertility.

Whether you deal with horrible PMS or PMDD, heavy periods or no period, infertility, acne, thyroid issues, PCOS, or endometriosis—or any other problem linked to hormonal imbalances—each step in this programme will help you identify and address the root causes that have consigned you to Period Purgatory. Keep in mind that each week of the programme should have a cumulative effect on the next. After all, your hormones don't operate in a vacuum. They are heavily influenced by your food choices and blood sugar, gut health, liver detoxification, stress levels, and thyroid function. Each week, you will be supporting your hormones from a new angle, so you can really move the needle on your health.

We'll start with a focus on using food as hormone medicine, supporting blood sugar and gut health. Then, in subsequent weeks, we'll shift our focus to liver detoxification, stress management, and thyroid optimisation. Six weeks from now, you'll have the tools you need to continue to nurture the true hormonal balance your body was designed to sustain.

In week one, you'll focus on eating foods to support your hormonal health. This is the basis for everything you'll incorporate in the weeks to come. If you don't have the nutrients you need to produce hormones properly or the understanding of how different foods affect your body, you won't have a sturdy enough foundation to build on.

Good nutrition is fundamental to hormonal health, and the foods we eat play a big role in how our hormones behave. In fact, the number one cause of hormonal imbalances, period problems, and fertility issues is a lack of the right nutrients in our diets.

Your period may come once a month, but what you eat throughout the month can and will make an immense difference in how you experience it. Remember, your body is doing the best she can with the raw materials you're giving her, so the better-quality materials you provide, the better able your body is to produce the hormones you need. No matter what your period problem or hormonal imbalance, you will no doubt benefit from a boost in nutrition.

There are few things in life that people hold stronger personal opinions about than food. It defines our cultures and family traditions. It's at the centre of our social engagements. It can even reflect our political and environmental ideologies. In almost every way, we truly are what we eat.

I point this out because, as we begin to talk about nutrition and its impact on our health, it's important to understand that a one-size-fits-all approach to food is not possible. This is due to not just our cultural diversity but, more important, our biological diversity, the biochemical factors that influence our individual behaviour, immune function, mental health, personality, allergic tendencies, tastes, and ability to process different chemicals. We're all unique and respond to different foods in unique ways. Your way of eating for hormonal health will be specific to you, and may shift and change over the course of your life, as you, say, get pregnant, pass through the postpartum time, develop an illness, or even start perimenopause.

THERE'S NO ONE "RIGHT WAY," ONLY YOUR WAY

The modern-day approach to nutrition has left a lot of people feeling weary and confused. Thousands of diet books have been published, each proclaiming to have discovered the ultimate diet for all humanity. All these diets are missing one critical factor: the individual. Without a deep knowledge of the individual, her genetics, gender, age, lifestyle, and body type, no diet on the planet can ever claim to be perfect for her.

Studies have shown that the same food impacts different people in different ways. For example, in one study, researchers fed eight hundred people an identical meal and then tested the participants' post-meal blood sugar levels. Far from being the same, the levels varied significantly from person to person. These variations were the result of the participants' many individual differences. And in fact, the same study found that personalised diets were much more successful at stabilising an individual's post-meal blood sugar levels.[1]

My mission is to show you how to tune back in to your body's innate wisdom, which means checking in often to see if something is (or is not) working for you and not relying on a specific diet or diet guru for answers. I want you to pay attention to how you feel physically and emotionally when you eat certain foods, with the goal of defining a way of eating that makes you feel energised, happy, strong, and healthy.

Note that I refer to "finding a way of eating," not to "following a diet." I strongly dislike the word *diet*; diets can box us into a very limited way of eating. I've seen many vegans introduce animal-based foods into their diet so they can rebuild their depleted hormones and regain a missing period. Conversely, I've seen meat eaters switch to a vegan diet and thrive. Then there are women who lose their periods on a low-carb diet, and others for whom that diet is the key to getting their periods back on track. Amazing, right?

Just as important, the word *diet* has come to suggest the need to conform to society's vision of the ideal body size and shape. Hearing someone talk about their diet conjures up images of my mum on her monthly SlimFast regimen in the 1990s, or of me as a teenager trying crazy ways to lose pounds, like taking diet pills and limiting myself to 1,500 calories a day. It was complete madness. I remember a number of times when I would eat nothing after 3 p.m. so I could wake up a couple of pounds lighter. Oh, my god! Fad diets and diet culture in general are dangerous to our health and hormones.

There is no one weight or body shape that promotes a healthy period. Actually, for many women, their "goal weight" is more likely to throw off their periods than to balance their hormones. I used to think if I could just be 55 kg, my life would be complete. (No joke!) After I forced my body into that weight, I had to work very hard to stay there—I was constantly hungry, eating a lot of carrot sticks and hummous (bleh), and spending an inordinate amount of time on the treadmill. Surprise, surprise, my period was irregular and sometimes even skipped months.

Can you relate? If so, my question for you is: are you going to continue to beat your body into submission, or are you ready to accept her and know that this is the home you were given this time around, and allow yourself to believe that true health goes far beyond your weight? There is so much diversity when it comes to our body sizes, and no amount of cultural conditioning is going to change our genetics. Choosing to let go of any rigid expectations of how your body should look is extremely important to do as you begin to explore the effect of food on your hormones. Trusting your body and how you are nourishing her is an essential part of finding your best health and periods.

Fat is not just sitting there taking up space and making it difficult to zip up your favourite skinny jeans. Body fat, also called adipose tissue, is hormonally active, and helps manage blood sugar, growth, blood cell production, and appetite.[2] Fatty tissue acts like an endocrine organ[3]—it produces oestrogen—which is why we need adequate body fat to sustain normal menstrual function. Too little body fat and you might experience symptoms of low oestrogen, such as irregular ovulation and periods, long cycles, amenorrhoea, and brain fog. On the other hand, too much body fat can cause a variety of period problems. This is why many women who are overweight or obese tend to struggle with oestrogen excess and its symptoms, such as heavy and long periods, PCOS, and anovulatory cycles.

With these principles in mind, I've incorporated various elements from a couple of different dietary theories to create the Fix Your Period way of eating and living. As you read more about fixing your period with food, you'll notice that there are no diet labels here, no Paleo, plant-based, keto, low-carb, and so on. To feed your hormonal health, let's keep it simple: you'll see lots of veggies, sustainably sourced animal proteins, gluten-free grains, plenty of healthy fats, fermented foods, and fruits. It's time you figured out what and how you should eat to optimise *your* hormones.

All this yumminess is a lot to take in. So, for now, don't stress about how much of this or that to eat. Just read up on all the amazing options you have. Later in this chapter (see "Week One Protocol: Feed Your Hormones"), I'll share an easy way for you to start revamping your plate for hormone health and getting all the key nutrients you need.

CARBOHYDRATES

I have always disliked the saying "You can't have your cake and eat it, too." I mean, life's too short not to eat cake. But while I'm all about the cake, I am also all about making sure you're setting yourself up for hormonal stability with the food you eat. And unfortunately, if it's eaten too often, cake doesn't make for happy hormones.

The essential component of grains, fruit, milk products, and vegetables, carbohydrates make up the largest portion of many of our diets. They're a great source of energy that can be used quickly and without much effort, which is why they're such an easy go-to when we're hungry. Carbohydrates also support thyroid function and thyroid hormone production; give the signal to your brain and adrenal glands that your body has had enough calories, which calms your stress response (and couldn't all of us use some of that?); and are a good source of fibre and resistant starch, which is fine dining for your healthy gut bacteria.

However, not all carbs are created equal. I can't stress enough that the best choices in carbohydrates are those found in whole foods. (And no, I don't mean the food store chain!) The less processed and packaged your food is, the better it will be for your body and your hormonal health. Simple or refined carbs such as white sugar, white flour, and the products made from them, such as pasta and baked goods, are typically the worst-quality carbohydrate to consume. On the other end of the spectrum, vegetables are the shining star of the carbohydrate world: low in sugar, high in fibre, and with a wide variety of vitamins, minerals, and antioxidants, compounds that help prevent or repair damage done by the unstable atoms in your body known as free radicals.

Your hormone-balancing programme should be filled with the most health-supporting carbohydrate sources possible. The first healthy carb that will soon become abundant on your plate may become your new happy hormone BFF: leafy greens.

Leafy Greens

Popeye was right. Leafy greens will really do your body good. They are the most nutrient-dense foods on the planet, yet are totally underrated—and missing from most people's daily diet. It's time to up-level your greens intake in a big way. After all, they are one of the few foods that can almost immediately affect your health.

There are many different types of leafy greens, and each of them contains an array of nutrients that not only impact your overall health but also have a pretty profound effect on the health of your reproductive organs—and all are essential for optimal hormone production and regulation:

- Beet greens
- Broccoli (tenderstem and purple sprouting)
- Dandelion greens
- Kale
- Mustard greens
- Red/green leaf lettuce
- Rocket
- Romaine lettuce
- Spinach
- Spring greens
- Swiss chard

I want you to start thinking of greens' effect on your body the way you think of the Amazon rainforest's effect on the planet. Just as the rainforest cleans the air, the abundance of nutrients found in leafy greens (chlorophyll in particular) helps remove potentially harmful toxins from your blood, makes new red blood cells, improves circulation, strengthens the immune system, and reduces inflammation. Indeed, when it comes to period problems, the nutrients in greens are gold:

CALCIUM. This mineral not only is supportive of our bones and teeth, but can also be a big help in reducing PMS symptoms such as anxiety, depression, fatigue, and pain.[4] In fact, low levels of calcium in the luteal phase have been found to cause or worsen PMS.[5] Oestrogen supports intestinal absorption of calcium,[6] so having sufficient oestrogen in your body is necessary for the integrity of your bones. It's crucial for women with amenorrhoea or low oestrogen to make sure they are getting adequate calcium through food and possibly supplementation.

MAGNESIUM. Magnesium has been shown to reduce bloating and breast tenderness and also helps to build progesterone.[7] It reduces PMS-related anxiety and sleeplessness and works amazingly well for period pain and migraines.[8]

IRON. Iron contributes to healthy egg production, stable energy levels, and healthy menstrual blood flow.[9] (Hint: too-heavy or too-light periods can be a sign of insufficient iron levels.)

POTASSIUM. This powerhouse mineral and electrolyte allows your body to make energy from the foods you eat, reduce bloating, and relieve menstrual cramps.

VITAMIN A. This vitamin helps maintain healthy, acne-free skin and may even help reduce heavy periods.[10]

VITAMIN B$_9$, OR FOLATE. Folate is well known for its prevention of neural tube defects in foetuses when taken before and during pregnancy, but it also acts as a mild antidepressant by indirectly helping to produce serotonin and dopamine.[11] Folate has also been shown to increase progesterone in premenopausal women,[12] protect cervical cells, and even reverse cervical dysplasia.[13]

VITAMIN C. Also known as ascorbic acid, vitamin C helps to increase iron absorption, which can help a missing period return and also may reduce anaemia caused by heavy bleeding.[14] It is the only vitamin shown to raise progesterone levels.[15] In addition, it helps protect your eggs and the cells of the cervix, thus reducing the risk of cervical dysplasia and cervical cancer.[16]

VITAMIN E. A powerful antioxidant, vitamin E has been shown to reduce chronic pelvic pain in women with endometriosis[17] and may reduce menstrual pain caused by primary dysmenorrhoea.[18]

VITAMIN K. An important nutrient for proper clotting of the blood, in some cases, vitamin K may be used to slow or stop excessive bleeding.[19]

Let's not forget the fibre in leafy greens. When the liver breaks down oestrogens, those metabolites are sent to the colon for removal. Eating more fibre encourages regular bowel movements, ensuring that those oestrogen metabolites are removed from the body and do not recirculate and wreak hormonal havoc. (Not to mention all the other advantages of regularly getting your poo on.) Can you believe how many benefits to your menstrual cycle are contained in just one bunch of leafy greens?

GREENS SPOTLIGHT: DANDELION GREENS

Packed with all the nutrients and minerals of other leafy greens, dandelion greens (the leaves and the root) also contain a high amount of potassium. This makes them one of the best diuretics on the scene, able to alleviate premenstrual bloating and breast tenderness. They are also a powerful liver detoxifier, aiding in the deactivation and excretion of oestrogen from the body, which is very important for women with oestrogen dominance.

Cruciferous Veggies

Some leafy greens such as kale, spring greens, mustard greens, and rocket are cruciferous vegetables. Other cruciferous vegetables include broccoli, cauliflower, cabbage, broccoli sprouts, and brussels sprouts. Cruciferous vegetables contain a compound called indole-3-carbinol (I3C), which dramatically enhances the body's ability to neutralise carcinogens and promote a healthier pathway for breaking down oestrogen in the body, thus protecting against various forms of cancer. It does this by inducing liver detoxification enzymes that help neutralise potentially harmful oestrogen metabolites and xenoestrogens (oestrogen-like environmental chemicals).[20]

I3C breaks down into the metabolites diindolylmethane (DIM) and sulforaphane glucosinolate (SGS). DIM supports phase one of liver detoxification (breaking down hormones and neutralising toxins). SGS has similar effects to DIM, but it supports phase two of liver detoxification (further processing hormones and toxins so they can be removed from the body). For the phases of liver detox, see Chapter 7. The best way to get I3C is in whole food form, through lots of cruciferous veggies.

When it comes to cruciferous vegetables, though, there are two important things to consider. First, these vegetables contain naturally occurring compounds called goitrogens. Goitrogens (specifically, in the case of cruciferous veggies, glucosinolates) can interfere with the proper functioning of the thyroid gland, making it harder for it to absorb iodine and slowing the conversion of T_4 into T_3, the active form of thyroid hormone.

Yet I believe the detrimental effect of glucosinolates in cruciferous veggies has been blown out of proportion. The amount of glucosinolates in most of these vegetables is not high enough to inhibit thyroid function. However, if you have hypothyroidism it's best to play it safe, so I recommend cooking your cruciferous vegetables (in particular, spring greens, brussels sprouts, and Russian kale[21]) to break down the glucosinolates and reduce the goitrogenic effects of these foods.[22]

Second, oxalic acid, or oxalate, a compound that occurs naturally in cruciferous greens (e.g. brussels sprouts, turnips, and leafy greens such as spinach, spring greens, parsley, and beetroot greens), can bind to calcium in the digestive process and inhibit absorption of this mineral. Boil or steam these foods to reduce the negative impact of oxalates on the body.

Or, if you experience pelvic pain, you may want to limit them. Scientifically, there has been only a weak correlation between vulvodynia (chronic pain around the vaginal opening) and oxalates, but anecdotally, I've seen diets high in oxalates—are you eating a raw spinach salad every day and putting spinach in your morning smoothie?—contribute to pelvic pain conditions such as vulvodynia and interstitial cystitis (also known as painful bladder syndrome). When women I've seen in my work went on a low-oxalate diet, they saw an improvement in or a complete resolution of symptoms such as persistent vulvar pain, urinary frequency or urgency, and incomplete emptying of the bladder. This was also found in a small study of women who went on a low-oxalate diet and calcium citrate treatment.[23]

CRUCIFEROUS VEGGIES

- Broccoli
- Brussels sprouts
- Cabbage
- Cauliflower
- Chinese cabbage
- Pak choi
- Radishes
- Turnips
- Watercress

Sprouts and Microgreens

Sprouts are germinated seeds, a plant in its infancy. And though small, they are packed with a ton of nutrients. It's easy to grow them at home, so you have a cheap and convenient way to support your hormones.

Broccoli sprouts have an extremely high concentration of the compound sulforaphane, which has super-anti-inflammatory powers.[24] It changes the way your liver metabolises oestrogen, redirecting it to a healthier pathway.[25] Because of this redirect, sulforaphane literally stops breast and ovarian cancers (and other cancers) from forming and growing, and massively reduces or eliminates PMS-related symptoms, acne, ovulation bloating and pain, and a host of issues related to oestrogen dominance.[26]

Microgreens, the next growth stage after sprouts, are the tiny leaves that appear on the plant. They can be grown from a variety of seeds, such as cabbage, spinach, broccoli, rocket, and Swiss chard. You may have seen them as a pretty garnish on meals in restaurants, but they're far more than food décor. In fact, a few studies have found microgreens to contain higher concentrations of nutrients than their grown-up counterparts.[27]

Microgreens, with their milder flavour, are a great option if you have a hard time with the pungent or bitter taste associated with dark leafy greens. To meet your daily greens quota, try them in smoothies or on top of salads, chilli, or soup.

Sweet Veggies

All varieties of vegetables play a key role in the process of becoming friends with your hormones, but there's a special place in my heart for sweet vegetables, especially because on many occasions including them in my diet has prevented me from gorging on sugar-filled foods. You'd be amazed at how easily a side of beetroot or sweet potato can stop those crazy cravings in their tracks.

Add these veggies into your regular food rotation—especially during the week before your period, as their natural starch content helps produce serotonin, the happy neurotransmitter that offsets anxiety and tension in the premenstrual time. They'll help you beat cravings and improve how you feel overall physically and emotionally. They are sweet, obviously; are full of fibre; and contain a lot of menstruation-supportive nutrients such as calcium, magnesium, and vitamins A, C, and a number of the B vitamins.

SWEET VEGGIES

- Acorn squash
- Beetroot
- Butternut squash
- Carrots
- Cassava or yucca
- Jicama
- Kabocha squash
- Parsnip
- Plantains
- Pumpkin
- Spaghetti squash
- Sweet potatoes and yams

Pulses: Beans and the B Vitamins

Pulses' (beans) nutritional stock is pretty high in my books. They're super healthy, super versatile, and super affordable. Just like sweet vegetables, they help you stay fuller longer and provide sustainable energy. Pulses are full of fibre, protein, and minerals, and their antioxidant capacity is off the charts!

The *B* in *beans* could stand for "B vitamins." That's great, as every woman should make it her mission to get adequate B-complex vitamins at all stages of her life, but especially B_6 and B_9, which play an important role in menstrual cycle support. In addition to being B_9 powerhouses—200 grams of most varieties of beans contains more than half your daily requirement—beans contain:

B₁, B₂, AND B₃, which have been shown to help PMS symptoms.[28]

B₅, which may help reduce cortisol overproduction and increase levels of adrenal steroid hormones and progesterone. This could be helpful for women with hypothalamic–pituitary–adrenal (HPA) axis dysfunction or low progesterone,[29] which often appears in the form of missing periods, irregular cycles, or lack of ovulation.

B₆, which improves symptoms of oestrogen dominance by helping the liver break down and deactivate oestrogens and by supporting the formation of progesterone.[30] This can help lengthen the luteal phase of your cycle and improve irregular menstrual cycles. Vitamin B_6 in its active form, pyridoxal-5-phosphate, has been shown to help reduce the symptoms associated with premenstrual syndrome, including premenstrual depression.[31] B_6 is also involved with the production of serotonin, which controls your mood, appetite, and sleep patterns. It also supports the production of GABA, what I call the anxiety-calming neurotransmitter. B_6 can improve irregular cycles, oestrogen dominance, progesterone deficiency, anxiety, and poor egg quality—so yeah, when it comes to your menstrual cycle, B_6 is kind of a big deal, and why B_6-rich foods are a must for a better period experience.[32] Bring on the B_6!

B₉, OR FOLATE is all kinds of wonderful for your period. (Remember the "Leafy Greens" section of this chapter.)

If pulses are so good for you, why do diets such as the Paleo and low-carb diets, eliminate them? The original argument is that pulses are harmful because they contain compounds called lectins, which have been linked to inflammation, leaky gut, and malabsorption of nutrients. That's true, but soaking and cooking beans reduces the lectins.[33] Cooking (in particular, pressure-cooking) deactivates the vast majority of lectins and offsets their negative effect on our bodies. Sprouting and fermenting beans also helps reduce the effect of lectins. One food with lectins you should be careful of, though, is peanuts: a lot of people eat them raw or in the form of raw peanut butter. Additionally, peanuts are susceptible to mould contamination, which could be why they are one of the most common allergens.[34]

SOYBEANS

Most people consume too much of the overprocessed forms of soy, such as soy milk, soy protein products, and soy-based cheese. Today, soy is the number one genetically modified crop in the world,[35] and in the United States, roughly 94 per cent of soy is genetically modified.[36] Also, the herbicides often sprayed on GMO crops wreak serious havoc on your hormones. Here's the lowdown: when it comes to soy, buy organic and consume only small amounts of whole and/or fermented soy, or avoid it completely. Fermentation greatly reduces the level of phytic acid, a storage form of phosphorous that inhibits the absorption of iron, calcium, magnesium, copper, and zinc. Fermentation does increase histamine levels in the end product, so if you have histamine intolerance, you may want to avoid fermented soy products.

Soy can cause menstruation issues because it contains isoflavones, the most potent phytoestrogens in the plant world. Phytoestrogens are naturally occurring compounds that can have a similar impact on your body as the oestrogen your body produces. Most women I've worked with become highly oestrogen dominant when they consume too much soy. Others experience a lightening and shortening of their periods as the phytoestrogens act as a kind of anti-oestrogen, blocking more potent oestrogens from binding to their receptors.[37]

If you eat soy-based foods on a regular basis or see soy listed on the ingredients label of something you eat often, and you notice menstrual cycle symptoms such as heavy periods, painful periods, breast tenderness, heightened emotional PMS symptoms, irregular periods, digestive issues, or skin problems such as acne, then it might be time to cut out soy and see how you respond. (Sit tight, we will do this in week three of the programme.)

So, unless you have a bean allergy, pulses can be eaten two to three times a week in small amounts, about 50 to 100 grams per serving at a time—on top of salads, in side dishes, or in soups. They are a good source of carbs, but not a great replacement for more nutrient-dense animal protein sources. Pay attention to whether you experience wind, bloating, or other digestive symptoms after eating them, and adjust your diet accordingly. These symptoms might indicate a condition such as small intestine bacterial overgrowth (SIBO), low stomach acid, or a food sensitivity. (We'll delve into these in Chapter 6.)

Gluten-Free Whole Grains

This is yet another contentious food group. While some people swear by strict adherence to a grain-free diet, I've found that, for most women, avoiding grains is neither desirable nor practical, and often not even necessary. We must be diligent in finding the right foods for our bodies without succumbing to the idea that we have to cut out entire food groups forever.

When it comes to grains, whole grains are the good grains, nutritious little gems that contain fibre, B-complex vitamins, essential fatty acids, and a wide range of minerals. Whole grains provide sustained and high-quality energy because the body digests them slowly. They also contain strong antioxidant properties, which protect your body and your reproductive organs from damage by free radicals.

As for the "bad" grains, refined grains such as white flour have typically been stripped of their outer layers, the bran and germ, which contain all the vitamins, minerals, and protein. What is left is the carbohydrate-dense endosperm, which is then refortified with synthetic forms of the B vitamins and minerals lost in the refining process. So, when it comes to your period and overall health, it is in your body's best interest that you keep refined grains to a minimum.

So, why do I recommend only *gluten-free* whole grains? Gluten, a protein found in grains such as wheat, barley, rye, kamut, spelt, and farro, makes these grains difficult for many people to digest. Studies show that about a third of people in the United States have some level of gluten sensitivity.[38] And then there's coeliac disease, which is an autoimmune disease with a response triggered by eating gluten. Every time we eat gluten, it creates microscopic tears in our gut lining. Eventually, these tears stop healing, and this can lead to persistent intestinal permeability.[39] Intestinal permeability, also known as leaky gut, is a main cause of virtually all autoimmune diseases, including Hashimoto's disease, Graves' disease, and even type 1 diabetes.[40] All these diseases will impact your hormones and subsequently your menstrual cycle.

In addition to gluten, you should pay attention to the way ingesting corn makes you feel, and avoid it if you experience gut issues. Corn contains a type of gluten known as zein. While it's not exactly the same as wheat gluten, there are similarities that can cause cross-reactive symptoms in people who are gluten intolerant or who have coeliac disease.

About 92 per cent of US corn is genetically modified[41] and sprayed with Roundup, which contains glyphosate (in the UK glyphosate is still used but is under review). This potent herbicide contributes to the toxin load that disrupts our endocrine system and thus our hormones. (I will discuss this more fully in Chapter 6.) There is a staggering array of corn products on the market. Look at any product label in the supermarket and you'll see some kind of corn-based ingredient in it—no doubt partly why corn is one of the most allergenic foods out there.

The only way to avoid genetically modified, herbicide-contaminated corn is to make sure the corn products you eat are organic. Or you can just avoid corn altogether. I love a good taco with tortilla chips as much as anyone, but if you've spent a long time not feeling great, feeling better is of more importance. I'll dive into this topic in Chapter 6, as the effects of these chemicals on gut health, and therefore hormone health, are profound. For now, start to observe your corn intake and see if it leads to bloat, acne, water retention, irritable bowel syndrome (IBS), or any other symptoms.

GLUTEN-FREE GRAINS

- Amaranth
- Black rice
- Brown rice
- Kasha (toasted buckwheat)
- Millet
- Quinoa
- White rice

Fruit

Fruit is a nutritious, healthy source of carbohydrates loaded with many beneficial antioxidants and other nutrients to support your hormone health. In this programme, I want you to focus on fruits low in fructose. If you've heard of the glycaemic index (a scoring system for foods that measures how quickly they raise blood sugar and insulin levels), you may be wondering why I'm cautious about fructose, as it ranks low on the glycaemic index (GI). First, fructose is still sugar, and too much of it negatively impacts your hormones. So, don't be fooled by the label "health food" when it is given to sweeteners high in fructose, such as agave nectar. Second, no matter where it may rank on the GI, too much fructose will put a lot of stress on your liver and can lead to non-alcoholic fatty liver disease and a breakdown in liver function. This can lead to serious hormonal imbalances. Don't get me wrong, high GI foods are a problem, too, and we'll delve into them more fully in Chapter 5.

Fruits with more than 4 grams of fructose per serving are considered high-fructose foods. I suggest limiting your consumption of these fruits, especially if you have a fructose intolerance, blood sugar issues (e.g. high or low blood sugar), insulin resistance, diabetes, or PCOS. Luckily, lots of fruits are low in fructose, and the fibre in these fruits keeps your body from absorbing their sugar all at once.

LOW-FRUCTOSE FRUITS	HIGH-FRUCTOSE FRUITS
Apricots	Apples
Berries (raspberries, strawberries, blackberries)	Cherries
	Dried fruit
Cantaloupe	Grapes
Grapefruit	Kiwi
Nectarines	Pears
Oranges	
Peaches	
Watermelon	

Eat fruit whole, keeping the fibre and micronutrients intact. A medium-size navel orange is loaded with fibre and vitamin C and contains approximately 9 grams of sugar total. Compare that to an 240 ml glass of orange juice containing about 21 grams of sugar (about 4 teaspoons) and a lot less fibre. Would you eat 4 teaspoons of sugar in the morning with your breakfast? I doubt it.

FAT

The 1990s called and they want their low-fat diet back. In case you didn't know, high fat is totally the new cool, and low fat is so out. Remember those SnackWell's Devil's Food Cookie Cakes? No joke, I used to eat an entire box in one sitting. After all, they were fat-free. Yes, I was one of those girls who obsessively stuck to less than 20 grams of fat a day so I wouldn't put on weight. I was starving, so it's no wonder my hormones were completely screwed up by the time I was seventeen.

Women have roughly 10 per cent more body fat than men on average because—wait for it—we make babies, and as you now know, our bodies are always trying to get us pregnant.[42] This extra fat storage is necessary for nourishing a foetus during pregnancy and then sustaining that baby once she is born. We require a certain amount of dietary fat to function at our best, and if we don't get enough of it, we're gonna get ourselves in trouble. Dietary fat supports your menstrual cycle and fertility,[43] and our livers use healthy fats to make cholesterol, a building block for some of our most important sex hormones, such as progesterone, oestrogen, and testosterone.

We've spent most of our lives being bombarded with the message that fat is really bad for us. Well, I'm here to tell you that eating fat will not make you fat or give you high cholesterol. You just have to eat the right fats. And when, after a long period of time without it— hey, it could be some people's entire lives—you start eating enough fat, miracles happen: your brain starts working, you lose the brain fog, your emotions calm down, and you're able to make decisions. In addition, fats help you feel satiated by stimulating the release of leptin, the hormone that tells the brain you're full, which helps prevent you from overeating.

Most of the women I see in my practice are not eating enough fat, or enough of the right fats.

So, for your menstrual and reproductive health, add healthy fat to each meal to facilitate increased absorption of critical fat-soluble vitamins such as A, D, E, and K, the star players in hormone regulation and fertility.

Here are signs your body needs more fat:

- You get headaches and brain fog and are plagued by indecision.
- About thirty to sixty minutes after meals you experience tiredness or sleepiness and want to take a nap.
- Your period has its own agenda. Either it's missing (for three months or more) or is extremely irregular, showing up every 35 to 90 days.
- You could eat and eat some more, and are never full. Often, you're starving again one to two hours after your meals.
- You have intense cravings for sugar. ("It's 3 p.m. Pass the M&Ms!")
- Your hands and feet are always cold, your hair is frizzy, and your skin feels like it's perpetually parched.

If you find yourself saying yes to any of these symptoms, you will most likely benefit from eating more fat. But how much? We'll get to that in a moment. First, let's take a look at the fats you need in your life now and the ones that should be banished for good.

The Lowdown on Fats

SATURATED FAT. Saturated fat is found in high quantities in animal meat, full-fat dairy, and other foods such as butter, coconut, and lard. This type of fat is always solid at room temperature, making it easy to differentiate from other fats. For years, we were told it was the worst kind of fat, complete with stories of sky-high cholesterol, clogged arteries, and heart attacks. Plenty of studies out there lay the blame for cancer, heart disease, high cholesterol, and obesity squarely at the feet of the saturated fat found in animal products. Thankfully, those studies have been debunked in recent years, but the cultural paranoia persists. Even non-animal saturated fats, such as coconut and palm oil, were nudged out of our diets years ago and replaced by seed oils such as soy, corn, and rapeseed. Here's the deal, though: saturated fat is essential to life. It helps your body absorb fat-soluble vitamins A, D, E, and K. Saturated fat protects your liver from damage by free radicals, and specific types of saturated fats strengthen your immune system, support metabolism, and provide some of the best materials for building steroid hormones.

MONOUNSATURATED FAT. Monounsaturated fats are highest in foods such as avocados and olive oil.

POLYUNSATURATED FAT. Polyunsaturated fats are found in seafood, nuts, and seeds. Two of the most important polyunsaturated fats are the omega-3 and omega-6 fats.

OMEGA-3 AND OMEGA-6 FATTY ACIDS. Fats are made up of chains of fatty acids, which are the basic building blocks of body fat and all the body's hormones. Our bodies can produce most fatty acids from the food we consume, but there are two kinds it can't produce: omega-3 and omega-6. These are called the essential fatty acids because, well . . . they're essential to our survival. Foods that contain them should be consumed regularly.

Omega-3 fatty acids are super important when it comes to hormonal health. Omega-3s can help reduce menstrual cramping and PMS symptoms.[44] The brain is high in omega-3 fatty acids, which have been shown to help the brain cope better with stress and to reduce the negative effects of chronic stress.[45]

These are the types of omega-3 fatty acids you should know about:

- Alpha-linolenic acid (ALA) is found in plant foods such as chia seeds, flaxseed, and walnuts. ALA can be converted to the two other omega-3 fatty acids, EPA and DHA.
- Eicosapentaenoic acid (EPA) and docosahexaenoic acid (DHA) are found primarily in cold-water fatty fish such as anchovies, herring, mackerel, salmon, sardines, and trout and in shellfish such as mussels and oysters.

When it comes to omega-6 fats, all are not created equal. Some are great for you, while others aren't. For instance, the natural forms found in coconuts, seeds, and nuts are what you want to be eating. Meanwhile, highly refined and processed peanut and rapeseed oil are extremely high in omega-6 fats and likely oxidised and damaged by the processing; this could trigger an inflammatory response and lead to hormonal havoc.

EAT THESE OMEGA-6 FOODS

Coconuts and coconut oil

Pumpkin and sunflower seeds

Pine nuts and pistachios

Borage oil, black currant seed oil, and evening primrose oil

AVOID THESE OMEGA-6 FOODS

Processed plant and seed oils such as rapeseed, corn, cottonseed, peanut, safflower, soybean, and sunflower

We evolved as human beings consuming omega-6 and omega-3 fatty acids in approximately a one-to-one ratio, but nowadays that ratio is anywhere between ten to one and twenty to one.[46] Yikes! The modern-day popularity and overuse of vegetable oil is a major cause. Most restaurants cook with omega-6-rich rapeseed, corn, cottonseed, safflower, soybean, and sunflower oils, making food much more omega-6 rich. Plus, most processed foods are made with them. The widespread practice of feeding a combination of corn and soy to domestic livestock has made our meat more omega-6 rich, too, while lessening the amount of omega-3 in it.

What's the impact on our health of so many inflammatory omega-6s? For one, chronic inflammation leading to severe menstrual cramps, migraines, endometriosis, fibromyalgia, and other conditions associated with chronic pain.

Omega-3 fatty acids are the building blocks for the anti-inflammatory prostaglandin E_1 (PGE_1), while omega-6 fatty acids are used to produce the pro-inflammatory prostaglandin E_2 (PGE_2). When we have more omega-6 in our diets than omega-3, our bodies produce more pro-inflammatory PGE_2 and less PGE_1. This puts the body in a chronically inflamed state. In fact, women with dysmenorrhoea have higher levels of PGE_2 compared with women without menstrual cramps. Also, those levels are highest in the first 2 days of one's period, which is typically when symptoms are at their worst.[47]

In addition, omega-3 supplementation is associated with lower androgens. Higher androgens are commonly linked to PCOS.[48] DHA stabilises moods; deficiencies in it contribute to premenstrual mood swings, depression, and postpartum depression.[49] Omega-3s from fish have been shown to lessen menstrual cramps because they reduce inflammation in the reproductive organs.[50]

To support our hormonal health, we need to bring our ratio of omega-3 to omega-6 back into balance by actively lessening our omega-6 intake and increasing our omega-3, specifically DHA- and EPA-rich food sources.

PLANT SOURCES OF OMEGA-3 FATTY ACIDS

A common misconception is that we can get enough omega-3s from plant sources such as flaxseed, chia seeds, and walnuts. While the body can convert some ALA (the type of omega-3 found in plant sources) to EPA and DHA, the most bioavailable and beneficial omega-3 fatty acids, for most of us this conversion is inefficient at best.[51] One study found that less than 5 per cent of ALA is converted into EPA, and less than 0.5 per cent of ALA is converted into DHA.[52] As if that weren't bad enough, high levels of dietary omega-6s inhibit this conversion process; [53] plus the conversion requires adequate levels of nutrients such as zinc, iron, and vitamin B_6.[54]

HOW TO INCORPORATE FATS INTO YOUR DAY-TO-DAY

Fats to Eat in Ample Amounts

- Cod liver oil or fish oil
- Cold-pressed, unrefined coconut oil
- Extra-virgin olive oil
- Fats from grass-fed animals (e.g. lard, tallow, and duck fat)
- Butter from grass-fed animals (butter contains very little dairy, but if you're sensitive to dairy, you can use ghee)
- Ghee from grass-fed animals
- Organic full-fat A2 cow dairy (this is far less inflammatory than A1 dairy)
- Organic full-fat goat/sheep dairy (full-fat cheese, full-fat raw milk, kefir)
- Organic grass-fed beef
- Free-range eggs
- Wild-caught fish such as herring, mackerel, salmon, sardines, shellfish, and trout

Fats to Eat in Moderate Amounts

These are all great sources of fat, but it's not necessary to eat a whole avocado or 150 grams of almonds each day. Plus, you'd likely get a major stomachache if you ate all those nuts. See the week one protocol at the end of this chapter for more specific guidelines on how best to incorporate these foods.

- Almonds
- Avocados
- Brazil nuts
- Cashews
- Chia seeds
- Coconut milk and coconut butter
- Ground flaxseed and flaxseed oil
- Hazelnuts
- Hemp seeds
- Nut butters (e.g. almond and cashew) and seed butters (e.g. sunflower and pumpkin)
- Olives
- Pine nuts
- Pumpkin seeds
- Sesame seeds (unhulled) and tahini
- Walnuts

Fats to Avoid

RANCID, OR OXIDISED, FATS. This is exactly what it sounds like: fat that has gone bad when exposed to more heat, light, or oxygen than it's meant to withstand. This commonly occurs in unstable, highly processed polyunsaturated oils such as rapeseed, corn, soy, and sunflower. However, it can happen to any oil due to improper storage (overexposure to light, heat, or air) and being kept for too long.

TRANS FATS. This is an unsaturated fat that's been exposed to high heat to become saturated in a process called hydrogenation. Trans fat is typically found in commercial baked goods and fried foods and should be avoided, as it disrupts sex hormones, significantly increases inflammation, and interferes with fertility.[55] Seriously, margarine, a trans fat, is just one molecule away from being plastic. If you put it in the sun, it will not melt. So, like a bad boyfriend, lose the trans fat.

NUTS AND SEEDS: NUTRIENT POWERHOUSES FOR A BETTER PERIOD

Mother Nature did good when she created nuts and seeds. They are little nutrient powerhouses filled with healthy fatty acids, minerals, and protein. Though I've placed them under "Fats to Eat in Moderate Amounts," that doesn't take away from how good they are for you. We just need to be cognisant of actual serving sizes for these foods. Each type of nut and seed has a different nutritional profile, but generally speaking, nuts and seeds contain various B vitamins, copper, vitamin E, iron, manganese, magnesium, phosphorus, selenium, and zinc.

- Brazil nuts are super high in selenium, a superstar mineral for your menstrual cycle. Selenium is found in large quantities in healthy egg follicles and plays a critical role in the later stages of follicle development.[56]
- Walnuts are the queens of plant-based omega-3s, providing more omega-3 fatty acids than any other nut.
- Pumpkin seeds are small but mighty. Just 30 grams contain significant amounts of copper, iron, manganese, magnesium, phosphorous, and zinc. While all these nutrients are crucial, I want to give a shout-out to zinc, which helps the follicles in the ovaries mature each month.[57] It also improves PCOS-related issues such as insulin resistance and high testosterone.[58] Additionally, zinc supports thyroid hormone production, and because of its anti-inflammatory effect, it even helps lessen period pain.[59]

PROTEIN

Protein seems to be *the* topic of the diet and wellness world these days. Some experts encourage us to eat zero animal protein, while others urge us to make it the main focus of our meals. To say this is confusing is an understatement! I've been a health coach for many years, and sometimes even I'm overwhelmed by all the noise.

Protein is a real hustler. In addition to creating your organs, muscles, nails, and hair, protein helps your cells communicate and facilitates muscle contraction and the transmission of nerve signals. Protein also makes up immune molecules, blood cells, hormones, and enzymes, and even assists your cells in making new proteins. And it is an essential structural component of all hormones, which means you've got to consume sufficient protein to make enough hormones. Wow! With protein performing all these roles, it's easy to see how essential it is to eat an adequate amount of the stuff.

Protein is made up of chains of amino acids. Your body needs twenty different amino acids, but you can manufacture only eleven of them. The remaining nine are called essential amino acids because you can't make them and need to get them from your diet. Foods that have all nine essential amino acids are called complete proteins. Animal proteins such as red meat, poultry, fish, eggs, milk, cheese, and yoghurt are all complete proteins. Complete plant-based proteins include lentils, quinoa, and soy.

You don't need to get all nine amino acids from one food. Other protein sources, while not complete, provide adequate nutrition when combined with another plant protein. For example, a meal of brown rice combined with spinach, beans, cauliflower, carrots, and tahini makes a complete protein combination. It also isn't necessary to eat a complete protein at every meal, as long as you are getting all the amino acids over the course of the day. As with fats, the type and quality of the protein makes a difference. Higher-quality proteins such as grass-fed meats, free-range eggs, wild-caught fish, and organic vegetables facilitate better hormone function.

Not enough protein or a low-protein diet (about 50 grams or less per day) messes with levels of growth hormone, thyroid hormones, and insulin—and drives the body towards fat storage, increasing both body fat and fatty liver.[60] Also, keep in mind that the only natural source of vitamin B_{12} is animal protein, so if you're plant-based or vegan, you should be supplementing. B_{12} plays many critical roles in the body, such as facilitating oestrogen detoxification and thyroid hormone production.[61] These two mechanisms alone have far-reaching effects, including keeping our moods in check, normalising our oestrogen levels, and lessening persistent fatigue.

PLANT-BASED PROTEIN

If you're relying on plant-based sources of protein, you may not be getting as much protein as you think. Many plant-based sources have decent amounts of protein, but they are not as easily digested and used by your body as animal proteins. This is because some plant protein sources (e.g. soy, wheat, corn, oats, lentils, and kidney beans) contain anti-nutrients, which have been shown to decrease protein absorption in the small intestine by up to 50 per cent.[62] So, be sure to eat a varied and abundant diet of high-quality protein.

GOOD SOURCES OF ANIMAL PROTEIN

- Grass-fed red meat (venison, lamb, beef) along with liver and/or pâté
- Free-range chicken
- Organic turkey, pork, and duck
- Free-range eggs
- Wild-caught fish and other seafood, such as sardines and shellfish

GOOD SOURCES OF PLANT PROTEIN

- Amaranth (complete)
- Beans (pulses)
- Chia seeds (complete)
- Fermented soy products (such as tempeh; complete)
- Hemp protein powder (complete)
- Hemp seeds (complete)
- Lentils
- Nut butters
- Pea protein powder
- Quinoa (complete)
- Soy (complete)
- Spinach
- Spirulina (complete)
- Walnuts

DAIRY

Do you eat dairy products? If so, I've got five questions for you:

1. Do you experience ovulation pain or period pain?
2. Do you have acne?
3. Do you experience bloating, gas, upset stomach, or IBS-like symptoms on the regular?
4. Do you often feel phlegmy or experience sinus congestion or sinus infections?
5. Did you experience frequent ear infections, need grommets, have repeated colds or flus, or have your tonsils removed as a child?

While high-quality dairy products can provide nutrients, especially fat and protein, if you regularly experience any of the symptoms just listed, I recommend reducing or removing conventional, non-organic dairy. I know that cutting back on or giving up any food can be difficult, especially a food many of us consume every day, but here's the scoop: dairy isn't doing your hormones or your period any favours.[63]

Most dairy in the United States comes from factory farms, where cows are fed products not natural to their diet, such as grain, corn, and soy. This creates significant inflammation in their bodies. They are also injected with rBGH (recombinant bovine growth hormone), a bioengineered hormone that forces the cows to produce more milk than they normally would. While its link to hormone problems is somewhat controversial, it has been banned in many countries, including the United Kingdom, Canada, Australia and the European Union.[64]

This overstimulation of the cow's udder causes it to become infected, thus requiring antibiotics. As a result, these added hormones and antibiotics reside in the milk. Once we ingest that milk, they interfere with our female hormonal system.[65]

For what it's worth, when I stopped consuming pasteurised cow's milk products years ago, my period pain pretty much disappeared. I've seen the same happen with countless clients. Many women also notice clearer skin—sometimes their acne disappears completely[66]—a decrease in stomach problems, and a resolution of their sinus issues. Nowadays, I stick to mostly goat's or sheep's milk cheese, sometimes treating myself to raw cow's milk cheese and the occasional ice cream or two in the summer. It's called "balance," people.

Given the benefits of ditching the dairy, I recommend you remove it from your diet for twenty-eight days and see how you feel. Before you freak out about the milk in your tea or the goat's cheese on your salad, take a deep breath. If you aren't ready to live without dairy, I get it. I love cheese as much as you do!

Here are some suggestions for easing into the process:

IF YOU DECIDE TO CONSUME MILK PRODUCTS, make sure they are full fat, organic, and free of rBGH, antibiotics, and pesticides. You can find these options at farmers' markets and in many supermarkets in the UK.

CONSIDER RAW-MILK DAIRY PRODUCTS. This is controversial, but consider that raw milk has not been through pasteurisation and homogenisation, which means that it still has beneficial intact vitamins and bacteria as well as enzymes, including lactase, which is the enzyme needed to break down the lactose in milk. People describe it as being much easier to digest and not causing the same physical responses such as allergies, colds, and stomach upset as pasteurised commercial dairy. Also, consider fermented dairy, such as raw-milk kefir, which has a lot of naturally occurring good bacteria and is easier to digest for many people. It's important to source raw milk from a reputable farm or producer who tests their milk for contaminants and makes those results public.

KNOW YOUR CASEIN. A1 casein is a protein found in milk from Holstein cows. It stimulates the production of inflammatory cytokines in many people.[67] A2 casein, which comes from Jersey cows and goats or sheep, does not appear to have the same inflammatory effect and seems to be easier to digest. In fact, when my clients swap out conventional cows' milk dairy products for goat or sheep cheese, their chronic colds, sinus issues, period pain, and acne subside. Try sourcing dairy from grass-fed Jersey cows, or goats or sheep.

CHOOSE MILK SUBSTITUTES. If you're all in, and are going to quit dairy, there are a number of milk substitutes you can try to ease the transition, such as rice, oat, hemp, and coconut milks; almond and other nut milks; plus yoghurt and other dairy-like products (cheese) made from these milk substitutes.

WEEK ONE PROTOCOL: FEED YOUR HORMONES

Now that you know which nutrient-rich foods support your hormone health and which processed ones don't—corn oil, I'm looking at you—you can start bringing more of the good ones into your diet and crowding out the bad. This week, you'll pile your plate high with the good stuff and chew your way to better nutrient absorption and digestive health.

Make Your Plate

How much of each type of food should you be eating to support proper hormone production? Keep it simple. At every meal (breakfast, lunch, and dinner) your plate should look something like this: half carbohydrates, one quarter fat, and one quarter protein (see Figure 6 below).

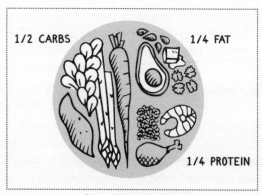

Figure 6: Make Your Plate

CARBOHYDRATES. Your plate should consist mostly of leafy green vegetables and other nutrient-dense, high-fibre veggies (like the cruciferous and sweet veggies). Greens have traditionally been a side dish, but I want you to rethink that. Start to view greens as your main dish and everything else as a side dish. If you don't consume greens regularly, start with 60 grams of cooked greens a day, which is not very much. Eventually work your way up to 240 grams a day or more if you'd like, sometimes consuming them raw, other times cooking them. I love steaming and sautéing greens; it softens them up while preserving their raw crunchiness. You can also include gluten-free whole grains, but they shouldn't be your only source of carbs. Pulses should be eaten two to three times a week in 100 to 200 gram servings. As for fruit, try two pieces of medium-size fruit a day.

FAT. Saturated fats, monounsaturated fats, and polyunsaturated omega-3 fatty acids should make up the majority of your fat consumption, starting with one to two golf ball-sized portions per meal, depending on your body's needs. (See "Specific Considerations" box on page 114.) Put avocado slices on your salad, add a small handful of pumpkin seeds into your soup, or enjoy a tablespoon or two of grass-fed butter on your sweet potato. This may not seem like a lot, but healthy fats are extremely dense sources of energy and nutrients.

PROTEIN. I recommend 75 to 100 grams of animal and vegetable sources of protein each day, depending on how active you are. This can be split up between meals and snacks. A very simple guideline: eat a serving of protein about the size and thickness of your palm at each meal. If you feel hungry within thirty to sixty minutes of finishing your meal, try eating more protein at your next meal and see how you feel.

Use the plate percentages just given as a rough guide. The goal is to feel satisfied and full, with no cravings for four to six hours or until your next meal. This requires some experimentation, but I've observed that the 50/25/25 ratio works really well to get most people on track towards keeping their energy high and moods stable, and ultimately have rockin' hormones. (Note: I never recommend reducing your fat intake to less than 25 per cent of your total food intake in a day.)

SPECIFIC CONSIDERATIONS

IF YOU HAVE HYPOTHALAMIC AMENORRHOEA OR HAVE NOT HAD A PERIOD FOR MORE THAN THREE MONTHS, you will need to up your general calorie intake and increase your carbohydrates, protein, and fat consumption. If a period is missing in action, I generally recommend eating a minimum of 2,500 calories a day. Because protein is an important building block for sex hormones (and for balancing blood sugar, which takes your body out of fight-or-flight mode), animal protein might be required every day or at each meal. In addition, you may need to consistently increase your fat intake at meals in order to get your period back. This may be more than the two golf ball-sized portions of fat I recommended on the previous page.

IF YOU HAVE IMBALANCED BLOOD SUGAR, INSULIN RESISTANCE, DIABETES, OR PCOS, eat animal protein at each meal to help stabilise blood sugar. You may need to experiment with your carbohydrate intake as well, possibly reducing it and increasing your protein and fat intake. I don't recommend a vegan or vegetarian diet for anyone with blood sugar instability or these conditions, unless you are carefully tracking your blood sugar and getting a wide variety of foods at each meal.

Chew Your Food

Digestion begins with the simple act of chewing. Are you even aware of your chewing or the number of times you chew your food? Well, it's one of the most important things you can do for your hormonal health—seriously. Chewing properly leads to greater assimilation of nutrients by initiating the release of digestive enzymes that break down food. If you don't chew your food well, digestion is compromised (and there's no point in eating good food if it's going to go to waste). Large food particles make it more difficult for the stomach to completely digest food, which causes an increase in bacteria in the intestines. This bacterial overgrowth can cause gas and bloating, constipation and diarrhoea, and abdominal pain and cramping. Eventually this will lead to nutritional deficiencies and hormone problems.

This week, make it a priority to chew, chew, chew. Try counting the chews in each bite, aiming for twenty to thirty. It might be a challenge at first, but the benefits of properly chewing your food are so great that doing so is a must for anyone who wishes to overcome hormonal problems. After chewing properly, you will likely experience less burping, windiness, bloating, and stomach pain—and you'll start to notice how little everyone else chews, which will freak you out!

I may have just flipped your understanding of food left, right, and centre, but by starting to focus on hormone-supportive foods and re-vamping your plate, you've taken a massive step forwards on the path to balanced hormones and better periods. We've started with food because it is the foundation for your organs, blood, bones, skin, hair, and, most important, your hormones. Eating high-quality food on a regular basis is akin to building a foundation out of concrete rather than sand. No matter where you are in the menstrual life cycle, you will benefit immensely from the changes you make now.

My best advice this week is to begin eating lots of hormone-friendly foods, get used to eating them in the right proportions at each meal, potentially cut out or cut back on dairy, and start chewing your food more mindfully. Then simply take note of, with genuine curiosity rather than judgement, how your body responds. Think of it as a personal experiment to see what works for you.

This is just the beginning, but achieving consistency in your meals now will make the next step (balancing your blood sugar) and the rest of the programme that much easier. And the longer you stick with it and the more consistent you are, the better results you'll have.

5

WEEK TWO

STEP OFF THE BLOOD SUGAR ROLLER COASTER

Now that you've begun revamping your meals and getting into the practice of chewing your food, it's time to add another important piece of the hormone-balancing pie and focus on correcting blood sugar imbalance.

Blood sugar problems are traditionally thought of as something that only diabetics and overweight people need to be concerned about. But here's the straight truth: every single one of us should be thinking about our blood sugar.

Sugar and other refined carbohydrates (think anything made of flour) can seriously affect your endocrine system and wreak hormonal havoc. Yes, that biscuit is impacting your ovaries. No, I'm not kidding. Don't get me wrong, your body can handle some sugar—glucose, or blood sugar, is the body's main fuel source, after all—but too much sugar and too much of the wrong kinds of sugar can raise blood sugar levels too high. And what goes up must come down. The subsequent crash will not only bring your blood sugar levels too low, but will also wreck you in the process. Hello, 3 p.m. energy slumps and 2 a.m. wakeups!

Before I got into health coaching, I didn't understand how stressful the mismanagement of my own blood sugar was on my body. Sure, eating a giant piece of cake or skipping a meal didn't make me feel good, but why was it such a big deal? Well, your body uses insulin to keep an even stream of glucose flowing into your cells, so they can convert it to energy. When you sabotage that balance, you risk short-term issues such as energy crashes, stomach upsets, sleep problems, anxiety, and long-term conditions such as polycystic ovary syndrome, endometriosis, dementia—women develop Alzheimer's at double the rate of men—and even cancer.[1] An ongoing dramatic rising and falling of your blood sugar really screws up your hormones and period, and plays a role in disruptive PMS and PMDD symptoms. We all think that being knee-deep in a tub of ice cream at this precarious time of the month helps, but it just makes matters worse. This is why getting your blood sugar under control is one of the first steps you can take as part of your hormonal health revamp.

I know. Reducing or quitting sugar isn't easy. I really get it! Wine and brownies are hard to resist. Luckily, there are some fairly simple ways to tame your wayward blood sugar, including small shifts such as eating breakfast with more high-quality protein and fat. You can step off the blood sugar roller coaster, where your blood sugar and insulin spike and crash continually, and onto a level playing field, where your blood sugar and insulin stay stable (at least most of the time).

SUGAR, THE LEGAL DRUG

I refer to sugar as the legal drug because of its powerful influence on mood and physical health. Have you ever felt yourself getting angry for no logical reason or even throwing a tantrum after eating a sugary treat? *That* is the power of sugar.

The average person in the UK is consuming 90 grams of sugar daily, three times the recommended amount, according to a report by Public Health England (it recommends 30 grams per day). That is over 32 kg a year. The average American consumes approximately 68 kg (150 pounds) of sugar per year![2] Compare that number to two hundred years ago, when the average person ate under 1 kg (2 pounds) of sugar *every year.* And the sugar back then came from sugar cane and beets and was not the high-fructose rocket fuel our bodies run on today. This dramatic change in our diet is the single greatest health concern in the developed world, and unfortunately, it has now spread to developing countries, making it one of the biggest global health crises we face.

Our addiction to sugar is usually talked about in connection with the rise in obesity, heart disease, and diabetes, but its impact on the body extends far beyond these Big Three. The focus on diabetes and obesity, while warranted, can trick people into thinking that their blood sugar is under control if they're at a normal weight or have not been diagnosed as a diabetic. Not the case. Even fitness fanatics and size 6 women can unknowingly be under the influence of big bad sugar. Unbelievably, 35 per cent of the American population is either diabetic or insulin resistant,[3] meaning their cells are resisting or ignoring the message insulin sends to move blood sugar from the bloodstream and into the cells, causing blood sugar levels to remain chronically high. Yes, insulin resistance increases the risk for diabetes, but it needs to be addressed even before diabetes is an issue—for the sake of your period, your fertility, and your hormones.

The World Health Organization recommends that we limit the amount of added sugars to no more than 5 to 10 tsp, or 25 to 50 grams, a day.[4] That's way below what most people are consuming. When reading labels, think of "added" and "refined" sugars as just what they sound like: additional sugars added to foods to increase their sweetness or palatability. These sugars have usually been manufactured or processed in some fashion to make them extra sweet—meaning, they are not in their natural from-the-earth state. Such sugars include white granulated sugar, brown sugar, corn syrup, high-fructose corn syrup, honey, and maple syrup. (Though these last two are in their natural state, they are still used for extra sweetness and behave in the body the same way processed sugar does.) Added sugars are found in just about every processed food out there, from juices and breads to energy drinks and yoghurts.

Compounding the problem of added sugars in almost everything we eat, we feel the need to reward every single good job or important event with sweet treats. After a few years of this "rewarding" we start to associate sweet things with feeling good physically and emotionally. This leads to a reliance on sugar that is akin to drug dependency.

Sugar makes us feel better because it stimulates the release of dopamine in the brain.[5] It is well documented by now that the cravings, withdrawal, and relapse symptoms in sugar addicts are similar to those of users of cocaine and heroin. And in fact, evidence suggests that sugar is more addicting than cocaine. In one study, cocaine-addicted rats were offered a choice between sugar and cocaine, and they chose sugar a massive 94 per cent of the time![6]

The negative impact on our bodies is just as severe. Some scary effects of sugar overconsumption include difficulty concentrating; an increase in calcium and magnesium excretion;[7] constipation; headaches; depression; anxiety; insomnia; candida overgrowth; chronic yeast infections;[8] recurrent bacterial vaginosis;[9] acne and other skin problems, such as acanthosis nigricans,[10] rashes, psoriasis, and eczema; premature gray hair; and breast and cervical cancers.[11]

And yes, hormonal imbalances. Don't forget, like cortisol, insulin is a tier 1 hormone and has a downstream effect on your tier 2 and tier 3 hormones. Because of this, consumption of refined carbohydrates and sugar is directly connected to oestrogen dominance; progesterone deficiency; and cortisol, melatonin, and thyroid hormone dysregulation in many women. My disruptive oestrogen dominance symptoms, and those of most of my clients, virtually disappeared when we got our blood sugar under control. Hallelujah!

The Role of Carbohydrates

So, where is all this sugar coming from? Look no further than carbohydrates. But as we covered in the previous chapter, all carbs are not created equal. The type of carb and the kind of sugar it contains makes a huge difference.

Complex carbohydrates are found in starchy vegetables and grains. Your body breaks them down into glucose, a simple carbohydrate and the form of sugar found in your bloodstream that is used as energy. The complex carbs in starchy vegetables and grains take longer for the body to digest and, so, don't cause dramatic spikes in blood sugar levels.

When eaten with the right amount of protein and fat, these carbs create smaller, more manageable rises in blood sugar. This is partly because protein and fat are slow energy sources for the body, and thus must go through a three-step breakdown process before they can be used. This, in turn, causes a more gradual rise and fall in insulin levels, allowing the body time to use up the energy rather than having to store it immediately.

Two types of simple carbohydrates, or sugars, glucose and fructose, are found in fruits and non-starchy vegetables. Before your body can use it, fructose needs to be broken down into glucose by your liver. Too much fructose can put an undue burden on your liver—a big part of the reason I suggest trying low-fructose fruit in week one. Even so, fruits are also loaded with fibre, which helps slow digestion and prevent blood sugar spikes. Anyway, most people aren't overloading on sugar because they are eating too much fruit; it's because they are eating too many refined or processed carbs.

Refined, or processed, carbohydrates are sugars and grains that have been altered in some way, and thus stripped of their vitamins, fibre, and other health-supporting nutrients. We're talking about added sugars, all kinds of flour, refined grains, plus all the foods made with these ingredients (e.g. sweets, baked goods, soft drinks, breads, and pastas).

Eating too many refined carbohydrates and sweetened or processed foods packed with added sugars is at the root of our blood sugar problems, and one of the main causes of most of today's chronic inflammation-based diseases.[12]

HOW YOUR BODY USES SUGAR

Our blood can only handle a certain amount of glucose at any one time, so what happens when we eat too much?[13] That's where the pancreas comes in. In response to the glucose in the bloodstream, this large gland behind the stomach releases insulin, the blood sugar regulating hormone. The insulin shuttles the glucose from your bloodstream into your cells, so it can be used for energy.

If your cells don't need this glucose right away, insulin carries the excess glucose to the liver, where it is stored as glycogen. Just as a car burns petrol, your body burns this glycogen for fuel between meals and during exercise. Unfortunately, if you consistently eat sugar and refined carbohydrates in excess, the liver fills up, and the excess glucose is converted to fatty acids (triglycerides). These fatty acids enter your bloodstream and get stored in your fat tissue, to be used later for fuel between meals, if you need it.

If all goes well and you don't eat those extra grams of sugar too often, you have a good chance of having balanced blood sugar.

What Balanced Blood Sugar Looks Like

But what does balanced blood sugar look like? Well, you'll know that your blood sugar is balanced if you:

- feel consistent energy throughout the day, with no marked crashes or bouts of sleepiness;
- experience minimal to no cravings for sugar or caffeine;
- experience no cravings for sweets or sugar after a meal;
- are able to fall asleep and stay asleep without waking up once or more during the night;
- wake up with energy for the day ahead;
- experience stable moods (yaaas!); and
- feel little or no physical pain (e.g. joint pain, headaches, or period cramps).

THE BLOOD SUGAR ROLLER COASTER

So, what's the blood sugar roller coaster? When you eat too much sugar, you flood your system, causing a huge spike in blood sugar levels. The pancreas responds by making more insulin to move the sugar into your cells. All this insulin moves the sugar out of the blood a lot faster than normal. The result is a dramatic drop in your blood sugar levels, also known as reactive hypoglycaemia. This drop in blood sugar makes you irritable, anxious, foggy-brained, and "hangry," and causes a craving for more carbohydrates (usually in the form of refined sugars) or caffeine, to bring your blood sugar levels back up to normal as quickly as possible. And up and down you go.

What Unbalanced Blood Sugar Looks Like

You'll know you have unbalanced blood sugar if you experience:

- crazy energy highs and crashes (one minute you're wide awake; the next, unable to keep your eyes open);
- sugar and caffeine cravings first thing in the morning, mid-morning, mid-afternoon, and after dinner;
- feelings of extreme hunger thirty to sixty minutes after a meal;
- trouble either falling asleep or staying asleep throughout the night;
- difficulty waking up in the morning (e.g. you want to keep hitting Snooze); or
- moodiness, meltdowns, anxiety, or panicky feelings.

What happens when we continue on this blood sugar thrill ride? Spoiler alert: it doesn't end well. Eventually, this vicious cycle will

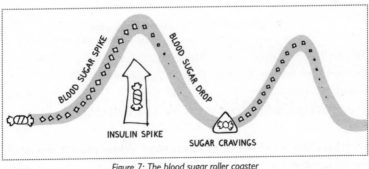

Figure 7: The blood sugar roller coaster

create what's known as insulin resistance. But what does that even mean, and why is it so bad?

Our muscles and fat cells do an excellent job of accepting all that glucose and converting it to energy or storing it away, but there is only so much they can do. Eventually, our cells reach their capacity and can no longer take on any more glucose. In essence, the cells become resistant to the effects of insulin, which leads insulin to no longer work properly. It's kind of like insulin is ringing the cell's doorbell, but no one is opening the door to let it in. So, it leaves the glucose package at the door.

This results in too much glucose in the blood, which signals the pancreas to compensate by increasing its insulin output, as more and more insulin is needed to get glucose out of the bloodstream and into the cells. The result? High levels of both glucose and insulin in your blood. This inability to properly move sugar out of the blood and into the muscles and fat cells is known as insulin resistance.

Meanwhile, the cells in your body and brain are starved for glucose to make energy. You feel tired, hungry, foggy, and depressed, and you crave more sugar *all the time*, even though there is plenty in your bloodstream. Insulin resistance is serious business, often giving rise to diabetes, gestational diabetes, and obesity.[14]

My point here is that it is *so* crucial to keep your blood sugar balanced at all times (or as often as possible). This is because insulin is a tier 1 hormone, and as you now know, all your hormones are in constant communication with one another. So, if your insulin production has run amok, your other hormones will soon follow suit.

What Insulin Resistance Looks Like

After a long period of chronic blood sugar dysregulation, insulin resistance may develop. On top of all the symptoms listed under "What Unbalanced Blood Sugar Looks Like," insulin resistance symptoms also include the following:

- Your belly fat (or muffin top) is growing and seems impervious to exercise or weight loss attempts;

- You experience a brain fog that doesn't seem to lift ("Where did I put my keys again?");
- You feel persistent fatigue that doesn't improve no matter how much you sleep (i.e. almost like jet lag);
- You feel unfocused, forgetful, absent-minded, and scatterbrained; and/or
- Your consumption of sugar or sweets doesn't relieve your cravings.

BLOOD SUGAR, INSULIN, AND YOUR MENSTRUAL CYCLE

As you can see, just about every cell in your body is affected by excess blood sugar and insulin. And your ovaries are no exception. In fact, your ovaries have a very interesting relationship with high blood sugar and insulin, both of which can induce ovulatory dysfunction and even PCOS in women who are genetically predisposed to the syndrome.[15]

There are insulin receptors on the ovaries.[16] Say what? Yup, that's right. Excess insulin raises LH, which causes the ovaries to produce more androgens (such as testosterone) and less of the oestradiol and oestrone they usually make.[17] And when ovaries produce excess testosterone in lieu of oestrogen, the entire feedback loop between your brain and ovaries gets interrupted, and your eggs are not able to grow adequately and, ultimately, be released.[18] Cue sporadic ovulation or lack of ovulation. *No bueno* for your menstrual cycle (see Figure 8 on page 126).

High insulin also lowers sex hormone-binding globulin (SHBG),[19] which is designed to bind up testosterone so that it's not available all at once. When SHBG goes down, it allows more free testosterone into the bloodstream, which can compound the problem.

Once you have higher levels of androgens, you may start to develop some of the symptoms of PCOS. This doesn't necessarily mean you have PCOS. Some women are genetically susceptible to PCOS, whereas others aren't. For instance, my blood sugar and insulin were all over the place when I was younger, and while I was never diagnosed with anything, I had some of the hallmark signs of PCOS: very irregular cycles with periods every three to four months, excess body hair, and hair loss on my head. However, once I worked on cleaning up my diet and stabilising my blood sugar in my early twenties, my ovulation was restored and my cycles regulated, my body hair growth slowed significantly, my hair loss stopped, and I never again developed any symptoms associated with PCOS. I've observed similar results in many of my clients over the years.

However, some women don't see a full resolution of their symptoms with these lifestyle interventions—a sign they need further testing to determine if they have PCOS and need additional treatment. No matter your genetics or diagnosis, though, one thing's for sure: balancing your blood sugar is an excellent first step towards reining in out-of-control hormones.

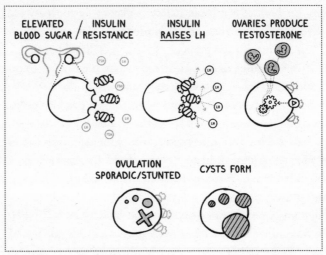

Figure 8: The blood sugar and insulin connection to higher ovarian production of testosterone and ovulation disruption

Insulin and Oestrogen Dominance

Now let's look at how insulin is connected to oestrogen dominance, or oestrogen excess, which is when oestrogen becomes dominant over its sister hormone, progesterone. Think of a seesaw, with oestrogen hanging out on the higher end and progesterone on the lower end. This imbalance is linked to PMS; painful, heavy, and long periods; breakthrough bleeding;[20] long cycles; PCOS;[21] endometriosis;[22] and fibroids.[23]

Insulin resistance raises the activity of an enzyme called aromatase, which is responsible for converting circulating testosterone into oestradiol. This means that high levels of insulin can raise oestrogen and pave the way for oestrogen dominance. Unfortunately, aromatase lives in your fat cells, so the more body fat you have, the more oestrogen you'll have, too.[24] This is why women who are overweight are more prone to conditions related to oestrogen dominance, and why weight loss can improve both insulin resistance and oestrogen dominance.

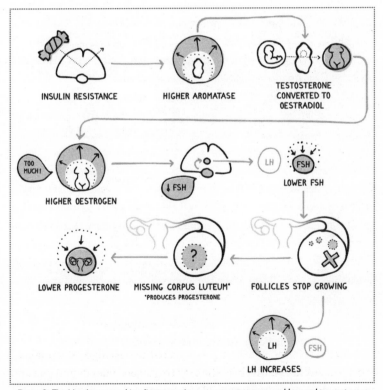

Figure 9: The blood sugar and insulin connection to excess oestrogen and lowered progesterone

Excess oestrogen in the body tells the hypothalamus that there's plenty of oestrogen to go around. Based on this intel, the hypothalamus then talks to the pituitary gland, telling it to slow down FSH production. Remember, FSH directs your ovary to stimulate and grow follicles that will produce oestrogen as they grow. So, if your brain thinks there is lots of oestrogen, it will slow down FSH production because it assumes the follicles in the ovaries are in full swing, making plenty of oestrogen.

When FSH production is suppressed, FSH is unable to complete its job of grooming the little follicles, and their development is stopped in its tracks. This is how ovarian cysts start to form. To compound the problem, some women end up with higher levels of LH relative to FSH over time. Why? As I said before, insulin resistance raises LH levels.[25] Research suggests that one of LH's jobs is to prevent further growth of the non-dominant follicles on the ovary once a dominant follicle has been chosen.[26] So, with elevated LH levels, your follicles basically don't have a chance in hell of getting to the point of ovulation. And even if a follicle manages to get to the point where it's ready and waiting for ovulation, those systemwide elevated LH levels don't allow for a high enough spike in LH to kick off ovulation.

After a while, ovulation generally begins to sputter, becoming delayed, and may stop occurring completely. When ovulation doesn't occur, there is no corpus luteum to make progesterone for the second half of the cycle. This leads to lower progesterone levels. And without enough progesterone, oestrogen steps into the dominant role, moving ever higher on the seesaw, and all those annoying symptoms crop up or worsen. You're probably wondering how so many things can go wrong when insulin levels go haywire. Insulin is just one hormone, right? Right. But remember, insulin is a top-tier hormone, reigning like a queen over all the other hormones in your body, and they have to do what it says.

Insulin, Inflammation, and Menstrual Cycle Pain

In the land of hormones, insulin resistance and inflammation go hand in hand. Perpetually elevated blood sugar and insulin create a bad environment for your sex hormones, but also cause the immune system to produce excess inflammatory chemicals, creating inflammation throughout the body. Unchecked inflammation is the root cause of almost every chronic disease as well as much of the pain we experience related to our cycles, including migraines, ovulation pain, and menstrual cramps. Reduce inflammation by stabilising your blood sugar, and the pain associated with your period will improve. Ta-da!

We're all familiar with the inflammation you can actually see if, say, you bang your knee on the coffee table and it gets red and swollen. (Ugh, don't you hate when that happens?) Well, elevated blood sugar and insulin levels from eating problematic foods like refined carbs and sugars trigger the same reaction inside your body as hitting the coffee table does for your knee. It's an invisible kind of inflammation that happens in your brain, gut, joints, reproductive organs, and elsewhere. Daily exposure to them is kind of like hitting your knee on the coffee table every single day. The inflammation will never get a chance to heal because you keep exacerbating it; instead, it spreads throughout your body like wildfire. And the inflammation can go on for very long periods, unbeknownst to us, because we don't see it.

So, what does this have to do with period pain? Prostaglandins, lipids with hormone-like effects, are found in every organ in the body. Their main job is to deal with infections and injuries. There are two types of prostaglandins, pro-inflammatory and anti-inflammatory, and we need both in the appropriate amounts. Insulin resistance and excess inflammation reduce anti-inflammatory prostaglandins while increasing pro-inflammatory prostaglandins, which becomes a big problem for our uteruses. When the pro-inflammatory prostaglandins are activated, they trigger inflammation, pain, and fever in the injured part of the body in an attempt to heal the damaged area. When there is bleeding involved, prostaglandins stimulate the formation of blood clots and contract the muscles around the damaged area to prevent blood loss. This is a good thing when you have an injury such as a big cut on your leg. It's not so great when you have your period.

In a way, our bodies perceive our menstrual bleeding as a kind of injury and take steps to heal it. The shedding of the endometrial lining triggers the release of a large number of prostaglandins. Those released at the source of the bleeding, in the uterus, will often stimulate muscle contractions—the cause of the painful cramps many women experience at this time in their cycle. This goes for ovulation pain as well. Prostaglandins are partially responsible for stimulating the release of an egg,[27] so if you notice worsening pain at ovulation, this is a potential sign of underlying inflammation.

But here's the deal: because prostaglandins are located throughout our entire bodies, their impact during this time is not restricted to our abdomens. Women are at higher risk of developing a migraine or tension headache in the 2 days leading up to their period, and at highest risk between days 1 and 3 of their period.[28] Prostaglandins are a major cause of migraines throughout the course of the menstrual cycle, and levels of certain inflammatory prostaglandins are higher during migraine attacks.[29] In particular, PGE_2, a pro-inflammatory prostaglandin, increases significantly during a menstrual migraine.[30]

I know firsthand how debilitating period-related pain can be, whether it's cramps, ovulation pain, or headaches, and how it can stop you in your tracks, making your normal daily routine impossible to manage. By balancing your blood sugar and ultimately lowering inflammation, you can significantly minimise your period cramps and ovulation pain and decrease the likelihood of those dreadful menstrual migraines. Sounds good, right?

A WORD ABOUT ALCOHOL

The cultural narrative concerning women and alcohol is that we need it just to get through life. This is evidenced by the trend in rewarding ourselves after a long day of work and parenting with a glass or two—or three; who are we kidding?—of wine. We see this in movies, on TV, and in the many memes that joke about "mummy juice." Alcohol has become a completely acceptable way for women to cope with life's overwhelming, frustrating experiences.

Unfortunately, alcohol can and does really mess with your hormones. (Sorry, ladies. I'm sure this is not what you wanted to hear, but you need to continually check in with yourself to expose what's no longer working in your life. And you won't get a handle on your period if you're getting loaded on a frequent basis.) Alcohol consumption causes a major blood sugar and insulin spike and, according to research, can actually increase oestrogen production and reduce progesterone production.[31] In addition, alcohol can increase the conversion of testosterone into oestrogen, which can increase chances of oestrogen dominance.[32] Drinking at night or before bed might help you fall asleep, but it disrupts your melatonin production, will likely mess with both the amount of high-quality, healing REM sleep you get and your ability to sleep through the night (because of the way the liver metabolises the alcohol during the second half of the night).[33]

Women often ask about a somewhat healthy source of alcohol or how much they can drink without consequences. Most people don't like my answer. The truth is, there isn't a miracle alcoholic beverage that won't have an impact on your health in one way or another. At the same time, for many people (me included), cutting out alcohol completely is unrealistic. So . . .

If You're Going to Drink No Matter What

It's up to you whether to drink, but if you do:

TAKE ACTIVATED CHARCOAL. Used in hospitals for alcohol poisoning, activated charcoal works by absorbing and filtering toxins from the stomach. Take one or two capsules before you drink. This is not a miracle fix, but it will help support your body's detoxification process.

EAT SOMETHING. Eat a meal (following the plate guidelines from Chapter 4, of course) or a high-protein snack before drinking, so the alcohol doesn't have such a profound effect on your blood sugar.

CHOOSE YOUR DRINK WISELY. The worst drinks are sugary cocktails and mixed drinks, for obvious reasons, and beer because of the gluten and carbohydrate content. Your best bet would be organic red wine, which is far superior to conventional red wine, as grapes are one of the fruits most heavily sprayed with herbicides. Also, red wine contains resveratrol, a powerful antioxidant.

LIMIT YOUR CONSUMPTION. Sticking to three drinks or fewer per week is your best bet.

CONSIDER WHY YOU'RE DRINKING. If you're drinking because you've had a rough day and want to unwind, or because you feel it will help you get through the hideous premenstrual time or painful cramps, then I suggest you take a look at these reasons and seek out alternative ways to care for your emotional and physical health. Unless you do, alcohol and its toxic effects on the body will continue to hijack your health.

EXERCISE AND BLOOD SUGAR MANAGEMENT

When it comes to exercise, there's good news and bad news. The good news is exercise has been found to enhance insulin sensitivity.[34] In fact, exercising in short, intense bursts with breaks in between, called high-intensity interval training, or HIIT, helps to clean up excess blood sugar and improve insulin regulation.[35] Similarly, resistance training, such as weight lifting, also has great benefits for insulin sensitivity.[36] Done in moderation, it helps remove fat from your muscles ("burn" fat), allowing them to use glucose better.[37] Resistance training and HIIT are often done in conjunction with each other and can be beneficial in addressing insulin resistance.

If you're groaning as you read this, take heart: there is some evidence that exercise doesn't have to be strenuous to improve insulin problems. Yoga also appears to be good for blood sugar management and insulin sensitivity.[38]

Now here's the bad news. Too much exercise causes problems with insulin. Are you running marathons or going to spin class five times a week and not losing any weight? Or, worse yet, are you exercising like crazy but *gaining* weight? (WTF, right?) It might seem counterintuitive, but this kind of intense exercise has a negative impact on insulin resistance. This is because extremely intense exercise raises cortisol levels and triggers inflammation.[39] Both these responses work great in the short term, but in the long term they drive your body into survival mode.

Here's how it works: first, your body releases energy from its stores, and you feel awesome. But then your body worries that it won't have enough energy to function, so it *increases* those energy stores, especially in visceral fat. It also increases cravings for carbohydrates. And those higher cortisol levels produced by intense exercise raise your blood sugar. All this results in inflammation, insulin resistance over time, and problems for your hormones and your period.[40]

Survival mode means your body is scrambling to conserve energy stores at all costs. So, if you're working out *hard* every day and wondering why the heck you aren't losing weight, now you know. If this sounds like you, you'll want to chill out on your exercise routine.

> **CAUTION:** If you have amenorrhoea (especially hypothalamic amenorrhoea) or you're in a low-oestrogen state, you may have to stop your intense exercise routine (spinning, boot camp, weight lifting classes, and intense HIIT) completely, or replace it with yoga, Pilates, or gentle walking.

Many clients have told me that when they kicked their alcohol habit, they slept more hours and had more consistent energy, fewer or zero PMS symptoms, more resilience, and an improved ability to deal with things that weren't working in their lives. (Hello! This is major.)

THE PMS—HORMONAL CRAVINGS CONNECTION

Do you feel full-on ambushed by your premenstrual cravings for sugar, chocolate, and baked goods every month? Or maybe your snack of choice is crisps, French fries, or some other salty goodness. It's not so hard to avoid these indulgences before ovulation, but after ovulation happens, all hell breaks loose! It is well known that we women have a pretty hard time battling our sugar and salt cravings the week before our periods. But why? And for goodness' sake, what can be done about it?

Two things are happening that are important for you to know about. First, higher oestrogen in the follicular phase correlates with increased insulin sensitivity, meaning insulin works better, or you need less of it, to control blood sugar in the first half of your cycle.[41] Once oestrogen drops post-ovulation, progesterone rises. Higher progesterone can affect insulin sensitivity negatively, which means you're more prone to blood sugar swings (hyperglycaemia to hypoglycaemia) and more sensitive to drops in blood sugar in the second half of your cycle.[42]

What might this look like? Oh, you know, food cravings, mood swings, brain fog, and bouts of fatigue. The key takeaway here is that before ovulation, we might be more able to tolerate a skipped meal, or a biscuit. But in the second half of our cycle, we need to be much more diligent about when and what we eat, so as to keep our blood sugar in balance. In the second half of your cycle, really limit your sugar, alcohol, and processed grain intake, and eat lots of fibre, protein, and healthy fats.

Second, when oestrogen drops after ovulation, so do levels of mood-related neurotransmitters in the blood—specifically, serotonin, dopamine, and norepinephrine.[43] This is because oestrogen has a modulating effect on these neurotransmitters.[44] Aggravating this problem is the fact that many women are oestrogen dominant, so the drop in oestrogen is more severe, resulting in a more drastic mood and energy shift. Or they're in a low-progesterone state, which means they don't feel that progesterone's full positive effects in the second half of their cycle.

This can cause significant cognitive and mood problems such as anxiety and depressed feelings, disrupted sleep, increased pain, and low energy. (Red alert: PMS and PMDD!) When your energy and mood bottom out and you feel jet-lagged from sleepless nights, cravings for carbohydrates and sugar start to set in. These foods will boost your neurotransmitter levels for a hot minute, but will inevitably cause a crash, which sends you spiralling into the depths of premenstrual potato crisp despair.

Once you and your blood sugar become pals, though, you'll notice the cravings start to die down and your mood more easily stabilise in the second half of your cycle. Hallelujah!

Wait, Is PMS the Same as Being "Hangry"?

Are you noticing the similarities between emotional PMS symptoms and blood sugar and insulin dysregulation? When you're in a state of reactive hypoglycaemia, or low blood sugar, after a high-carb or high-sugar meal, the symptoms are basically identical to the more prominent PMS symptoms: insatiable hunger, cravings, anxiety, fatigue, irritability, and brain fog.

Nutrition plays a major role in the treatment of PMS.[45] A nutritional analysis published in the early 1980s stated that PMS patients consumed 62 per cent more refined carbohydrates and 275 per cent more refined sugar than women not suffering from PMS.[46] This is why parting ways with the cupcakes and eating more protein, fat, and blood sugar-stabilising carbohydrates will allow you to step off this roller coaster.

WEEK TWO PROTOCOL: BALANCE YOUR BLOOD SUGAR

Ready to start feeling ah-mazing in your body again? During the next week you'll develop eating habits to support your quest for blood sugar balance by testing your blood sugar and following my 7-Day Blood Sugar-Balancing Meal Plan. I'll arm you with everything you need to test your blood sugar on your own—this will be especially exciting for all you biohacking babes—and eat the foods to keep you and your glucose even-keeled throughout the day. No more peaks and troughs around here. And we'll amp up your magnesium, an essential and mighty mineral for all things period-related.

Test Your Blood Sugar

Testing your own blood sugar is the ultimate period hack because it will clearly tell you how the food and beverages you consume are affecting you on the cellular level. If that isn't taking back control of your health, I don't know what is.

Pay attention to the symptoms you feel after you eat or drink and compare them to the lists "What Balanced Blood Sugar Looks Like" and "What Unbalanced Blood Sugar Looks Like," which appear earlier in this chapter (pages 122 and 123). Start to get a clearer picture of how the food you're eating is impacting your blood sugar levels and use that data to make targeted changes to what you're eating and drinking to keep your blood sugar steady in the weeks and months to come.

To start the healing process, you'll first need to get comfortable testing your blood sugar using a glucose testing meter. This bio-hacking tool provides a great way to know for sure what your fasting blood sugar is, whether you're keeping your blood sugar balanced after meals, and, if not, which foods are causing your blood sugar instability. The glucose meter, test strips, and lancets you'll need can all be purchased separately or in a test kit. (These are all available online.) The replacement strips can be expensive, so before you decide which meter to buy, compare prices.

TESTING SCHEDULE

Test your glucose for at least three consecutive days, but to get a clear picture of how you're responding to different foods and drinks that you'd normally consume, it's most helpful to do it for seven consecutive days. Adhere to the following testing schedule:

BEFORE YOUR FIRST MEAL. The best way to test your fasting glucose is first thing in the morning, after eight hours of not eating.

IMMEDIATELY AFTER YOU EAT. Then test again, to determine how the food has affected your blood sugar.

EVERY FIFTEEN MINUTES UNTIL AN HOUR HAS PASSED. You'll test four times in the hour after your meal, at 15, 30, 45, and 60 minutes after eating. Always test after breakfast, and alternate between testing after lunch and dinner, to get a good idea of what's happening at different times of the day.

TWO HOURS AFTER YOUR MEAL. Test your blood sugar again.

OPTIONAL: AFTER EATING CERTAIN FOODS. You can test after eating certain foods to isolate their effect on your blood sugar. If any food

raises your levels over 20 to 25 points, it is not a good food for you
and should be avoided.

Be sure to record the numbers in your workbook (find it a fixyour-
period.com), a notebook, or on a spreadsheet so you have a record of
the results. Also make a note of the time you tested and what you ate.

WHAT TO LOOK FOR

- Fasting blood glucose levels should preferably be between 70 mg/
  dL and 85 mg/dL. If your fasting glucose is consistently between
  100 mg/dL and 125 mg/dL, you might be prediabetic. If this is the
  case, make an appointment with your doctor immediately.
- Post-meal blood sugar should go up only about 20 to 25 points,
  and should rise to no higher than 110. For instance, if your fasting
  glucose was at 85, you wouldn't want it to be higher than 110 after a
  meal. A level higher than that could indicate both the beginnings of
  insulin resistance and a higher risk of metabolic syndrome. If your
  levels go up by more than 20 to 25 points after you eat, you need to
  home in on what is causing the spike. Your blood sugar level should
  never go above 130 mg/dL thirty minutes to two hours after a meal.
- Your blood sugar levels should go back to your previous fasting
  number (or close to that) one hour after eating.

NOTE: Most people will see the spike between thirty and forty-five
minutes after they eat. (This is why you test every fifteen minutes
for up to one hour after eating: to catch the spike.)

DIRECTIONS FOR TESTING BLOOD SUGAR

Estimated time, start to finish: about 2 minutes

1. Wash hands. Invisible debris on fingers can result in erroneous
   readings. Avoid using alcohol-based hand cleaners/sanitisers,

especially if you're checking regularly. They can dry your fingers and cause calluses.

2. Rinse fingers under warm water to increase blood flow.
3. Prepare supplies.
   A. Spring-loaded device with sterile lancet for sticking finger
   B. Glucometer
   C. Test strips
   D. Tissue paper or cotton pad for blotting blood
4. Choose a location on your finger to get a blood sample. Rotate areas to prevent calluses. The fleshy pads of the fingertips are easiest and often the least painful.
5. Collect blood sample.
   A. Cock the spring-loaded device and prick any finger. Follow the instructions provided by the manufacturer.
   B. Gently squeeze finger; avoid using a pumping action.
   C. Touch the blood to the test strip.
6. Obtain the glucose reading.
   A. The glucometer will blink or count down once the blood has been absorbed by the test strip.
   B. Record the number from the glucometer in your notebook or on your spreadsheet.
7. Clean up.
   A. Safely discard used lancet, tissue paper, or cotton pads in the rubbish.

TROUBLESHOOTING

UNSTABLE BLOOD SUGAR. Unstable blood sugar can be a sign of multiple other imbalances in the body, especially if you have already adopted a hormone-friendly way of eating and are still seeing high or weird numbers after certain meals. If this is the case, it could indicate:

- one or more food sensitivities;
- levels of high or low cortisol and unmanaged stress;
- leaky gut or bacterial dysbiosis such as candida; and/or
- another immune response or autoimmune disease.

If there is no observable pattern to your levels, and the unstable blood sugar doesn't seem related to a specific food, make an appointment with a doctor to evaluate any underlying issues that may be causing unexpected blood sugar spikes and drops.

FAULTY READINGS OR GLUCOMETERS. Every now and again, you may get a faulty reading, showing an extremely high or extremely low number. If this happens once, restart your glucometer and take the reading again with a new test strip, making sure you follow the steps correctly. If extremely high or extremely low readings happen consistently, consider exchanging your glucometer for a new device, or replace its batteries to see if the numbers change.

Follow the 7-Day Blood Sugar-Balancing Meal Plan

Move over, turkey sandwiches. Protein + complex carbohydrates + healthy fats + fibre = the foundation for optimal hormonal health. We're talking high-quality protein that is organic or free range, complex carbohydrates such as gluten-free grains, healthy sources of fat such as avocado and olive oil, and fibre in the form of vegetables. Trust me, girlfriend, eating meals that adhere to this plan is going to be a game-changer for your hormones. Follow this meal plan, and you'll feel the difference in just seven days. Each day includes breakfast, lunch, and dinner.

Breakfast is one of the most important meals of the day. Each day you'll have a protein-rich breakfast that fuels you through the entire morning—no 10 a.m. coffee breaks here. This will set you up for stable blood sugar throughout the day. I've included my favourite breakfasts in the meal plan.

DEVELOP GOOD BLOOD SUGAR-BALANCING EATING HABITS

As part of the meal plan, you'll also follow a few good blood sugar–balancing habits:

- Wait to eat your next meal until you feel a little hungry, but do not wait until you are starving or experiencing irritability, shakiness, fatigue, or sugar cravings.

- Make sure you're eating enough at each meal to keep you satisfied for at least three to four hours. Undereating will make it extremely difficult for you to balance your blood sugar. If you have dysregulated blood sugar, you may have to eat sooner.
- Avoid drinking caffeinated beverages before breakfast.
- Eat a high-protein and high-fat breakfast within one hour of waking up.
- Go for a thirty-minute walk after dinner to help you digest your food and take your mind off wanting pudding.
- Fast from dinnertime until breakfast. Aim for a minimum of twelve hours between dinner and breakfast. But if you feel hungry before those twelve hours are up, please eat.
- Always eat in a calm environment. No eating while driving or walking.

Your mantra this week is: regular meals equal regular periods.

If you feel hungry sooner than four hours after eating, in the mid-morning or mid-afternoon or after dinner, grab a small snack with protein in it, such as an apple with almond butter, a chia seed pudding, or a few slices of avocado wrapped in turkey, to prevent your blood sugar from dipping too low. If you're craving carbs, coffee, or a glass of wine (it happens), try taking a walk, do a quick ten-minute meditation, have a cup of tea or ice-cold sparkling water with lemon or lime, or take a B-complex supplement to perk up your energy—or all the above.

Tuning in to how long you feel steady and energised after eating will help you figure out your perfect meal schedule. Paying attention to the signals your body sends you will take some trial and error, so adopt an attitude of experimentation.

GET MORE MAGNESIUM INTO YOUR DIET
If I had to recommend one mineral to women, it would be magnesium. It has such a profound effect on our periods because it plays a part in more than three hundred enzyme reactions in the body. Magnesium appears to become depleted by cyclical changes in the

female sex hormones during the luteal phase, which plays a role in PMS symptoms such as migraines and bloating.[47]

Some examples of magnesium-packed foods you are likely already incorporating from the recommendations in week one include dark leafy greens, especially spinach and Swiss chard, pumpkin and sunflower seeds, almonds, cashews, black beans, avocados, and cacao or high-cacao-content dark chocolate. Aim for 350 mg of magnesium every day. It takes just two cups of spinach or Swiss chard, a half cup of black beans, half an avocado, and 30 grams of pumpkin seeds to get your daily magnesium needs met. So easy!

I'm also a big fan of supplementing with magnesium. You can try magnesium glycinate or malate, or a combination of both. These are the most well-absorbed forms of magnesium and will lessen the likelihood of stomach upset or diarrhoea. Magnesium citrate is not as well absorbed and can cause diarrhoea, but it works well if you are prone to constipation. Follow the dosage instructions on the label of the product you purchase.

Balancing your blood sugar is one of the most important steps you can take to fix your period. There is a laundry list of ways elevated blood sugar affects you: sporadic ovulation and periods, cramps, migraines, cravings, difficulty losing weight . . . I could go on, but you're probably already convinced: it's time to become a blood sugar-balancing rock star!

7-DAY BLOOD SUGAR–BALANCING MEAL PLAN

DAY	1	2	3
PRE-BREAKFAST	475–600 ml water or **Detox Lemon Elixir*** 20 minutes before breakfast	475–600 ml water or **Detox Lemon Elixir*** 20 minutes before breakfast	475–600 ml water or **Detox Lemon Elixir*** 20 minutes before breakfast
BREAKFAST	**Breakfast Goddess Bowl***	**Low-Sugar Berry Smoothie Bowl*** with 1 scoop of collagen or protein powder mixed in	**Breakfast Goddess Bowl***
LATE-MORNING SNACK (IF NEEDED)	**1–2 Power Balls***	Half an apple, sliced, with 1 tbsp sunflower seed butter and 1 hard-boiled egg, if needed	**1–2 Power Balls***
LUNCH	Baked chicken breast (size of palm or a little larger) and 1–2 servings **Crunchy Cabbage Salad*** and 75 g roasted sweet potatoes	Leftover **Pan-Seared Wild Salmon*** on a bed of baby rocket, 75 g chopped veggies of your choice, 50 g fresh olives or avocado; top with olive oil and lemon juice or vinaigrette of choice	**Curried Chicken Salad with Cashew Cream Mayo***
AFTERNOON SNACK	Up to 75 g tahini with celery, carrots, and cucumber	**1–2 Power Balls***	Half an avocado with sea salt and 2 tbsp pumpkin seeds
DINNER	**Pan-Seared Wild Salmon*** and **Crazy Simple Sautéed Greens***	Your choice of **Chicken Soup Three Ways*** variations	**Kale Salad with Pomegranate or Figs*** and a bowl of **Creamy Carrot Soup***
BETWEEN MEALS	Water or green, mint, or ginger tea	Water or green, mint, or ginger tea	Water or green, mint, or ginger tea

* This recipe can be found in appendix A.

4	5	6	7
475–600 ml water or **Detox Lemon Elixir*** 20 minutes before breakfast	475–600 ml water or **Detox Lemon Elixir*** 20 minutes before breakfast	475–600 ml water or **Detox Lemon Elixir*** 20 minutes before breakfast	475–600 ml water or **Detox Lemon Elixir*** 20 minutes before breakfast
Coconut Yoghurt Parfait with Pomegrante and Pistachios* with 1 scoop collagen or protein powder mixed in	**Breakfast Goddess Bowl***	**Low-Sugar Berry Smoothie Bowl*** with 1 scoop of collagen or protein powder mixed in	**Breakfast Goddess Bowl***
Half an avocado with cucumber slices and one hard-boiled egg	1–2 **Power Balls***	Half an apple, sliced, with 1 tbsp sunflower seed butter and 1 hard boiled egg, if needed	1–2 **Power Balls***
Leftover **Kale Salad with Pomegrante or Figs***	**Curried Chicken Salad with Cashew Cream Mayo*** and 1 serving of **Parsnip Fries***	Leftover **Turkey "Mole" Chilli with Butternut Squash***	Baked chicken breast (size of palm or a little larger) and 1–2 servings **Crunchy Cabbage Salad***
75 g of mixed nuts including almonds, Brazil nuts, cashews, and walnuts	Up to 75 g tahini with peppers, carrots, and courgettes	1–2 **Power Balls***	**Chocolate Chia Pudding***
Baked chicken breast or wild salmon (size of palm or a little larger) and 1–2 servings **Mix-and-Match Salad***	**Turkey "Mole" Chilli with Butternut Squash***	Dinner out with friends: choose something with a mix of whole-food carbs, natural fat, and protein, and ENJOY!	**Ginger-Lime Cod en Papillote*** and **Crazy Simple Sautéed Greens***
Water or green, mint, or ginger tea	Water or green, mint, or ginger tea	Water or green, mint, or ginger tea	Water or green, mint, or ginger tea

6

WEEK THREE

FIX YOUR GUT, FIX YOUR HORMONES

Welcome to week three! Over the past two weeks, you've been feeding your hormones a variety of delicious and dynamic foods. These nutrient-dense menstrual cycle-supporting foods serve to keep your blood sugar from swinging wildly all over the place so you can reinvigorate your sex hormones and breathe new life into your period. While you don't have to adhere to the 7-Day Blood Sugar-Balancing Meal Plan (pages 142–143) moving forward, to keep your blood sugar stable your goal should be to continue eating with its principles in mind.

This week we're going to focus on one of the most exciting areas in health research these days: the gut. It seems as if every day a new study comes out linking our gut health to some common condition that scientists never before imagined could be connected to our digestive system. Everything from obesity to endometriosis has been traced back to the delicate balance of microorganisms, enzymes, and substances in our guts, making the old adage "Go with your gut" more relevant today than ever.[1] Period problems are no exception.

Regardless of which hormones you're looking to bring into balance, or the period issues you're trying to correct, your gut health needs to be a top priority as your gut plays an integral role in how *all* your hormones behave in your body.

Amazingly, your gut produces hormones and neurotransmitters— hey, melatonin, thyroid hormone, and serotonin!—and is home to a certain group of gut bacteria called the estrobolome, which helps regulate oestrogen levels in the body. It also contains more of the immune system than any other part of the body, meaning it plays a crucial role in the development of the autoimmune diseases that directly impact the endocrine system.[2]

Unfortunately, due to our increased use of antibiotics, the added stress in our lives, and our less-than-stellar diets, our gut health, on the whole, has never been worse. Take me, for example.

Gut health hell—that was my experience of high school and college. Chronic constipation was the worst of it. It was normal for me to go four or five days, sometimes up to a week, without having a bowel movement. I experienced perpetual bloating, serious heartburn issues, and non-stop stomach aches. Like so many women, I suffered from f*cked-up digestion all the way into my early twenties, yet had no clue it was linked to underlying gut issues, chronic system-wide inflammation, and all my hormonal woes.

Of the women I see in my practice, about 90 per cent have some kind of gastrointestinal challenge, ranging from food sensitivities and allergies to leaky gut, chronic constipation, diarrhoea, and IBS. This is hardly surprising given that your body needs adequate quantities of vitamins, minerals, and antioxidants to create hormones, which means that at the end of the day, you are only as healthy as the food you can digest and absorb. You can eat an impressive array of high-quality foods, but if your gut isn't functioning optimally, it won't make much difference to your hormones. Unless you can break that food down and deliver its essential nutrients to the rest of your body, your diet can't help you.

It's time to upgrade your gut function.

LET'S GET REAL ABOUT POO

Before we get into the ins and outs of the gut-hormone connection, we need to discuss bowel movements and the secrets they can reveal about our hormones. Yup, that's right, a subject you've always considered gross, inappropriate, and highly embarrassing might just give you some insights into your period troubles. When it comes to educating women about their health, poo is one subject that is not discussed enough. And because no one talks about it, women have no idea it's not normal to have a bowel movement only a few times a week, or to need to run to the loo after meals.

The brain directs the digestive process. In fact, the vagus nerve, the main line running from your brain to your digestive system, oversees the entire process of rest and digest. When you experience heightened emotional or physical stress, the fight-or-flight response kicks in, and suddenly digestion is low on the body's list of priorities. The cortisol produced by the adrenal glands in response to stress changes how the gut works, disrupting the entire digestive system, from the brain to the gut barrier to the microbiome.[3]

Usually, one of the first signs of stress impacting digestion is bowel movement irregularities. When you're in survival mode, your body isn't focused on absorbing and using the nutrients you've just consumed, and it certainly can't think about the next trip to the loo. Instead, it either dumps that food really fast (diarrhoea) or holds on to it (constipation) for a later time, when things have calmed down.

If you don't go to the loo daily, your overall toxic load goes up. This in turn hinders hormonal production and equilibrium. It can also lead to an imbalance in gut bacteria that changes the way you process oestrogen.[4] However, diarrhoea that comes on after a meal or that has you running to the bathroom frequently isn't okay, either. Loose stools let us know that we aren't digesting and absorbing nutrients well, which can be detrimental to our health and hormones in the long run.

So, what's happening with your poo? Whenever you go to the loo, get in the habit of recording your bowel movement's texture, colour, and smell, and note the presence of any undigested food, how long it took you to excrete, and how long it has been since your last bowel movement. Ideally, you should have at least one bowel movement each day that is:

- one long, smooth piece that is easy to pass;
- medium-brown with no visible food particles; and
- not putrid smelling, sticky, or greasy.

If your bowel movements don't look like this or you experience any constipation or loose stools, pay close attention to what changes as you embark on the protocol in this chapter and those in the weeks to come. Your poo will be the perfect indicator of what's happening in your gut and hormonally, and what changes need to be made or sustained to reduce inflammation and experience better periods.

PERIODS AND POOS

When we talk about the psychological and physiological changes we experience in each phase of our cycle, our poo tends to get overlooked, but our menstrual cycle has a very direct and predictable effect on our GI tract.

It's extremely common for women to have regular bowel movements in the first half of their cycle, but then, as soon as ovulation hits and progesterone levels begin to rise, they get constipated until their period comes. One of the properties of progesterone is that it's a muscle relaxant. In fact, it's commonly given to pregnant women to delay labour and pre-term birth because it can effectively reduce uterine muscle contractions.[5] When your muscles are relaxed, it becomes more difficult for the bowel to contract, thus making it harder to move things along. As your progesterone levels drop in the day or two before your period, your constipation should subside.

This progesterone drop triggers an inflammatory response that releases prostaglandins, which stimulate muscle contractions in the uterus and cause your uterine lining to shed.[6] Due to its close proximity to the uterus, the bowel is one of the first organs to be affected by prostaglandins. Once they infiltrate the bowel, their effect is the same as it is in the uterus. They influence bowel contractions, and you might end up with loose stools or diarrhoea right before your period begins or on the first day of bleeding. Sometimes it is much-needed relief after weeks of constipation. But too much of a good thing is a bad thing. When you have excess prostaglandins, one bowel movement could turn into being stuck in the bathroom all day. And this is a problem.

While progesterone may predispose you to constipation in the second half of your cycle, and its subsequent drop before your period might mean loose stools, just know that once you start healing your gut, you'll likely begin to see an improvement in both of these super-disruptive problems.

Gut Dysbiosis, Leaky Gut, and Hormonal Health

The two most common ways the gut malfunctions are gut dysbiosis (unhealthy gut microbiome) and leaky gut (when your gut lining becomes too permeable).[7]

The gut microbiome comprises more than one hundred trillion bacteria, viruses, and yeast cells with between five hundred and a thousand species of microorganisms living in your colon alone.[8] The type of bacteria in your gut plays a huge role in determining your health and your body's ability to derive nutrition from your food. The trick to having a healthy gut microbiome is to have a diverse set of bacterial species in your gut and the right balance of healthy bacteria (versus opportunistic or pathogenic bacteria) in the right place.

As the diversity of the gut microbes decreases and there are too few beneficial bacteria, this imbalance allows the opportunistic or pathogenic bacteria to overgrow, leading to dysbiosis, which translates to "not living well together." It can cause symptoms such as:

- gassiness or bloating, no matter what you eat;
- food sensitivities;[9]
- brain fog;
- chronic bad breath;
- inflammatory bowel diseases such as Crohn's and ulcerative colitis[10] or irritable bowel syndrome, with symptoms such as stomach cramping, diarrhoea, and constipation;[11]
- fatigue or low energy;
- autoimmune conditions such as Hashimoto's,[12] coeliac disease,[13] type 1 diabetes,[14] and multiple sclerosis;[15] and
- obesity.[16]

Think of *gut dysbiosis* as an umbrella term for the many conditions brought on by an imbalance in the types of microorganisms in the intestinal tract. These conditions include SIBO (small intestinal bacterial overgrowth); fungal, bacterial, or candida overgrowth; other types of yeast and mould; *Helicobacter pylori*, or *H. pylori* (think stomach ulcers); and parasites. All these conditions need to be tested for, diagnosed, and treated by a doctor.

Your gut bacteria can become unbalanced for many reasons. Carb- and sugar-heavy Western diets,[17] alcohol consumption,[18] and chronic stress[19] are common culprits, as are antibiotics, which eradicate the good gut flora along with the harmful pathogens. Antibiotics also increase gut permeability and are associated with IBS and Crohn's disease.[20] The inability to digest a group of carbohydrates and sugar alcohols known as FODMAPs (i.e. fermentable oligosaccharides, disaccharides, monosaccharides, and polyols; I know, such a mouthful) is also a frequent cause of dysbiosis. Oral contraceptives disrupt the gut microbiome, setting the stage for major conditions such as Crohn's and ulcerative colitis.[21] Additionally, oral contraceptives also tip the balance of the microbiome in favour of more yeast and harmful bacteria. This sets up an environment for bacterial vaginosis and yeast infections.[22]

The human body is sometimes described as a "tube within a tube": our digestive system is simply a tube running through our body that separates what's in our guts from the rest of our body. *Leaky gut* is just what it sounds like: the lining of the gut has become compromised, and bacteria, food particles, and other toxins "leak" through it and into the bloodstream. This gut lining is essential to our survival, as it prevents toxins and pathogens we consume from entering the body and causing damage to our organs.

The lining of the gut is about one cell layer thick.[23] Can you believe that? At this point, you might be asking: if it's so important to keep the contents of our guts separated from the rest of our body, why is our gut lining so thin? This barrier is highly selective and allows only useful material through, while at the same time blocking harmful substances. And when stuff that isn't supposed to get through gets through, it triggers an immediate response from your immune system, which deploys cells to combat the invaders. Think of them as a line of immune system soldiers waiting on the other side of your gut wall, ready to attack any foreign invaders who dare pass through it and into the bloodstream.

One of the first symptoms of leaky gut is a food sensitivity—as in suddenly being unable to eat dairy or wheat without feeling bloated or getting a headache or a runny nose. Eventually, an immune system that is continually in attack mode creates a cascade of food sensitivities and allergies,[24] immune system abnormalities, and, ultimately, autoimmune disorders.[25] In fact, research suggests that leaky gut is related to almost every disease of Western civilisation.[26] Yikes!

What causes leaky gut? A lot of the usual suspects. The primary culprit is chronic physical and emotional stress, as high levels of cortisol increase intestinal permeability and create an inflammatory response in the gut.[27] Inflammatory foods and beverages such as wheat,[28] corn, refined carbohydrates, soy, dairy, conventionally raised meats, sugar, and alcohol[29] also play a large role. (I know, I know. Why are sugar and alcohol always the cause of our woes? If cake and wine could fix all our problems, I'd be the first in line to eat them.)

We can't forget common medications such as birth control pills,[30] certain antibiotics,[31] and non-steroidal anti-inflammatories, or NSAIDs, such as ibuprofen, naproxen, and aspirin.[32] Finally, we come to genetically modified foods. The herbicides routinely sprayed on GM foods are designed to kill crop-eating insects by damaging the lining of their guts. Humans are likely not immune to this effect, and consumption of GM foods sprayed with glyphosate herbicide may trigger a similar response in our own guts.[33]

You may have thought your oestrogen levels were determined solely by what's happening with your ovaries. But that's not entirely true. Both gut dysbiosis and leaky gut impact your hormones, particularly oestrogen, in significant ways. After all, the gut is intricately connected to how much oestrogen circulates in your body at any given time. When oestrogen is created and released from the ovaries and other tissues, it travels through the body, interacting with a number of different systems. Once it has faithfully fulfilled its duties, it ends up in the liver, where it is "deactivated." The liver then dumps the deactivated oestrogen hormones into the intestine, where they're broken down further before being eliminated from your body in your poo.

A group of bacteria called the estrobolome helps break down oestrogen when it enters the intestine.[34] The bacteria in your estrobolome produce an enzyme called beta-glucuronidase, which has the ability to "reconjugate" oestrogen—that is, return oestrogen to its activated state.

In people with healthy microbiomes, the estrobolome bacteria easily break down the oestrogen, allowing the body to dispose of it. But in people with unhealthy microbiomes, these beneficial bacteria become somewhat ineffective, allowing the beta-glucuronidase-producing bacteria to dominate. This leads to a higher level of beta-glucuronidase, which *reactivates* too much of your oestrogen, ultimately reversing all the liver's hard work.

Your body cannot excrete active oestrogens, so they are reabsorbed through the gut wall and go back to hanging out in your bloodstream. Once back in the bloodstream, these reactivated oestrogens do all the things they were doing before. Over time, too much beta-glucuronidase will recycle too much of your oestrogen and lead to oestrogen dominance.[35] It's no surprise that researchers have established a connection between a dysfunctional estrobolome and conditions such as endometriosis; PCOS; and endometrial, ovarian, and breast cancer, which are all connected to improper detoxification of oestrogen.[36]

On the other hand, lower beta-glucuronidase means less oestrogen is reactivated and sent back into the bloodstream. In someone with healthy ovarian oestrogen production, this is all good. But in someone with low ovarian oestrogen production, lower reabsorption of oestrogen in the gut will only exacerbate the problem of oestrogen deficiency.

And wouldn't you know it, ovarian hormone production is compromised by gut dysbiosis and leaky gut. A compromised gut microbiome can lead to the production of lipopolysaccharides (LPS for short), potent toxins that are released from the cell walls of gram-negative or pathogenic (disease-causing) bacteria when they die.[37] An example of gram-negative bacteria is *E. coli*. These toxins affect the internal gut environment, and if they pass through leaky intestinal walls, they can prompt an inflammatory immune response as well as inflammation in the ovary (particularly the corpus luteum) that disrupts ovarian production of progesterone.[38] This can cause all the problems associated with lowered progesterone, like luteal phase defect and short cycles, PMS, heavy periods, and breast pain.

GLUTEN AND LEAKY GUT

When it comes to food that can directly affect your gut's permeability, gluten stands out from the crowd. A protein found in wheat, barley, and rye, gluten is the sticky stuff in these grains—the name is derived from the Latin word for "glue"—that helps make nice fluffy breads, pastries, and cakes. One of the main components of gluten is gliadin, which, when consumed, triggers the release of zonulin from the gut lining. Zonulin is like a little woodpecker making holes in the gut lining by weakening the tight junctions in the intestinal barrier and inducing intestinal permeability. This eventually leads to leaky gut.[39] Once these "doors" in the gut lining have been opened, all sorts of invaders can sneak into the body, including gluten, and trigger the immune system's foot soldiers to start attacking.

People with coeliac disease, a very serious autoimmune condition, experience severe damage to their gut, which reduces their ability to absorb nutrients. Coeliac disease affects approximately 1.4 per cent of the global population and appears to have increased in prevalence over the last three decades.[40] The more controversial non-coeliac gluten sensitivity is a condition in which a person sensitive to gluten and other proteins found in wheat develops symptoms, but coeliac disease and a wheat allergy have both been ruled out. Many of the symptoms of non-coeliac gluten sensitivity and coeliac disease overlap those of leaky gut;[41] however, it is possible to be diagnosed with coeliac disease and not have stomach problems.[42]

So, just because you don't have gut health concerns, don't think you're in the clear. In fact, coeliac disease is connected to impaired fertility or unexplained infertility;[43] a higher rate of miscarriages; complications during pregnancy and low birth weight;[44] delayed puberty or onset of menstruation;[45] irregular periods; early menopause; and secondary amenorrhoea, a cessation of periods in women who previously had normal periods.[46]

I've seen multiple cases where the only problem was amenorrhoea or unexplained infertility, and once gluten was removed, the gut was healed, and nutrients were replaced, the women got their periods back or got pregnant naturally.

Coeliac disease and non-coeliac gluten sensitivity are serious conditions. If you have been diagnosed with one of them, avoid gluten. If you suspect you have them, I strongly recommend you work with a qualified functional medicine or naturopathic doctor to confirm this through testing. If your trouble is neither coeliac disease nor non-coeliac gluten sensitivity, you could have a related condition, such as small intestine bacterial overgrowth (SIBO), parasites, or fungal overgrowth.

What about the rest of us? Should we avoid gluten, too? As with all food-related questions, the answer is not simple. You may tolerate gluten just fine (or think you do), but consuming gluten harms your gut barrier. Because modern wheat has way more gluten than ancient varieties, and because in the U.S. it is sprayed heavily with pesticides and herbicides that do a number on our gut health and immune system, we're more sensitive to gluten today than ever before. So, gluten or no gluten? Here's my take: eating gluten regularly is like scratching a cut on your leg every day so it never heals properly. Eventually you end up with a bigger, more infected cut. Same goes for your intestinal lining: foods containing gluten will keep "scratching" it.

That being said, I have some good news: your gut lining is so badass that it completely regenerates itself every five to seven days.[47] By eliminating gluten from your diet, you can begin to restore those tight junctions between the cells of your intestinal lining and prevent leaky gut.

Gut Health, PMS, PMDD, and Mood

Did you know that the gut has five hundred million neurons, five times as many as are located in the human spine? These neurons compose what is referred to as the enteric nervous system, also known as our "second brain." The main role of this "brain" is to manage our digestive process from start to finish, from swallowing to breaking down food, to nutrient absorption and eventually elimination.

But that's not all it does. Our gut brain is connected to our actual brain through what is known as the gut-brain axis.[48] The vagus nerve, a cranial nerve which runs from the brain to the digestive system, facilitates bidirectional communication between the brain, the rest of the nervous system, and the gut.[49] This back-and-forth communication between the brain and the gut is why you get that "butterflies in your stomach" sensation when you're nervous or get a sharp feeling in the pit of your stomach when you receive bad news. It's also why gut problems such as inflammation, gut dysbiosis, and leaky gut can lead to problems associated with the brain such as anxiety, depression, and other mood disorders.

In other words, if you have gut inflammation, there is likely to be brain inflammation, which will affect your moods and emotional state.[50]

Given the constant cross talk between our gut and nervous system (including our brain), it's no surprise that this complex interplay could also influence the hormones related to our emotional state and menstrual cycle. I see it in my practice all the time—when my clients implement a gut-healing protocol, they experience a significant improvement in not only their period problems, but also their anxiety, depression, PMS-related mood swings, and even PMDD. Some preliminary evidence suggests that PMS and PMDD are associated with reduced vagus nerve function, meaning that supporting the function of your nervous system and your gut-brain axis with the gut-healing protocol I lay out a little later in this chapter can help with mood-related period disorders.[51]

I hope it's clear now what an essential role our healthy bacteria play in brain function, and why it's crucial to work on gut bacterial imbalances if you're struggling with anxiety, depression, PMS, or PMDD. As this research continues, we could very well begin to see doctors prescribing probiotics instead of anti-depressants.[52] Wouldn't that be something?

Leaky Gut and Chronic Pelvic Pain

According to Dr Jessica Drummond, founder of the Integrative Women's Health Institute, "Relieving any pelvic pain condition, including endometriosis, vulvodynia, or painful bladder syndrome, starts with improving your digestive function." This is because chronic pelvic pain-based conditions are often rooted in gut-related problems such as inflammation, dysbiosis, leaky gut, IBS, food sensitivities, and autoimmune disease.

To build on what we discussed in Chapter 3, evidence suggests that endometriosis is an inflammatory disease, and potentially has some autoimmune components. In one study, researchers concluded that endometriosis had almost all the hallmarks of an autoimmune disease and had been found to occur in conjunction with other autoimmune conditions such as multiple sclerosis, rheumatoid arthritis, and inflammatory bowel diseases (including Crohn's and ulcerative colitis).[53]

As you now know, leaky gut is a trigger for autoimmunity; it may also trigger some of the autoimmune characteristics of endometriosis. LPS, in combination with oestradiol, promotes pelvic inflammation and worsens endometriosis.[54] One study found that 80 per cent of the female subjects with endometriosis had SIBO, and another suggested that the health of the intestinal bacteria played a critical role in the development and progression of endometriosis.[55] In short, the health of the GI tract is connected to endometriosis, which is why the condition often overlaps with certain gut-related problems such as IBS.[56]

But the relationship goes both ways: endometriosis can directly affect the GI tract. Prostaglandins, which the uterus and endometriotic lesions release during menstruation, affect the smooth muscle of the bowel and cause symptoms such as intestinal cramping and diarrhoea. The endometrial cells can even invade the wall of the intestines. This can interfere with the gut's ability to keep waste products moving, risking SIBO, yeast overgrowth, and bacterial imbalance, all of which will only intensify the symptoms of endometriosis.

Vulvodynia is characterised by chronic pain in and around the vulva; it can feel like burning, stinging, or just soreness during sex; when wiping, inserting a tampon, or just sitting; or any or all the time (unprovoked). It is estimated to affect around 16 per cent of women age eighteen to sixty-four, which is shocking because most people have never heard of it.[57] A medical diagnosis for vulvodynia has been hard to nail down, as the condition has been linked to nerve damage, autoimmunity, and chronic yeast infections; it also appears to have a psychological element, with vulvar pain heightened by anxiety, depression, stress, and past sexual abuse.[58] Suggestions for its treatment are as numerous as the theories behind its cause, which is why there's no one-size-fits-all approach to treating it.

So, does it all come back to the gut? At least in part, yes. This is why I often recommend a gut-healing protocol to women experiencing ongoing pelvic pain, and have seen remarkable results, ranging from a reduction in pain that allows a client to start living life again to a complete resolution of symptoms.

An Unhealthy Gut, Too Much Histamine, and Your Period

Are you plagued by headaches, fatigue, bloating, itching, insomnia, irritability, and gut issues during the middle of your cycle (almost like you're experiencing PMS during ovulation)? Or maybe you're experiencing cramps and have tried addressing them in numerous ways (changing your diet, taking supplements, exercising, doing pelvic physical therapy), yet nothing seems to work? The reason may be something called histamine intolerance, a condition exacerbated by gut health issues *and* oestrogen.

Histamines get a bad rap for the "itchy, sneezy, watery eyes" problems they cause for so many of us during allergy season, but they actually serve a valuable function. When your body encounters a common allergen such as pollen or pet dander, it triggers the release of histamines from immune cells known as mast cells. The histamines go to work dilating your red blood vessels and thinning them out, which clears the way for your immune system's white blood cells to get to the site of the problem. (It kind of reminds me of a police escort helping VIPs get to their destination faster.)

This immediate inflammatory response leads to the symptoms we all know so well: itchiness, puffiness, sneezing, swelling, and hives— all of which are caused by histamine release. The problem arises when your body produces too much histamine and/or is unable to clear it out efficiently. What results is more histamine than the body needs and the condition known as histamine intolerance or a more serious condition known as mast cell activation syndrome (MCAS).

Besides pollen and cat dander, you know what else triggers the release of histamines? Oestrogen. Oestrogen triggers the release of histamines from mast cells in the uterus and ovaries.[59] The more oestrogen we have roaming around our body, the more histamines are produced. Unfortunately, the more histamines we have, the more oestrogen is produced—and around and around we go in this vicious circle. The oestrogen connection is why you may feel really terrible at ovulation, when oestrogen is highest in the body, and notice an improvement in your histamine-related problems during the second half of your cycle, when oestrogen drops and progesterone rises.

It's worth noting that histamine and mast cells may play a role in several period problems, including endometriosis[60] and heavy periods. For example, endometriotic lesions contain a high number of mast cells that contribute to pain and the abnormal immune response that drives the disease.[61] Mast cells are also present in the uterine lining and may also be involved in heavy periods by releasing heparin, which is a blood thinner and increases flow.[62]

What's the Letts notes version of all this? Healing leaky gut and dysbiosis reduces the production and burden of histamine and its negative effects. This is why women with endometriosis, heavy bleeding, period pain, and PMS-like symptoms around ovulation need to include a gut-healing protocol in their treatment plan.[63]

WEEK THREE PROTOCOL: HEAL YOUR GUT

Okay, so you've got raging hormones and a gut in need of an overhaul. The goal for this week is to start optimising your digestion by increasing the number and diversity of the good gut bugs over the pathogenic ones and plugging the leaks in your gut lining. You're already off to a great start thanks to your work in weeks one and two to incorporate loads of nutrient-dense foods in your day-to-day diet and eating for blood sugar balance. Now we're going to ramp things up by eliminating inflammatory foods and supporting each step of digestion to facilitate your gut healing.

In addition to following this protocol, I strongly recommend that you work with a functional medicine or naturopathic doctor, or another qualified health professional, to explore whether you have any serious underlying conditions such as SIBO, fungal or candida overgrowth, parasites, *H. pylori*, coeliac disease, or an inflammatory condition such as ulcerative colitis or Crohn's.

WHEN SOMETHING'S UP DOWN THERE

The bacteria in your gut directly influence the bacteria in your vagina, meaning that if your gut is overrun by harmful bacteria, it will likely lead to vaginal and even urinary tract infections. If you are experiencing any of the following problems, it's high time you took a deeper look at what's happening in your GI tract.

YEAST INFECTIONS. These are linked to an overgrowth of candida in the gut triggered by antibiotic use and a high-sugar/high-carb diet. Symptoms include a thick white vaginal discharge, itching, burning, and irritation.

BACTERIAL VAGINOSIS. Healthy vaginas are acidic thanks to beneficial bacteria known as *lactobacillus*, which produce lactic acid. A vaginal pH higher than 4.5, lower levels of *lactobacillus* bacteria, and an overgrowth of unfriendly microbes can cause bacterial vaginosis to develop. Symptoms include a fishy-smelling discharge that looks grayish or yellowish, itching, and burning. It is very important to get diagnosed and treated by a doctor; untreated BV can lead to pelvic inflammatory disease.

URINARY TRACT INFECTIONS. These are the worst! They occur when bacteria from the digestive tract (often *E. coli*) migrate from the anus into the urinary tract and cause infection in the urethra, the bladder, and even the kidneys. There is a direct link to the gut in this case. Symptoms include a strong urge to pee all the time, pelvic pain, cloudy urine, and a painful burning sensation all the time.[64]

Most conventional treatments do not address the deeper cause of these vaginal or urinary infections: gut dysbiosis.[65] I encourage you to work with your functional medicine doctor or naturopathic doctor to explore treatment options that do. Following this week's gut-healing protocol is a first step.

Begin the Fix Your Period Elimination Diet

You can take a million supplements to heal leaky gut and *all* the probiotics in the world to support your gut bacteria, but at the end of the day, if you continue to eat certain foods you're sensitive or allergic to, you'll never achieve the good gut health you desire. Such efforts are akin to putting a sticking plaster on a surgical wound.

Eliminating—for a short period of time—certain foods that are well-known immune system aggravators is one of the most effective ways to heal your gut. What's even more exciting is that an elimination diet of this kind can help quiet symptoms such as ovulation and period pain and diagnoses such as endometriosis, vulvodynia, and painful bladder syndrome, all considered chronic (long-term) conditions. Ultimately, when we eat to support our gut health, we also support healthy hormones. By eliminating inflammatory foods, you'll be well on your way to happier hormones and periods, too.

Here is how it works: for this week and the remainder of the six-week programme, you'll eliminate the foods that create the most inflammation. This will create a more hospitable environment for friendly microbes and effectively stop the chronic irritation of your delicate gut lining, leading to fewer undigested food particles leaking through and creating an immune response. These foods include wheat and other gluten-containing grains, corn, dairy, soy, peanuts, eggs, sugar, alcohol, caffeine, and inflammatory fats and oils. Check out the recipes in appendix A for lots of easy "Mix-and-Match" options to keep you full and satisfied.

TIPS FOR SUCCESSFULLY ELIMINATING INFLAMMATORY FOODS

CLEAN OUT THE CUPBOARDS AND FRIDGE. Get rid of those foods that are *so* freaking hard to resist. Toss 'em or give 'em away. (Don't binge on them, as tempting as it may be.) Remember, this is for only a short period of time—but you may find you feel so good you'll want to continue eating this way at least 80 per cent of the time.

REDUCE CAFFEINE CONSUMPTION. Over the next week, slowly reduce your consumption so you're off all caffeine by week two of the elimination diet. Try half caffeine/half decaf and gradually change the ratio until you're drinking decaf only. (Quitting cold turkey can cause pretty severe headaches and mood swings for many, so I don't recommend it.) Also, consider a coffee replacement,

FOOD GROUP	FOODS TO EAT	FOODS TO AVOID
PROTEIN	Grass-fed red meat (venison, lamb, beef) along with liver and/or pâté; wild-caught fish, sardines, free range chicken, turkey, pork, and duck	Shellfish and fish heavy in toxins (visit seafoodwatch.org for recommendations), eggs, processed meats such as ham and salami and hot dogs, and all soy products such as tofu, tempeh, soy milk, soy "meats," and edamame
GRAINS	Rice, quinoa, and buckwheat	Corn, all gluten-containing grains (wheat, barley, rye, kamut, spelt, and farro). If you've got an autoimmune condition and/or continual bloating, take out all grains
SWEETENERS/ SUGAR	Stevia, honey, maple syrup, blackstrap molasses, monk fruit. (When I say these are allowed, I mean add 1 tsp of honey to your tea or a splash of maple syrup to a smoothie. Any sugar consumption should be limited)	Brown, white, and cane sugar; evaporated cane juice; agave nectar; corn syrup and high-fructose corn syrup; all artificial sweeteners such as saccharine, aspartame and sucralose
LEGUMES, NUTS, AND SEEDS	Pumpkin, flaxseed, sesame, sunflower seeds, almonds, walnuts, Brazil nuts, pine nuts, and pulses. (If you experience wind, bloating, or abdominal pain after eating pulses, consider eliminating them, too)	Peanuts and soy
FATS AND OILS	Coconut oil, coconut butter, avocado oil, lard, tallow, duck fat, butter from grass-fed cows, ghee, extra-virgin olive oil, flaxseed oil, sesame oil, walnut oil, and MCT (medium-chain triglyceride) oil	Rapeseed oil, soybean oil, corn oil; sunflower, safflower, and cottonseed oils; trans fats or partially hydrogenated fats
DAIRY PRODUCTS	Coconut, almond, and hemp milk; coconut or cashew yoghurt, butter from grass-fed cows	Cow, goat, and sheep milks; soy milk, yoghurt, and cheese; oat milk; dairy-based cheese, yoghurt, and kefir
FRUIT	All fruit	If you have vulvodynia or interstitial cystitis, consider removing citrus fruits
VEGETABLES	All vegetables	If you have an autoimmune condition, consider removing nightshade vegetables (e.g. potatoes, tomatoes, aubergine, peppers)
BEVERAGES	Water, sparkling water, herbal teas	Coffee, caffeinated teas, alcohol, juice, and soft drinks

such as Dandy Blend, Teeccino, or Four Sigmatic's Mushroom Coffee with Lion's Mane (available online).

PLAN, PLAN, PLAN, AND PREP, PREP, PREP. Before you begin eliminating foods, take a day to prepare your meals, and schedule another prep day two to three days later. You should plan on two prep days each week for the rest of the gut-healing protocol. Chop and roast veggies in a big batch (broccoli, cauliflower, squash), as they will keep for two to three days in the fridge, even longer if you freeze them. Make stock or soup, roast a chicken or pieces of salmon, and roast some sweet potatoes. Create salads in kilner jars and store them in the fridge. Eating during an elimination diet and eating well in life are both about proper meal prep, so take some time this week to really think about what you're going to eat and plan it out. Trust me, *you can do this*! I believe in you. No matter how busy you are, if you plan ahead, all will be well.

TAKE CARE OF YOURSELF. Make extra time for rest and rejuvenation. Take steps to slow down, take any non-essential responsibilities off your plate, ask for support from loved ones, prioritise healthy sleep, and find emotional support where you need it. Taking a soothing bath, getting a massage, getting out in nature, taking a yoga class, or writing in your journal will help you move through any possible detox symptoms with more ease.

EAT AT HOME DURING THE FIRST FEW DAYS. Eating in the privacy of your own home relieves you of having to avoid specific foods at a dinner party, restaurant, or event, or explain your food choices to friends, coworkers, and family.

SYMPTOMS YOU MIGHT EXPERIENCE WHILE YOU DETOX

When your body starts to detox, you may experience some symptoms. Don't worry, these will subside pretty quickly (usually within one to three days).

- Headaches or migraines
- Fatigue

- Skin rashes or acne
- Mood swings
- Body odour
- Body aches or joint pain
- Irritation or annoyance with family members or friends
- Constipation (followed by better bowel movements as the protocol continues)
- Renewed energy and focus (usually by day three).

You may find that when you eliminate problematic foods, you have much more energy and mental clarity. Why? Well, you gave your digestive system a break from hard-to-digest foods and foods you may be intolerant to. Therefore, your liver, kidneys, pancreas, and stomach don't have to work as hard and aren't in constant distress. Your body can use that newfound energy to repair itself rather than constantly put out fires, which means better periods in the long term. Yay!

IF YOU HAVE A HISTORY OF EATING DISORDERS

If, after reading through the elimination diet protocol, you feel triggered or experience fear, or if any past restrictive eating patterns creep in, work with a coach or qualified health practitioner. Undereating can be detrimental to your stress levels and your hormone-balancing efforts. If it becomes a trend, it is important to seek help to make sure you're getting the nourishment you need.

SUPPORT YOUR GUT AS YOU ELIMINATE INFLAMMATORY FOODS
While on the elimination diet, you can assist your digestion in many ways. Go ahead and do all the following if you're so inclined, but even just one should have a positive impact. Note: You'll find all supplement recommendations in the supplements section of appendix C.

SUPPORT STOMACH ACID PRODUCTION. Stomach acid is generally viewed as a terrible thing, but good stomach acid production is key to keeping opportunistic and pathogenic bacteria at bay. Stomach acid further digests your food and allows for the breakdown of protein, vitamin B_{12}, iron, and calcium so they can be absorbed properly. Low stomach acid is one reason so many of us experience frequent heartburn, burping, bloating, wind, and even nausea after eating. By supporting stomach acid production, you'll experience:

- a reduction in bloating, wind, and burping after you eat;
- less of that uncomfortably full feeling after a meal (like your food is "just sitting there");
- a reduction in cravings after eating;
- a satisfied, energised feeling after eating, instead of feeling sleepy and stuffed; and
- more ease in the loo—your bowel movements should start to look smoother, without bits of food in them.

One easy way to boost stomach acid production is with bitter herbs. Also known as digestive bitters, these have been used in traditional cultures for thousands of years to improve digestion. Look for digestive bitters that have some of or all the ingredients commonly used in herbalism, such as beetroot, burdock, dandelion, fennel, gentian, ginger, goldenseal, licorice root, milk thistle, peppermint, wormwood, and yellow dock. Take a dose of bitters (following the label or directions from a herbalist) before each meal to help get your digestive juices flowing.

DRINK BONE BROTH. I'm going to go out on a limb here and say bone broth is one of the most healing foods in existence. It has been used for centuries in many traditional cultures as a healing, fertility-enhancing food. A mineral- and amino acid-rich infusion made by slow-cooking the bones of healthy animals with vegetables, herbs, and spices, this digestive aid contains high levels of gelatine, collagen, and amino acids such as glutamine, glycine, and proline, which all help support your gut mucosa and rebuild the gut lining.[66] I encourage you to make your own stock, using bones from grass-fed or free-range animals.

If you're not feeling the bone broth, I suggest you consume gelatine or collagen daily. Both provide benefits similar to those in the proteins found in bone broth, although in a slightly more processed form. Collagen can be easily mixed into smoothies, hot and cold soups, and even bone broth for additional healing power. Gelatine gels up when added to liquid, so it's often used in healthy gummies and puddings and to thicken soups and sauces.

CAUTION: Bone broth, collagen, and gelatine are high-histamine foods, so if you have symptoms of high histamine, consider skipping them.

TAKE A GUT-HEALING SUPPLEMENT. A comprehensive gut-rebuilding powder or supplement provides the maximum gut-healing benefit without the hassle of taking multiple supplements. The ingredients in a broad-spectrum gut-healing supplement usually include L-glutamine, zinc carnosine, quercetin, and herbs calming to the GI tract, such as slippery elm, marshmallow, and licorice root. You'll find recommendations in the supplements section of appendix C.

CONSUME PROBIOTIC-RICH FERMENTED FOODS OR TAKE A PROBIOTIC. Sauerkraut, kimchi, or any kind of fermented vegetable is a great source of probiotics and encourages neighbourly behaviour among the trillions of organisms that coexist in your GI tract. Add 1 to 2 tablespoons to meals each day. If you're not feelin' the fermented foods, you can take a probiotic.

Depending on the state of your gut, or if you're eating fermented foods or taking probiotics for the first time, you may notice symptoms such as fatigue, headaches, body aches, and skin irritations—a detox response commonly known as the Herxheimer reaction. This occurs when the new, healthy bacteria you introduce kill off unhealthy bacteria, which die, creating toxins the body needs to eliminate. There is basically a bacteria revolution happening in your gut!

If you take a probiotic, start with half a capsule a day for seven days to avoid adverse reactions. Just empty the half capsule on your food or tongue. If this dose is tolerated, you can increase the dose to one full capsule a day. However, if you notice an adverse reaction, such as described in the previous paragraph, I recommend cutting your dose in half for a week or so before slowly attempting to increase it again. The reaction shouldn't last long—if it persists for more than seven days, please see your doctor—and you'll feel a lot better the slower you go.

CAUTION: Fermented foods are high in histamines, so if you have symptoms of high histamine, consider avoiding them and take the probiotics instead. If you have SIBO or trouble digesting FODMAPs (i.e. fermentable oligosaccharides, disaccharides, monosaccharides, and polyols), fermented foods and probiotics may cause uncomfortable bloating, so you may have to skip both until you have resolved the underlying issue.

IMPROVE OESTROGEN ELIMINATION IN YOUR POO WITH CDG. Calcium D-glucarate inhibits the enzyme beta-glucuronidase, which helps improve excretion of oestrogen through the bowel and can lessen symptoms of oestrogen dominance such as heavy or painful periods as well as physical and emotional PMS symptoms. The recommended dose is 500 mg to 1,000 mg a day. Please see a trained practitioner for guidance.

A gut that is constantly upset, lacking the right amount of stomach acid, leaking harmful substances into your bloodstream, or overrun by opportunistic bacteria is not a place where food is digested properly or nutrients used effectively and efficiently to make hormones. Plus, an inhospitable gut disrupts your oestrogen levels, exacerbating many period problems, from PMS to heavy and irregular periods. By listening to our guts, we can begin to have a conversation with this little world within us, and grow to appreciate all it does for us. The closer we can become with our microbial helpers, the more we will be able to serve them so that they can serve us. So, make it a priority to reclaim your gut health. At each meal, remember that you are not just feeding yourself. You're feeding *one hundred trillion* little friends who love you and want to help you support your hormones in the best way possible.

7

WEEK FOUR

LOVE UP YOUR LIVER

Welcome to week four. You're halfway through the programme, and by now you should notice some of your symptoms easing as you've focused on eating foods that support hormone creation, stabilise your blood sugar, and promote gut health and healing. Now it's time to show your liver some love. This week we'll focus on understanding the way your liver and detox mechanisms play a key role in hormone balance and fertility, how to reduce your exposure to the foods and chemicals that dampen your liver's ability to do its job, and which foods to add in to maximise your hormone and liver detox powers.

Detoxing often brings to mind the latest cleanse requiring us to drink green juice for two weeks to purge our bodies of all the terrible things we've ever consumed, right? But the fact is, our bodies are removing harmful substances all the time. Everything we eat and drink and many of the things we inhale and absorb through our skin pass through the liver to be detoxified.

Think of the liver as both your body's housekeeper and its processing plant. It cleans your blood, breaking down chemicals, toxins, bacteria, and excess hormones into less harmful forms so they can be safely removed from the body. While it does this, it simultaneously breaks down beneficial substances such as carbohydrates, proteins, fats, vitamins, and minerals so that their elements can be remade into the compounds your body needs. Unfortunately, many people are overexposed to toxins and underexposed to the nutrients that support detoxification, which can cause the housekeeper to become overworked and underpaid. When this happens, harmful substances build up in the body, and your health and hormones suffer. In fact, your liver contributes significantly to the state of your overall and hormonal health. Let's put it this way: if your hormones are out of whack, it's likely your liver has something to do with it.

The good news is that your liver has an impressive capacity to heal, and there are many things you can do to get it back on track and doing its thing. The action steps for this week will help you support your overburdened liver and make it extra efficient for the sake of your hormones. But before we get into the ins and outs of this week's protocol, let's break down where all these toxins come from.

IS YOUR SHAMPOO MESSING WITH YOUR HORMONES?

Yes, it probably is. Our environment is saturated with man-made toxic chemicals that make our livers work overtime and that interfere with our bodies' complex and carefully regulated hormonal messenger system (so much so that they are known as endocrine disruptors). Did you know that there are tens of thousands of chemicals in existence, yet most have not been tested for safety, much less proven safe?[1] Or that the average woman is likely exposed to hundreds of chemicals each day? From triclosan in dish soap, to parabens in shampoo, to glycol in skin care products, and bisphenol-A (BPA) in packaging, these little chemical devils are everywhere! And they are *potent*.

So, let's take a look around the average home to see if we can uncover all the secret hiding places for these toxic monsters. Here are the first places we'll be looking:

Household Cleaners

Most household cleaners contain fragrances, foaming agents, preservatives, artificial colours—I mean, have you *seen* Windex?— and bleaching agents that are all harmful to humans in some way. The solvents found in window and carpet cleaners, called glycol ethers (e.g. polyethylene glycol, ethylene glycol, 2-butoxyethanol, and propylene glycol), are known to cause prolonged menstrual cycles, miscarriage, and fertility problems.[2] Triclosan and other antibacterial additives are potent xenoestrogens,[3] chemicals that mimic the hormone oestrogen and wreak havoc on your natural hormones. (More on those in a moment.) Triclosan has been shown to interfere with thyroid metabolism and the production of testosterone.[4] And this is just what's under your kitchen sink!

Keep in mind: You might not even be aware that one or more of these chemicals is in your favourite product. Companies are not required to list them on the label, and when they do, they often use generic-sounding words such as *cleansing agent* or *fragrance*.

Personal Care and Lifestyle Products

Now let's move on to what's under your bathroom sink: moisturisers, shampoos, soaps, and body lotions. What's most concerning is the sheer number of chemicals in our personal care products that are linked to reproductive problems and cancer. Some of the most common ones include: parabens, preservatives commonly used in cosmetics, which are xenoestrogens;[5] phthalates, industrial chemicals found in fragranced products (perfume or anything that's been made to smell nice), which pose serious risks to female reproductive function and male fertility and cause reproductive birth defects and hyperthyroidism;[6] oxybenzone, the ingredient in most chemical sunscreens, and a potent xenoestrogen linked to endometriosis;[7] and toluene, a chemical solvent found in many nail polishes that causes respiratory tract irritation and is a known neurotoxin (poison to your nervous system).[8] Do you get a headache or sinus issues in a nail salon? Well, toluene might be one reason for this.

Menstrual and Vaginal Care Products

Have you ever considered the ingredients in your pads, tampons, lubricants, douches, feminine care wipes, and creams? Well, you should, because these products are used on some of the most naturally absorbent tissue in the body: the vulva and the vaginal canal. Both have very thin tissue and a very rich blood supply, which makes these areas highly sensitive to toxin exposure. Most menstrual and vaginal care products contain a cocktail of fragrances, synthetic fibres, pesticide-soaked cotton, harsh adhesives, plastics, artificial colours, bleaches, and even petroleum-based foams. When your sensitive vaginal tissue is exposed to these products, toxins get absorbed quickly into your system. Basically, using these products is the worst thing you can do to your vagina!

This is particularly true for tampons, which are designed to be in direct contact with the vaginal wall for a prolonged period. One of the most dangerous toxins present in tampons is the bleaching agent used to whiten them: chlorine dioxide. This chemical leaves behind a harmful byproduct called dioxin, which the World Health Organization describes as "highly toxic" and able to "cause reproductive and developmental problems."[9] If you're thinking you're okay because you use tampons only once a month, and not that many of them, well, think again. It turns out that even small amounts of exposure to these products inside the vagina can be harmful.[10] And really, should we care that much about having pearly white tampons for the ten seconds we see them before they go into our vaginas?

I've heard countless stories from women about the awful symptoms they've experienced using these products, such as yeast and bacterial infections, inflamed and raw skin, and vaginal burning. (Our poor vaginas.) So, it's no coincidence that my clients have reported experiencing less-heavy periods and period pain and reduced infections after making the switch from conventional pads and tampons to organic cotton products or menstrual cups.

Food and Drinking Water

The main source of toxins in our food is the pesticides used in modern industrial agriculture. Organophosphate pesticides are used on almost all non-organic crops; on lawns and golf courses; and in public parks. These chemicals have been found to contribute to a wide variety of health problems, including infertility, obesity, developmental disorders, birth defects, and Alzheimer's disease.[11] Atrazine is a potent weed killer that's very common in tap water due to its widespread use. Possibly its most fearsome trait is its ability to turn male frogs into females, due to its oestrogenic effects, which makes it a potent endocrine disruptor.[12] Atrazine has been linked to increased miscarriage and infertility rates, low sperm count, and it may lower metabolism, contributing to diabetes and metabolic syndrome.[13]

Packaging is also a frequent source of exposure. Bisphenol-A, widely used in plastics (e.g. water bottles, baby bottles, plastic-lined tins, and other packaging), is highly oestrogenic, potentially causing high oestrogen levels in both men and women and contributing to birth defects in children.[14] But even when packaging is labelled "BPA-free," similar compounds that are equally oestrogenic may still be present, so watch out for plastic-lined packaging of any kind.

This brings us to our drinking water. Our water supply is the bloodstream of our environment. Everything that's produced in our world ends up, at some point, in our water, including many of the contaminants I've just described, plus antibiotics, hormones from birth control pills, and narcotics that are either peed out or flushed down the toilet. Yikes!

Chlorine and fluoride are routinely added to our water supply, with about two-thirds of the US population exposed to fluoridated water. In the UK the coverage of fluoridation is not consistent around the countries of the union. Northern Ireland and Wales do not use fluoride, and England is not universally served by fluoridation. You might have always been told that fluoride is good for your teeth, and while it has been shown to reduce cavities, it's problematic in other ways. Indeed, evidence suggests that it is toxic to the nervous and reproductive systems, kidneys, and thyroid.[15] Bottom line: filter your drinking water or, better yet, all water in your household.

You're probably like, "Okay, you can stop. Don't tell me any more!" Unfortunately, there's more.

THE IMPACT OF ENDOCRINE DISRUPTORS

Endocrine disruptors are an especially problematic group of toxins that negatively affect your body's natural hormonal equilibrium. (I've mentioned a few of them already, but they're important to highlight, as they are a major contributor to period problems.) These toxins are found in plastics, skin care products, preservatives, foods, insecticides, medications, and building supplies.

As their name implies, they disrupt the endocrine system and can be especially detrimental during pregnancy. Significant exposure to endocrine disruptors in the womb, in infancy, and in early childhood has been shown to have effects on sexual development, birth weight, mental capacity, and immune system development.[16] Endocrine disruptors have been linked to early puberty, impaired immune function, breast and endometrial cancer, birth deformities, obesity, and metabolism disorders.[17] Most endocrine-disrupting chemicals are fat soluble, meaning they do not get rapidly flushed out of the body, but rather, are stored in your body fat, which means they can hang out there for decades.

All endocrine disruptors impact the normal function of the endocrine system by mimicking naturally occurring hormones in the body, such as oestrogens, androgens, and thyroid hormones, tricking the body into thinking it has more hormone than it does. Because they can mimic a natural hormone, endocrine disruptors are able to lock on to a receptor within the cell in the same way the natural hormone would, preventing the natural hormone from getting into the cell.

The disruptor may give a signal stronger than the natural hormone, causing you to experience symptoms of an imbalance even when your lab work looks normal. For example, you might have symptoms of oestrogen dominance (e.g. PMS or heavy periods), but your blood work shows normal levels of oestrogen and progesterone.

Xenoestrogens

Xenoestrogens are one of the most abundant endocrine disruptors found in our world. They are basically oestrogen imposters, and function by mimicking oestrogen, which can cause symptoms of high oestrogen in both women and men. However, not all xenoestrogens are derived from toxic chemicals. Some, called phytoestrogens, come from plants and seeds. There is a lot of confusion over the difference between synthetic and natural xenoestrogens, so let's break it down.

SYNTHETIC XENOESTROGENS

Synthetic xenoestrogens are man-made chemicals that imitate oestrogen. They include birth control pills, dioxin, BPA, phthalates, parabens, pesticides, and chemical sunscreens such as oxybenzone, benzophenone, and PABA. These synthetic xenoestrogens accumulate in the fatty tissue and can cause symptoms of oestrogen dominance such as PMS, heavy periods, breast tenderness, irregular periods, low sex drive, and mood swings. They can also worsen conditions that are fed by oestrogen, like endometriosis, fibroids, and adenomyosis.

When it comes to synthetic xenoestrogens, BPA tops the list as one of the worst offenders. Consuming food containing BPA has been shown to increase appetite even while the stomach is full.[18] This is why BPA is considered an "obesogen," a chemical that promotes obesity.[19] What's most disturbing is that in animal studies, BPA has been shown to disrupt follicle and egg development (in females, pregnant females, and potentially their female foetuses; I kid you not)[20] and proper production of oestradiol in the ovaries. This can interfere with our menstrual cycle and have devastating effects on our fertility.[21] In one study, mice exposed to BPA in utero were found to stop producing viable eggs at a much younger age than normal.[22] Yes, this stuff is literally toxic to our ovaries.

PHYTOESTROGENS

Phytoestrogens, however, are *natural* xenoestrogens. Derived from plants, they are structurally similar to the body's natural oestrogen and able to bind to oestrogen receptors. Soy and flaxseed are well-known examples of phytoestrogens.[23] Phytoestrogens are much weaker than both your own oestrogen and synthetic xenoestrogens. And depending on your individual biology and natural hormone levels, they can have an oestrogenic effect or an anti-oestrogenic effect. When they bind to your oestrogen receptors, they can block more potent oestrogens from binding instead and, in some women, reduce symptoms of oestrogen dominance.[24] On the flip side, they can have an oestrogenic effect when natural oestrogens are on the lower side or in cases of amenorrhoea, which will have a positive effect on the menstrual cycle. They've also been shown to help with anovulatory cycles.[25]

ARE PHYTOESTROGENS THE "GOOD" XENOESTROGENS?

It depends. Here's where our biological differences come into play.[26] Some women rave about flaxseed working miracles to resolve their oestrogen dominance symptoms. Others complain that flaxseed makes them feel even more oestrogen dominant. The same goes for soy. Organic soy consumed in small amounts has been shown to reduce oestrogen dominance in some women,[27] but for others, even a modest amount of soy is too much and can lead to significant menstrual problems such as heavier periods or longer cycles.

Then again, I've seen flaxseed and soy consumption work miracles for some women in a low oestrogen state caused by anovulatory cycles or irregular ovulation. These women observed shortened cycles and more regular periods and even regained missing periods.

Bottom line: It's great that studies show that phytoestrogens help both reduce symptoms of oestrogen dominance and even resolve amenorrhoea, but at the end of the day it's less about the specific food than the interaction between the food and the specific woman. In other words, there's no one-size-fits-all approach to hormonal health, so it's important to experiment and find what works for your body.

YOUR LIVER IS A REAL WORKHORSE

As you can see, we are surrounded by chemical enemies. And while your liver is a workhorse when it comes to detoxifying your body, thankfully it has a few detoxification allies to help ease the burden. For example, the lungs remove carbon dioxide, and the skin blocks absorption of potentially harmful substances and releases toxins through sweat.[28] The digestive system eliminates food waste through bowel movements (and sometimes vomiting). The kidneys filter waste products from your blood multiple times a day, and your lymphatic system drains excess fluid from your tissues, pulling any stored toxins with it.

The Portal System: The Blood Toxin Conveyor Belt

Even with all this help, your liver remains the indispensable and undisputed champion of detoxification. Its role is so vital, in fact, and the substances it deals with so dangerous, that it even has its own circulation system, separate from that for the rest of the body, so that it can safely transport and filter toxins without harming other organs. This special circulatory system is called the portal system, and it's like a conveyer belt at a processing plant. Blood travels onto the belt from the spleen, pancreas, and gastrointestinal tract, where it gets filtered, with beneficial nutrients that can be reused by the body separated from waste chemicals that will be expelled. This expulsion process happens in three distinct phases.

Keep in mind that how well these phases work is determined by your genetics, your nutrient status, your overall exposure to alcohol, certain medications (acetaminophen in particular), and environmental toxins.[29] Some of us are more exposed to these elements than others, and others of us might have genetic variants that affect how well our livers do their job.

PHASE ONE
As the blood travels along the conveyer belt, enzymes in the liver convert toxic chemicals into less harmful forms. While these

enzymes can neutralise most traditional chemicals, rendering them harmless, many of the more potent toxins we're exposed to today, such as pesticides and BPA, can actually become more chemically active, and potentially more harmful, during this process. It is therefore extremely important that these activated toxins get through all the phases of the detox process and are properly jettisoned from the body. If, instead, they fall off the conveyer belt and reenter the bloodstream, they can do some serious harm, including causing damage to the RNA and DNA in our cells, which is pretty much as bad as it sounds.

In order for this phase to work the way it's supposed to, the liver requires a lot of antioxidants, amino acids, vitamins from nutrient-dense foods, and plenty of water. But even if you give your liver all the tools it needs to work optimally, if the conveyer belt is too overloaded with toxins, it won't be able to keep up. When the liver becomes overwhelmed like this, dangerous toxins will inevitably fall off the belt and reenter the bloodstream or continue down the line unprocessed, which leads to more overload and a knock-on effect in later phases. Yes, your liver is a workhorse, but there are limits to its strength and stamina, and we push those limits at our own peril.

PHASE TWO

Moving down the line, in this phase, the liver pairs specific amino acids and nutrients with the intermediate toxins from phase one, allowing them to be converted from fat soluble to water soluble. The liver does this because water-soluble compounds can be excreted by the body via bile or urine, while fat-soluble compounds cannot. If there are deficiencies in these amino acids and nutrients, or if the liver is simply overloaded, many of these toxins will remain in their fat-soluble form. This will prevent them from being expelled and, instead, like a group of escaped convicts, they will race back into the body and hide away in our fat cells. Some of their favourite hideouts are our brains and our hormone-producing glands, as these fatty organs make appealing havens for fugitive toxins. If we allow too many of these outlaws to populate these organs, it can lead over time to serious brain issues and hormonal imbalances.[30] But when the liver is healthy and working well, the water-soluble toxins produced in phase two are packaged up and cleared for departure from the liver, at which point they enter the third, and final, phase of detoxification.

PHASE THREE

This third phase happens in the gut, where the cells in the intestinal lining and the bacteria in the colon further process them before they make their final journey out of the body. And then, at last, early one morning, in the quiet solitude of a sacred space, these once-dangerous toxins, now rendered harmless, are unceremoniously and quite literally flushed down the drain.

Signs the Liver Isn't Working Well

If you experience one or more of the following, it could mean your liver is in trouble:

- Routine headaches or headaches around ovulation or your period;
- PMS symptoms, decreased libido, and infertility;
- Disrupted sleep, especially between 2 and 4 a.m.;
- Asthma or allergies, especially if they are newly developed;
- Skin disorders, including eczema, acne, and rosacea;
- Unexplained weight gain, inability to lose weight, or excessive abdominal fat;
- Blood sugar disorders (as the liver plays a key role in blood sugar regulation);
- Nutrient malabsorption (look for undigested food in your stool or chronic diarrhoea, anaemia, or constant hunger and fatigue); and/or
- Mood swings, poor mental function, and lowered stress tolerance.

A Congested Liver and Oestrogen Excess

Our old friend oestrogen is highly susceptible to what's going on with the liver. Oestrogen is a "use it and lose it" hormone, meaning once it has done its job, it needs to be neutralised. Much of this neutral-isation happens in the liver, so your overall oestrogen levels are heavily reliant on this organ's ability to lose the oestrogen that has done its job. According to Dr Carrie Jones, "you need all the phases of oestrogen detox to work smoothly, otherwise you get a back-up in your system causing all those annoying period-related symptoms."

Remember, there are three main types of oestrogen: oestrone (E1), oestradiol (E2), and oestriol (E3). In the first phase of liver detoxifica-tion, in addition to handling toxins as just described, the liver breaks down oestradiol and oestrone into oestrogen metabolites, which pass through phase two and three as well.

Now, for those of you who aren't into science, hang tight for the next two minutes.

OESTROGEN AND PHASE ONE OF LIVER DETOX

In phase one, the oestrogen is broken down into three main metabo-lites. These are 2-hydroxyestrone (2-OH), 4-hydroxyestrone (4-OH), and 16-alpha-hydroxyestrone (16-OH).

Since 2-OH is considered the less harmful metabolite when compared to 4-OH, there is a lower risk of cancer if your oestrogen converts into 2-OH.[31] Then we have 4-OH and 16-OH, which are more potent, and are often referred to as "bad" oestrogens. While not a bad little metabolite per se, if 4-OH builds up too much, it can be converted into DNA-damaging and cancer-causing compounds.[32]

Meanwhile, 16-OH is considered a proliferative metabolite, which means it makes things grow. Proliferation might be a good thing when it comes to bank accounts and Instagram followers, but it's not so great when it comes to your cells. As Dr Jones says, "16-OH is good for bones but bad for boobs." Higher levels of 16-OH increase the risk of uterine fibroids, heavy periods and clots, breast tenderness and swelling, and breast cancer.[33] Still, you need 16-OH for good bone health, so like 4-OH, it's not bad in the right quantities, but too much of it can cause serious problems.

OESTROGEN AND PHASE TWO OF LIVER DETOX

In this phase, 2-OH and 4-OH are broken down further into 2-methoxy and 4-methoxy (the water-soluble forms), so they can be sent off to the gut for final breakdown and release. 2-methoxy is thought to be anti-oestrogenic, or a "good oestrogen."[34] It is considered a health promoter and helps prevent symptoms of oestrogen dominance such as PMS, sore breasts, and heavy periods, so the goal is to make sure that your 2-OH is adequately converting to 2-methoxy. The *COMT* gene makes an enzyme of the same name that plays a crucial role in this phase of liver detoxification and the production of 2-methoxy. *COMT* gene mutations can lead to a higher predisposition to "being oestrogenic," meaning that your liver doesn't break down oestrogens as efficiently as that of someone without a *COMT* mutation.[35]

OESTROGEN AND PHASE THREE OF LIVER DETOX

Phase three of detoxification occurs once everything is out of the vicinity of the liver. After the second phase of detoxification, the processed oestrogens are all safely packaged up and transported from the liver in the bile. They pass through the gallbladder and into the intestines. As you learned in Chapter 6, the bacteria in the colon further process these compounds so they can make their final journey out of the body through the colon. In other words, you gotta be pooing really well so you can make sure to get all that nicely packaged-up oestrogen out!

If all this is over your head, don't worry. What really matters are the steps you take to make sure oestrogens don't fall off the conveyor belt and get strewn all over the floor. The bottom line is that the more you protect and enhance your liver's ability to do its job, the easier it will be for oestrogens to be broken down into the right metabolites and pushed through the remaining phases so they can head to the sewage system (literally).

GENETICS AND LIVER DETOXIFICATION

I have not been blessed with superior detoxification genes. In other words, I have variants on many of the genes that contribute to healthy liver function. Yup, I'm a mutant, and you may be one, too. But don't panic. While this does suck and can put you at a disadvantage, you can do a lot to work with your less-than-ideal genetic makeup.

Genetic variations are commonly referred to as mutations, or single-nucleotide polymorphisms (SNPs, pronounced "snips"). A woman can have many different SNPs, which she can learn about by doing a genetic test. Some SNPs have no bearing on your health, while others might determine your response to things such as caffeine or your suscepti-bility to certain diseases. Just because you have one of these variants, it doesn't necessarily mean they are "turned on" or that you will ex-perience problems. One of the most common SNPs associated with detoxification and hormone imbalance is MTHFR. (It sounds like a bad word, doesn't it?) The MTHFR gene has had a lot of attention for its effect on mental health, but you should know about its implications for reproductive health, too.

When the MTHFR gene is mutated, it alters a very important process called methylation. Methylation controls every response in the body, from how you convert food into energy, to detoxification, to DNA repair, to how you respond to stress.

Important for your liver, the MTHFR gene is responsible for the breakdown and utilisation of B vitamins, which are crucial to phase one of liver detoxification and brain function. (Hey there, anxiety and PMS!) Additionally, people with an MTHFR variant may not make enough glutathione, one of the body's most powerful antioxidants and detoxifiers, and are thus more susceptible to liver dysfunction and toxic overload.

If you have an MTHFR variant, you might find yourself severely fatigued, depressed, anxious, and in chronic pain.[36] You may also experience diffi-culty getting or staying pregnant. Unfortunately, many women discover they have an MTHFR mutation only after trying unsuccessfully to get pregnant or having one or several miscarriages.[37]

Not sure if this applies to you? If you have symptoms that remain unresolved, get genetic testing and work with a trained practitioner to make adjustments to your supplementation or diet to support your health and hormones further. No matter what your genetic makeup, the recommendations to support your liver in this week's protocol will help you.

WEEK FOUR PROTOCOL: LOVE UP YOUR LIVER

If you're inundated with period problems, you may feel overwhelmed, and discouraged at the thought of healing your liver. But there is good news. First, you're already doing a lot of the things you need to do to support your liver's recovery. Second, when given the right support, your liver has a tremendous ability to heal—after all, it is the only organ that can regrow.

Your next steps involve reducing your toxic load and beginning to introduce nutrients that will get your oestrogen detoxification humming along. While you continue your elimination diet and healing your gut, there is a lot you can do to make this happen.

Now, I don't expect you to make all these changes in one go. (I know it can be overwhelming.) What I do want you to do, though, is think hard about the undue stress you're putting on your liver and commit to supporting its function by making two to three changes this week. If you want to do more, go for it!

Reduce Your Toxic Load

By now you've likely caught on that toxic substances are everywhere, so outright avoidance is not an option—unless you're planning to move to a deserted island in the South Pacific (which wouldn't be a terrible idea). So, in limiting your exposure, your goal is to do what you *can*. This week, to reduce your exposure to endocrine disruptors and other harmful chemicals, choose at least one strategy in each category (Food and Drinking Water, Household, Personal

Care and Lifestyle, and Menstrual and Vaginal Care) of the "Choose Your Own Toxic Load Reduction Plan" table (see pages 184–185). To make it easier, I've organised the choices into good, better, and best options, so you can choose the ones that most closely suit you and your lifestyle (and on which you can most realistically be expected to follow through).

Support Your Liver's Natural Oestrogen-Detoxing Power

As you can see, liver detoxification and, more important, oestrogen detoxification is a carefully orchestrated step-by-step process that requires all hands on deck and a whole lot of resources. This doesn't have to be intimidating or complicated. Just remember that filling your diet with colourful, nutrient-dense foods (the same ones you need to create an optimal hormonal landscape) and adding supportive supplements will help you upgrade your liver's natural ability to process hormones.

DIET AND THE LIVER

I want to take a moment here to reemphasise the importance of decreasing your intake of refined carbohydrates. Sugar and refined foods not only mess with your blood sugar but can also cause fat buildup in the liver—25 per cent of the world's population has fatty liver disease—diminishing that organ's detox capacity.[38] The more you commit to keeping refined carbs off your plate, the easier it will be for your liver to do its thing, and the closer you'll be to feeling you can take on the world. Plus, if you consume the nutrients that will assist phases one and two of the oestrogen-elimination process so you have healthy amounts of the *right* oestrogens circulating in your body, you'll not only fix your period problems but also reduce your risk for oestrogen-driven cancers.

NOURISH EACH PHASE OF YOUR LIVER'S DETOX

During phase one of your liver's detoxification, you'll want to support the breakdown of oestradiol and oestrone into their respective

CHOOSE YOUR OWN TOXIC LOAD REDUCTION PLAN

GOOD	BETTER	BEST
FOOD AND DRINKING WATER		
Eat mostly whole foods, choosing organic versions of the Dirty Dozen* and eating hormone-free and/or antibiotic-free meats, fish, and dairy.	Eat mostly whole foods, ensuring that the majority of your vegetables, meats, fish, and dairy are organic, free-range, or caught wild.	Eat an entirely organic whole-foods diet.
Use a pitcher-style or countertop water filter for your drinking water.	Install a drinking water filter on your kitchen tap and one in your shower.	Use a whole-house water filter.
HOUSEHOLD		
Remove all synthetic air fresheners from your home and open your windows often.	Vacuum frequently with a vacuum equipped with a HEPA† filter and change your A/C and heater filters regularly.	Use a high-quality air purifier equipped with a HEPA† filter.
Remove bleach-containing cleaning and laundry products from your home.	Swap out each of your home-cleaning products for "green" products that don't contain bleach, synthetic fragrances, or other harsh chemicals.	Make your own cleaning products using water, vinegar, essential oils, baking soda, and other natural ingredients.
Kick your plastic water bottle, straw, and shopping bag habit once and for all. No excuses!	Replace plastic wrap with reusable food wraps and silicone lids; replace plastic containers with glass containers; and replace plastic sandwich and freezer bags with reusable silicone bags.	Avoid takeout foods that come in plastic containers and stop eating tinned foods; make fresh food instead.
PERSONAL CARE AND LIFESTYLE		
Swap your conventional lipstick or lip gloss—we ingest a lot of that stuff—face lotion, and liquid or powder foundation for a more natural line of products.	Swap your shampoo, conditioner, and hair styling products for organic versions.	Swap your conventional body lotion for an organic, chemical-free version, and switch to chemical-free sunscreen.
Stop accepting receipts; the coating on most receipt paper contains BPA.	Get rid of your plastic flip-flops and any other plastic shoes—yes, you can absorb chemicals through your feet!	Opt for organic dry cleaning to avoid the harmful chemicals used in the traditional process.
Exercise in a way that makes you sweat for 30 minutes at least once or twice a week. (Note: if you have hypothalamic amenorrhoea, ask your doctor if you should limit or avoid strenuous exercise.)	Exercise in a way that makes you sweat for 30 minutes three to four times a week. (Note: if you have hypothalamic amenorrhoea, ask your doctor if you should limit or avoid strenuous exercise.)	In addition to the exercise in columns one and two, use an infrared or regular sauna or steam room a few times a week. Afterward, replenish lost electrolytes by adding ¼ tsp Celtic sea salt or Himalayan salt to 475 ml water.

GOOD	BETTER	BEST
MENSTRUAL AND VAGINAL CARE		
Switch from conventional pads and tampons to organic cotton pads and tampons.	Try reusable organic cotton pads.	Switch to period underwear or a menstrual cup.
For the love of god, ditch the douches, ladies; they cause way more harm than good.	Make sure your vaginal wipes, cleansers, and lubes are free of harsh chemicals and synthetic fragrances.	Avoid vaginal wipes, cleansers, and creams altogether! Your vagina will thank you.

* Apples, celery, cherries, grapes, kale, nectarines, peaches, pears, potatoes, strawberries, spinach, and tomatoes ("Dirty Dozen," EWG's Shopper's Guide to Pesticides in Produce, https://www.ewg.org /foodnews/dirty-dozen.php)

† High-efficiency particulate air

metabolites, focusing on balancing the amount of oestrogen that goes down the 2-OH, 4-OH, and 16-OH pathways. During phase two, you'll want to support the COMT enzyme, which plays a critical role in breaking down those metabolites into the final water-soluble product that can be easily passed into the digestive tract for excretion.

So, how do you know if all this is happening as it should? Urine testing is the only way to know which pathways your oestrogen is going down and how well the COMT enzyme is working to further break down the resulting metabolites. (See appendix B for testing options.) In the meantime, let's talk about all the nutrient goodness you can add to your day to support your liver this week. I think you'll be quite encouraged, as you might already be eating a lot of these foods.

NUTRIENTS THAT SUPPORT PHASES ONE AND TWO

- A range of B vitamins from dark leafy green vegetables, pulses (if you tolerate them well), liver from grass-fed animals, green veggies such as broccoli and brussels sprouts, eggs, poultry, avocados, nuts and seeds, and wild salmon and other fish
- A range of antioxidants found in colourful fruits, vegetables, teas, herbs, and superfoods such as blueberries and cranberries;

artichoke, beetroot, cabbage, carrots, and greens; green tea; turmeric, chlorophyll, coriander, dandelion root, burdock root, and milk thistle

- Protein and amino-acid rich foods from healthy meats, eggs, poultry, wild fish, bone broth, or collagen protein
- Cruciferous veggies such as rocket, pak choi, broccoli sprouts, cabbage, cauliflower, spring greens, kale, radish, and Swiss chard
- Glutathione-building foods such as sulphur-rich garlic and onions; selenium-rich Brazil nuts and sardines; and bitter-tasting dark leafy greens such as rocket, chicory, and mustard greens.

NUTRIENTS THAT SPECIFICALLY SUPPORT PHASE ONE

- Vitamin C from berries, broccoli, cauliflower, grapefruit, oranges, peppers, spinach and other leafy greens, and tomatoes
- Vitamin E from almonds, avocado, and sunflower seeds
- Minerals such as copper, iron, manganese, selenium, and zinc from a healthy whole-foods diet or a high-quality supplement
- Coenzyme Q10 (coQ10) from healthy meat and poultry, organ meats, and oysters, or from a high-quality supplement.

NUTRIENTS THAT SPECIFICALLY SUPPORT PHASE TWO

- Vitamin B_6 from chicken, chickpeas, organ meats such as liver and kidney, wild-caught salmon and tuna, and spinach
- Magnesium from almonds, dark leafy greens such as kale and spring greens, pumpkin seeds, and whole grains such as buckwheat
- Choline from eggs, shrimp and scallops, liver, meat, chicken, and dairy products.

LIVER DETOXIFICATION SUPERSTAR SUPPLEMENTS

If you've fully integrated the recommended lifestyle and dietary changes but are still experiencing symptoms of oestrogen dominance or sluggish detoxification, consider adding in one of these super-star liver detoxifiers. I always recommend incorporating naturally supportive foods first, but the supplements included here are great when more specific liver support is needed.

GLUTATHIONE. As I said before, glutathione is one of the chief antioxidants in the body. It protects the liver from environmental damage and plays a key role in preventing a host of conditions linked to inflammation. Supplement options include one of the following:

- Liposomal glutathione;
- N-acetyl cysteine, a precursor to glutathione (recommended dose: 300 mg twice daily for one to three months); or
- Milk thistle herb, which protects the liver cells,[39] helps stimulate phase one detox, and increases glutathione activity (recommended dose: 280 to 420 mg a day for one to three months).

DIINDOLYLMETHANE (DIM) AND SULFORAPHANE GLUCOSINOLATE (SGS). These two scary-sounding things are cruciferous vegetable extracts that encourage positive oestrogen metabolism and detoxification. DIM can be useful for supporting phase one liver detoxification, and SGS is useful for support during phase two. Both are especially helpful for cases of oestrogen dominance and can make a big difference for women dealing with uterine fibroids, painful and swollen breasts, endometriosis, PCOS, PMS, PMDD, hormonal acne, period issues after getting off birth control, and heavy or irregular periods.

When it comes to supplement support of the liver detox phases, you'll want to work backwards. Begin with SGS supplementation and then, if you don't experience the desired results, move on to DIM. For SGS, the standard dosage recommendation is 100 mg every other day for twenty-eight days. For DIM, it's typically recommended to take 200 mg to 400 mg a day for twenty-eight days once the SGS supplementation is complete. If you've already introduced many foods and nutrients that benefit the liver and you're still experiencing symptoms, introducing these supplements is a great next step.

I recommend working with a naturopathic or functional medicine doctor, who can test you to figure out which phase of your liver detoxification needs support. You don't want to supplement with DIM and support phase one if in fact you need to support phase two; this will only overburden phase two and make your symptoms worse.

> **CAUTION:** If you have low oestrogen, it is not recommended to supplement with DIM as it can worsen symptoms of this hormonal imbalance.

I talk a lot about the liver with my clients, and now you know why: a healthy liver is essential for reducing your risk of hormonally driven conditions and degenerative diseases. Chemicals are everywhere and in just about everything, but don't be overwhelmed. The beauty is that by making small swaps and lifestyle changes like the ones you're making this week, you will encourage your liver's detoxification capacity and make a huge impact on your hormone recalibration efforts.

8

WEEK FIVE

STRESS HACKS IN THE AGE OF
CHRONIC OVERSTIMULATION

Welcome to the fifth week of your six-week programme. By now, I hope you're feeling more energised, calm, and centred; sleeping better; and feeling more optimistic about your menstrual cycle. You may already be noticing a decrease in PMS symptoms, cramps, or even premenstrual spotting. Better yet, your period this month may have been manageable—whoa!—or perhaps it returned after an extended hiatus? Woohoo!

By completing weeks one through four of this programme, you've already taken a load off the physical stressors your body has been combatting, such as too much sugar, skipped meals, and caffeine. Now it's time to focus on the emotional and environmental stress we encounter each and every day—because let's face it, we live in an age of chronic overstimulation, with little chance of avoiding stress altogether. In fact, Dr Libby Weaver, PhD, coined the term *rushing woman's syndrome* to describe the health consequences women face due to the unrelenting stress and perpetual busyness we all contend with every single day.

We all know the usual external sources of stress, such as overly demanding jobs, relationship turmoil, taking care of family, never-ending to-do lists, or life in a fast-paced or polluted city. However, three sources of stress are often overlooked. These include chronic infections (e.g. the Epstein-Barr virus and Lyme disease) and disease states (e.g. autoimmune conditions and cancer); childhood trauma (physical and sexual abuse, neglect, violence, and parental substance abuse, which leave scars that affect how you handle stressors in your adult life); and the things we don't even consider stressful in our day-to-day, such as that intense spinning or CrossFit class you do three times a week, EMF (electromagnetic frequency) exposure from your mobile phone and laptop or the streetlight that shines in your bedroom window at night. Combine these, and add in not knowing how to cope with all this stuff, and it's no wonder so many of us are frazzled, anxious, and overwhelmed.

Changing the way you deal with the stressors in your life, external and internal, past and present, is key to keeping your periods on track. Why? Because stress has an overwhelming impact on your entire endocrine system. Remember, when we experience an emotionally stressful event, it elicits the same physical response (i.e. a flood of cortisol) as an attacking lion elicited in our ancestors. As we know from Chapter 2, cortisol is one of the tier 1 hormones, which means it cascades down to impact all the other hormones. When you are stressed (i.e. when the "lion" is attacking), the release of cortisol has the unfortunate effect of causing your body to divert resources from bodily functions that aren't important in this "fight-or-flight" situation in order to give us the fuel to overcome or escape the threat.

The reproductive system is one of these "less important" bodily functions, and one of the first to be hit with these budget cuts. Chronically overwhelmed by stress, your body and brain determine that your life circumstances are too dangerous for reproduction, and the mere act of ovulation is marked as "low priority." No ovulation, no cyclical hormone fluctuations . . . and down the rabbit hole of period problems we go!

Because most of us live with chronically high levels of stress, we are forever grappling with one or more of these period-related issues.

Therefore, learning to handle stress like the goddess you are is essential for balancing your hormones and fixing your period.

If you're already stressed out just reading this, don't worry. I've got your back. In this chapter, we're going to rehab your adrenals, the endocrine glands that bear the brunt of your life drama, so you can move even closer to true hormone harmony.

THE HPA AXIS AND THE BODY'S STRESS RESPONSE

Shaped like almonds and barely bigger than walnuts, the adrenal glands are small but mighty. Located right above the kidneys, they are part of a very important trio called the hypothalamic–pituitary–adrenal axis, better known as the HPA axis. One of the main functions of the HPA axis is to coordinate our body's stress response.

When we encounter a stressor, the first part of the body to react is the brain. The brain stem releases norepinephrine, which sends a signal to the amygdala, a region in the brain responsible for mood and emotional responses such as fear and anxiety. This is what makes us alert—you gotta be on your toes for the danger you're facing, right? Thus when triggered, the amygdala in turn sends a signal to the hypothalamus, activating the HPA axis. The hypothalamus is the brain's distribution hub, filtering information and transferring it between the nervous system and the endocrine system. When the hypothalamus receives the distress signal from the amygdala, it immediately passes this information on to the pituitary via corticotropin-releasing hormone (CRH). The pituitary then releases adrenocorticotropic hormone (ACTH), which instructs the adrenals to release stress hormones, including epinephrine (adrenaline) and cortisol, to help the body overcome the threat it's facing. They also release DHEA, which acts as a regulatory hormone, buffering the effects of the cortisol (see Figure 10 on page 192).

You know when you get an adrenaline rush? Well, that's epinephrine being produced by your adrenal glands in response to the ACTH signal—think of it as the police arriving on the scene. Epinephrine

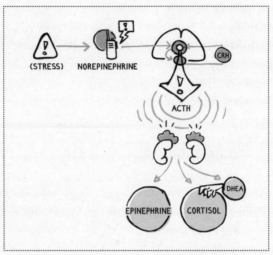

Figure 10: How the stress response happens in the body

plays a crucial role in your body's fight-or-flight response, raising your heart rate, dilating blood vessels in the muscles, increasing air flow to your lungs, spiking your blood sugar (to give you a boost so you can fight or flee as needed), and triggering the inflammatory response to prepare for wound healing after injury. The entire process happens so quickly that often we're not even aware of the situation before the HPA axis has been triggered. That's how awesome our bodies are.

In non-emergency situations, when the HPA axis is functioning normally, cortisol is released by your adrenal glands in a daily cycle as part of your circadian rhythm, quickly rising to peak levels within two hours of waking, to help you get things done, and dropping in the evenings as you prepare to sleep. Cortisol works in conjunction with melatonin (the sleepy-time hormone), which rises at night and then drops during the day.

When stress becomes chronic, however, this perfectly orchestrated pattern begins to shift. Sure, cortisol can power you through demanding situations, whether it's juggling a hectic morning schedule or managing a nerve-racking deal at work, but unlike its fellow stress hormones norepinephrine and epinephrine, cortisol sticks around as part of the body's longer-term response to stress. Over time, all that stress leads to overproduction of cortisol, with high levels all the time or lower levels during the day causing fatigue and brain fog, and higher levels at night driving down melatonin and inhibiting sleep.

Melatonin is responsible not just for helping you sleep. Its role is far more complex—but you probably already suspected that; when it comes to your endocrine system, nothing is so simple. There are melatonin receptors on your ovaries, which means that this hormone not only regulates your sleep/wake cycle but also plays a role in your menstrual cycle. In addition, melatonin is a powerful antioxidant and has been found to have quite profound effects on endometriosis.[1]

Evidence suggests that low and high levels of melatonin can disrupt the ovulatory process.[2] Take women who do shift work—they have disrupted circadian rhythms and melatonin levels and experience longer menstrual cycles and heavier, more painful periods than women who work daytime hours.[3] Lower levels seem to affect healthy follicle development and play a role in infertility,[4] and high levels can actually prevent the LH surge and halt ovulation, which is why supplementation is not necessarily a good idea and should always be done under a doctor's supervision.[5] So, as you can see, your body needs to make melatonin in the right amounts; working on getting better sleep is a good first step.

HPA Axis Dysfunction

While the body's natural reaction to stress is protective in the moment, the continual activation of the stress response system can cause damage over long periods of time. This is the main reason that ongoing stress is such a significant cause of many different diseases in our fast-moving modern world, where stress response mechanisms that were designed to be active for only brief and distinct periods are activated continually. In short, our poor HPA axis is doing *a lot* more work than it was designed to do, and the end result of this ongoing activation is called HPA axis dysfunction. The first warning signs of

HPA axis dysfunction are often sleep disruption, inconsistent energy, and ongoing and unshakeable fatigue.

Wait, isn't that called "adrenal fatigue"? Yes, you've probably heard the terms *adrenal fatigue* and *adrenal burnout*. While popularly used, they don't adequately encompass what happens to your HPA axis and your adrenals in the face of ongoing psychological and physical stress. Your adrenals don't actually become "fatigued" or "burnt out"; rather, as it is exposed to more stressors than it can handle, the entire stress response system is interrupted. This is why the terms *HPA axis dysfunction* and *HPA maladaptation* are used now instead.

So why is our modern-day environment causing so much darn disruption? Perhaps it has to do with our demanding and insane world. (Just a wild guess.) As a card-carrying feminist, it pains me to say that our biology makes women much more vulnerable to hormonal imbalances than men. Because our bodies are highly susceptible to the stresses associated with modern-day life, we must be diligent about how we manage our stress.

There is not a person on the planet who doesn't experience at least one form of internal or external stress—hardly surprising when you remember that everything from poor diet to physical injury to chronic illness, sleep problems, and mental and emotional burdens can contribute to HPA axis dysfunction. The trouble is we have so many stress inducers in our lives that we have completely normalised and adapted to most of them. That bagel and extra-large coffee you treat yourself to? Check. Late nights on your laptop drinking in the blue light from your screen? Check. Navigating never-ending to-do lists that don't seem to get shorter no matter what you do? Check. And this goes for things you think are healthy, too, such as exercise and dieting. Your body is the result of millions of years of evolution, and our modern society is just a blip on that time line. Your body doesn't know that marathons are now run for fun, or what the hell a spinning class is; it knows only that you're inexplicably pedalling your ass off. So, you can't blame it for thinking you might be running from a lion. The point is, even if you're not "feeling" stressed, you might not be off the hook.

The symptoms of HPA axis dysfunction are diverse and can often seem unrelated to one another. This is because there are cortisol receptors on almost every cell in your body, which means when your cortisol is off, it can have a system-wide effect. That being said, you'll know you've got HPA axis dysfunction when you:

- have difficulty falling or staying asleep;
- get a second wind late at night;
- feel "tired but wired";
- wake up feeling tired or groggy even after seven to eight hours of sleep;
- experience mid-morning and mid-afternoon energy crashes;
- feel "hangry" on a regular basis;
- experience memory and cognitive issues such as brain fog, fatigue, depression, and anxiety;
- are unable to handle life's stressors, feel overloaded and out of control most of the time, and/or have frequent meltdowns; and
- experience physical issues such as an inability to handle strenuous exercise or recover from it, a weakened immune system and frequent colds, and dizziness, especially when standing up quickly.

When it comes to hormonal imbalances, these are often among the first symptoms you will likely experience. How many of these feel familiar to you? Remember, cortisol is a tier 1 hormone, meaning it has a downstream effect on your other hormones. So, if the stressors that prompt its release are left unaddressed, you will start to experience multiple hormonal imbalances and additional symptoms that don't even feel related to your adrenals.

No doubt cortisol is a boss lady hormone, and it will always make a point of letting you know who's in charge.

HPA Axis Dysfunction and Your Sex Hormones

You are likely well aware that we live in a society that almost guarantees HPA axis dysfunction. However, you might not be aware of the

profound effect that our adrenal function—or, rather, dysfunction—
has on our sex hormones and menstrual cycle.

As you can see in Figure 11 below all our steroid hormones are
derived from cholesterol, which is manufactured into pregnenolone,
known as the "mother hormone" because it's the precursor to so many
of our important downstream hormones such as cortisol and DHEA,
progesterone, androgens, and oestrogens. DHEA, for its part, is like
the "bonus parent"—while it's a precursor to testosterone, oestrogen, and other steroid hormones, it is also derived from pregnenolone. Both these parent hormones are required in adequate amounts
to produce all their downstream hormone babies.

As I've described before, when we experience a stressful situation,
our body diverts energy from other bodily systems to give us the fuel
to overcome the threat and increase our chances of survival. The
hypothalamic–pituitary–ovarian axis (HPO axis), which controls the

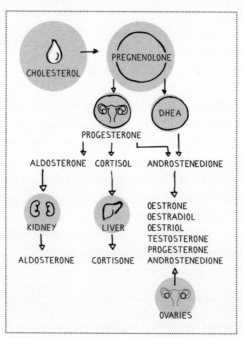

Figure 11: All steroid hormones are derived from cholesterol

female reproductive system, is one of the first to be affected, resulting in period and fertility problems.

HOW HPO AXIS DYSFUNCTION HAPPENS

Stress affects the HPO axis on multiple levels:

First, in the hypothalamus, cortisol has a dampening effect on the secretion of GnRH, which is responsible for triggering the pituitary to release gonadotropin hormones (FSH and LH).[6] Lower GnRH means lower FSH and LH, which will indirectly tell the ovaries to decrease their production of oestrogen, progesterone, and testosterone, thus slowing down or stopping the entire menstrual cycle.[7]

This is why ongoing activation of our body's stress system and higher levels of stress-related hormones are directly linked to anovulatory cycles or irregular ovulation. This can cause irregular periods or hypothalamic amenorrhoea in some women, or heavier periods and irregular bleeding patterns (e.g. spotting) in others.[8] Not to mention, testosterone is the primary hormone responsible for healthy sex drive, so when levels drop, your libido nose-dives. It's no wonder that a higher libido magically appears when many of us are on holiday. Over 40 per cent of the women who come to me for help identify low libido as one of their top symptoms and concerns, and cortisol dysregulation is usually the main culprit involved in the theft of their va-va-voom.

Second, similarly to its effect on GnRH, cortisol, in a further attempt to thwart the chance of ovulation and potential pregnancy, directly inhibits the production of FSH and LH in the pituitary.[9]

Third, if, by some miracle, enough FSH and LH make it to the ovaries, cortisol has come up with a way to block them by making the ovaries resistant to the effects of these hormones.[10] In other words, even if you think you're fine, when your body senses that you are in danger, it's like, "Hell, no, we are going to take lots of precautions and attempt to stop ovulation every step of the way."[11]

Fourth, according to Dr Sara Gottfried in her book *The Hormone Cure*, cortisol can bind to progesterone receptors, because the progesterone receptors are similar to the cortisol receptors.[12] If cortisol binds to the progesterone receptor, it is occupied and unavailable, and the progesterone molecule can't get into its own receptor. It's kind of like progesterone planes lined up at a busy airport waiting for a gate to open to unload passengers, but all the cortisol planes are in the gates and not moving. This has the effect of mimicking progesterone deficiency in the body, even if there is enough progesterone circulating in the blood, which means that on top of the symptoms I've just described, you might have problems with PMS, anxiety, and getting and staying pregnant.

Finally, in one study done on women undergoing in vitro fertilisation, it was found that cortisol was higher in the follicular fluid of eggs that were not fertilised and lower in eggs that were successfully fertilised, indicating that higher levels of cortisol may actually hinder egg maturation in the ovaries.[13]

Don't forget, your body evolved in prehistoric times. So, it doesn't know the difference between your daily eight kilometre run and coming face-to-face with a dangerous predator.

What all this means is when we face what the body considers an emergency situation, the last thing it wants to do is ovulate and procreate.

HPA Axis Dysfunction and Your Thyroid Hormones

Cortisol also suppresses your thyroid. To put it simply, when cortisol goes up, your thyroid hormones go down. Corticotropin-releasing hormone (CRH) inhibits thyrotropin-releasing hormone (TSH) from the hypothalamus, which then inhibits TSH production from the pituitary. And rising cortisol levels directly lower TSH production.[14] Elevated cortisol suppresses the 5-deiodinase enzyme. This in turn decreases the conversion of T_4 to T_3, which means you won't have as much of the active form of the thyroid hormone your body needs to function at its best. Not only that, but during times of long-term stress or illness, our body converts more T_3 into something called reverse T_3.[15] If T_3 is the fuel to fire up your metabolism, think of reverse T_3 as the extinguisher of that fire. It's meant to conserve energy during times of illness or scarcity and can lead to or even worsen hypothyroidism symptoms.

In addition to this, cortisol also raises blood sugar, which can lead to insulin resistance. Insulin resistance has been found to damage the thyroid cells and worsen Hashimoto's thyroiditis.[16] On the other hand, a *low*-cortisol state also increases susceptibility to autoimmune and inflammatory diseases such as Hashimoto's and rheumatoid arthritis.

And to really bring home the widespread negative impact of sustained high cortisol—it is also linked to high blood pressure, diabetes, increased belly fat, brain changes such as atrophy of the hippocampus (where memory is synthesised), depression, insomnia, and poor immunity.[17] I cannot stress (no pun intended) this enough: sustained high cortisol is not your friend, and it is therefore crucial that you address your stress in order to fix your period.

The women I work with who aren't ovulating or who are ovulating very sporadically due to high stress often feel that their bodies aren't working properly and have betrayed them. I remind them that if the body feels as if it's perpetually running from a lion, all of their efforts to fix their period will be in vain. Addressing both real and perceived stress will work wonders to regulate ovulation and periods, naturally restoring fertility. Once women understand that their bodies are actually working the way they're meant to, they can move out of the place of disempowerment and blame and start on the road to healing.

STRESS AND GUT FUNCTION

Stress can completely change how the gut works, affecting the time it takes for food to move through, what gets digested, how it gets absorbed, and even what bacteria are growing. This is why when you are under severe stress you may experience constipation or diarrhoea. In addition, the release of cortisol triggers the release of inflammatory cytokines from the immune system and plays a role in breaking down the gut wall, which increases intestinal permeability and leaky gut. One more reason it's so important to manage your stress![18]

WEEK FIVE PROTOCOL: SUPPORT YOUR STRESS RESPONSE

Many of the other components of the Fix Your Period programme are already helping you address internal stressors such as out-of-control blood sugar, exposure to environmental toxins, and poor gut health. Now I want to equip you with my favourite strategies for easing the impact of chronic overstimulation and revamping the way your body reacts to stress. Some of these strategies can be applied right away, while others take some true self-assessment first. The implementation of these practices may feel less tangible than the dietary changes you've been working on. However, much of the way stress affects our bodies is through the way we perceive it, so bringing awareness to your relationship to stress is imperative to reducing the cortisol dysregulation that's likely throwing off your period and fertility. With these strategies, you'll be able to step off the stress roller coaster, reclaim your hormonal health, and live in period paradise.

Learn Your Personal Stress Threshold

Awareness is everything. We each have a personal stress threshold, the maximum amount of stress we can handle before we break down physically and/or emotionally. Learning your threshold, acknowledging it as a line you should not cross, and recognising when you need to slow your roll or take a break will prevent you from falling off the stress cliff. To do so, put on your detective's hat and think back to times in your life that were immensely stressful, and remember how your body reacted.

I'll use myself as an example. When I am mega stressed—like right now, as I write this book!—I pay attention to warning signs from my body that I am approaching the point of no return, the threshold that, if crossed, will lead to some type of system-wide crash. For me, these are a stiff neck and mild to moderate upper- and lower-back pain. (Hey, cortisol!) If I keep powering through, ignoring the warning signs (my body's Check Engine light), these symptoms precipitate a full-on breakdown of my back. That sounds a little dramatic, but in these circumstances, making even the simplest movement will throw my back out and plunge me into so much pain that only my chiropractor and acupuncturist can help me.

If I'd hit the brakes a few days earlier by going to a yoga class or pulling out my MyoBuddy Massager (which looks like a big handheld sander) to massage my quads (which are super tight from my sitting too much), back, and neck, I would have avoided this catastrophe.

Countless clients of mine have investigated their own personal thresholds over the years. Here are some common warning signs they've shared:

- A scratchy throat or losing their voice, which turns into a knockdown, drag-out cold or flu;
- Increasing headaches that result in a full-blown migraine;
- Eye strain and dry and itchy eyes that turn into an eye infection requiring antibiotics;
- A pimple or two that turn into a full-face breakout that lasts for days or weeks;
- A day or two of diarrhoea that triggers an ulcerative colitis flare-up;
- Anxiety that worsens over days and weeks, leading to a full-on panic attack;
- Mild jaw pain that morphs into pain so bad you can't even open your mouth;
- A monster period requiring massive doses of painkillers; and
- A missed period with no ovulation in sight.

Think back to the last time your body "crashed" and try to remember the warning signs. Write them down to keep them top of mind. Otherwise, you'll likely blow through those red alerts next time and feel wrecked yet again. And when you feel the onset of those distress symptoms that mean you're about to hit your threshold, take action: say no, take the night off from social engagements, get support, or incorporate the other self-care techniques I've suggested in this week's protocol.

Understanding your body and its limits, and knowing that these signs of being overstressed are little nudges from your body that it's time to slow down, will help you avoid the physical and emotional damage caused by unmitigated stress and set you on your way to a happier period.

Set Boundaries

I believe in having strong personal boundaries because, hey, your mental health is worth it. But saying it and doing it are very different. Start by getting clear on how you want to feel each day and the pursuits or commitments that will help you get there. Make a list. Do you want to feel happy, joyful, free, cared for, loved, generous, optimistic, carefree, calm, blissed out, or at ease? Make a note of it. Then write down what helps you achieve those feelings. Maybe it's getting eight hours of sleep each night, meditating for fifteen minutes in the morning, having a date night with your partner, attending your kid's ballet class, reading a book for an hour each week, listening to your favourite podcast, preparing a healthy breakfast, or volunteering at your local food bank. You get the idea. When we start taking responsibility for how we want to feel and what it is we really want to do, we lay the foundation for self-fulfillment and happiness and crowd out feelings of frustration, resentment, and being overwhelmed.

Now that you have a clear sense of what will help you achieve your health goals, practise saying no to the activities that don't. Women are programmed to overcommit, overprovide, and people-please, often at the expense of our own health—wait, who am I kidding? It's *always* at the expense of our own health. It's easy to get pulled into what other people ask of you. So, this week when someone asks you to do something that you know will compromise the health of your adrenals and how you want to feel every day, practise saying, "Probably not . . . but let me think about it." Or, better yet, work up the courage to say no right away.

Take a hard look at your current commitments and to-dos and ask yourself, "Will doing this recharge my batteries or deplete them?" If it will deplete them, say no and don't do that thing anymore; find a smarter way of doing it; or delegate it. Don't feel guilty about opting out and putting your needs first.

Get Support

Not all challenges in life can be resolved without help. Instead of trying to overcome every obstacle on your own or giving up in despair, get comfortable asking for help. You won't look weak. Besides, in most cases, people are happy to help you with the things you need. Ask your partner to make dinner, ask a neighbour to do a carpool with you, call a close friend for moral support when you're having a rough day, delegate work tasks to your assistant. Don't spend your valuable energy bandwidth doing things you don't want to if you have the resources to hand them off to others. And don't be shy about leaning on your girlfriends. In fact, women naturally respond to stressful situations by seeking out the support and protection of other women. This is known as the "tend and befriend" stress response, and it is unique to women. "Tend and befriend" raises levels of oxytocin (the love and bonding hormone), which reduces feelings of fear and induces relaxation. This is part of the reason women have better health than men and possibly why they live longer.[19] So, make a date this week with your favourite gal pals; I have no doubt it will fill your tank.

Upgrade Your Sleep Habits

That old adage "I can sleep when I die" is not gonna cut it when you're trying to fix your HPA axis dysfunction. I can't stress it enough—again, no pun intended—but when it comes to adrenal recovery, sleep is everything. Yet, if you're stressed out, getting a good night's sleep may feel downright impossible. When we have HPA axis dysfunction, the interplay between cortisol and melatonin doesn't happen the way it's supposed to. Remember, cortisol puts you on high alert, and if your cortisol levels are soaring, especially at night, your melatonin will be simultaneously suppressed, and you'll be wide awake when you need rest the most.

The answer is to get your body's circadian rhythm back in sync. This twenty-four-hour internal clock that cycles between wakefulness and sleep is cued by light. So, in the evening, as light decreases, your cortisol levels drop and melatonin rises. In the morning, as light increases, melatonin should go down as cortisol goes up and the body shifts from sleep to wakefulness. This rise in cortisol first thing in the morning is known as the cortisol awakening response (CAR), and it represents your brain's ability to tell your adrenals to make cortisol as soon as your eyes open.[20] The set point for cortisol for the day, the CAR establishes your circadian rhythm. But if the CAR isn't working correctly, you miss out on a whole bunch of important things in the short term, such as consistent energy and blood sugar stability, and risk long-term conditions such as diabetes and depression.[21] (See appendix B for CAR testing options.)

The goal is to be in bed by 10 p.m., get an average of seven to eight hours' total sleep, and one and a half to two hours' deep sleep, what's needed for proper human growth hormone production. Think of deep sleep as the time for your night-time clean-up and repair crew to do its work. (Deep sleep can be measured using a wearable sleep tracker such as the Oura Ring or a Fitbit.)

Unfortunately, our modern world (especially its artificial light) has made it tough for us to achieve this goal and get some decent shut-eye. Here are a few things you can do to get your body back on track for upgraded sleep.

DURING THE DAYTIME

GET SUNLIGHT IN YOUR EYES. I don't mean stare at the sun, but it is important to get into sunlight, ideally first thing in the morning, in order to support your cortisol awakening response and your entire circadian rhythm. This includes opening the blinds or curtains as soon as you wake up, to get light in your eyes, or using a light box or light therapy lamp. Also, make sure to go outside without sunglasses and get sunlight in your eyes at least once a day.

GET GROUNDED. This may sound a little New Age-y, but scientific evidence suggests that walking barefoot on the earth, grass, or a beach can help reset your adrenal function and improve chronic fatigue.[22] The research suggests that the earth's electrons induce a relaxation effect when our bodies are in contact with it.[23] Science or not, it shouldn't come as a surprise that getting into nature has a healing effect on us!

AT NIGHT

STOP EATING AT LEAST TWO HOURS BEFORE BEDTIME. Eating right before bedtime activates the digestive system and raises blood sugar, which can disturb sleep. If you find yourself waking up at 3 a.m., it could be due to a late-night meal or snack. This blood sugar spike and subsequent crash during sleep might also cause you to wake up starving.

CREATE A BEDTIME RITUAL OR ROUTINE. Your body needs a signal that it's the end of the day and time to relax. Answering emails in bed at 11 p.m. doesn't send this signal. A bedtime ritual doesn't have to be complicated. For some people, it's as simple as settling down with a good book to read for a few minutes, enjoying a cup of hot herbal tea, reflecting on your day in a journal, or doing some gentle stretching or a guided meditation.

STICK TO A REGULAR BEDTIME. Having a regular bedtime builds on the bedtime ritual and helps to establish a healthy sleep pattern. Think about it, if your bedtime is different every night, that's not much of a pattern. Establishing a regular bedtime and sticking to it allows the body to plan its sleep cycle.[24] Even if you don't fall asleep right away, lying in bed at the same time each evening—set a reminder—will help create a pattern that will promote sleep. Tip: I reverse-engineer my bedtime ritual and determine how long it will take, so I know the exact time to get into bed.

SET A "LIGHT CURFEW" FOR ELECTRONIC DEVICES. Establish a rule for yourself: no electronic devices (computer screens, televisions, smartphones, or tablets) past 9 p.m. or while you're in bed. That's right. Banish them from the bedroom. The light these devices emit is heavy on the blue spectrum, which is particularly stimulating to the brain, keeping you awake.[25] Limit the other lights in your life as well. After 9 p.m., turn off as many lights in your house as possible and use candles instead. Also, light-blocking (e.g. blackout) curtains or blinds will keep your room nice and dark.

DON'T EXERCISE RIGHT BEFORE BED. I know this might go without saying, but please don't go for a run at 8:30 in the evening. Studies have shown that exercising for one hundred fifty minutes per week can significantly improve sleep[26]—but not when you do it right before hitting the sack. Exercising late in the day *increases* cortisol levels, so consider doing it in the morning or at midday, when your energy should be at its highest.

CHECK YOUR ALCOHOL AND CAFFEINE CONSUMPTION. Because it makes you drowsy, alcohol may *appear* to help you fall asleep, but it actually interferes with rapid eye movement (REM) sleep, the period of sleep when you dream.[27] Dream time is extremely important for HPA axis restoration. Caffeine artificially stimulates your adrenals to release cortisol and decreases the amount of melatonin released from the pineal gland—the exact opposite of what you want to have happen for good sleep. Best to pay attention to how caffeine makes you feel. If you're having anxious thoughts, get the jitters, or have difficulty falling and staying asleep, either have your caffeine earlier in the day or steer clear of it entirely.

Recharge Your Batteries

At the end of the day, we're all probably dealing with more stress than we may realise. Far from the tranquil days of our hunter-gatherer ancestors, we now live in a world full of constant pressures and hyperstimulation. For many of us, we've become accustomed, and in some cases addicted, to the rush we get from stressful situations. However, when we are overstressed to the point where our tank begins to run dry, warning lights will appear. If we don't give our bodies time to refill and recharge and continually push past our stress threshold, we'll inevitably end up in the breakdown lane with all kinds of problems. Remember, though, stress in moderation is your friend. It will give you the energy and confidence to overcome the many challenges you will face in your life. But like all friends, you need to respect its boundaries and limitations.

9

WEEK SIX

SUPPORT YOUR THYROID FOR HEALTHIER PERIODS

Welcome to the sixth and final week of the Fix Your Period programme. You're about to cross the finish line, which means it's celebration time. We've talked about the thyroid and its critical influence on period health all along, but as we round the corner into lasting hormone balance, it's time to give this influential endocrine gland the attention it deserves.

THE THYROID AND YOUR MENSTRUAL HEALTH

Your thyroid is deeply connected to your menstrual health. Though small in size, this butterfly-shaped gland impacts virtually every organ. In fact, each and every cell in your body has a receptor site for thyroid hormones, meaning these hormones have some influence on the function of virtually *all* your tissues and organs. Affecting everything from digestion to mental health to reproduction, your thyroid calls a *lot* of the shots in your body, so you need to treat it like the VIP it is—because if it isn't working flawlessly, it will only cause you grief.

Because of our hormonal makeup, women are five to eight times more likely than men to develop a thyroid disorder.[1] You may know of common symptoms such as unexplained weight gain; serious fatigue;

depression and mood issues; aches and pains; chronic colds and other illnesses; hair loss and/or brittle, strawlike hair; cold hands and feet; and dry skin. What most women don't know, and are often not told, is that their anovulatory cycles, low sex drive, PMS, painful periods, excessive menstrual bleeding, irregular periods, amenorrhoea, recurrent miscarriages, and infertility can also be caused by an underactive or overactive thyroid.

While thyroid problems may affect us more than men, they do not discriminate by age. They can develop in childhood; as a reaction to our being on the birth control pill; during or after pregnancy; and in perimenopause. Most people develop *hypo*thyroidism, or an underactive thyroid, while far fewer people develop *hyper*thyroidism, an overactive thyroid.

Understanding the symptoms of an overactive or underactive thyroid, getting the right tests to determine if you have a thyroid condition, and maintaining a thyroid-friendly lifestyle are the final steps to fixing your period (and fertility) problems and really seeing noticeable shifts in your overall health.

HOW YOUR THYROID WORKS

The thyroid is located in the lower front part of your neck, just above the collarbone. Shaped like a butterfly, it's about 5 cm long and 2.5 cm high. It produces a number of hormones that act throughout the body, influencing metabolism, growth and development, and body temperature.

An important part of thyroid function is to convert iodine into thyroid hormones. Thyroid cells are the only cells in the body that use iodine, and they combine it with the amino acid tyrosine to make triiodothyronine (T_3) and thyroxine (T_4). The raw material for T_3, T_4 accounts for 80 per cent of the thyroid's hormone production. Some T3 is produced in the thyroid and your body also converts T4 to T3 in the liver, gut, kidneys, and brain. T_3 is the type of thyroid hormone that your cells recognise, so it's safe to say that this conversion process has to work well in order for you to feel happy, energetic, and that life is good.

This delicate balance of T_4 and T_3 levels is regulated by the hypothalamic–pituitary–thyroid (HPT) axis. Yes, yet another axis in the body. When more T_4 and T_3 are needed from the thyroid for use in the body, the pituitary gland releases a hormone called thyroid-stimulating hormone, or TSH, which signals the thyroid to produce more thyroid hormone. When thyroid hormone levels rise high enough, TSH production slows down. And like a typical feedback loop, when T_4 and T_3 levels drop, TSH levels rise (see Figure 12 below).

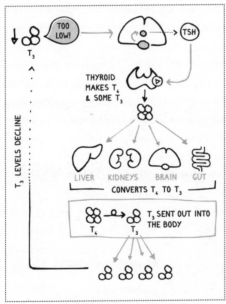

Figure 12: The HPT axis and how the thyroid works

WHEN YOUR THYROID IS DYSFUNCTIONAL

If your thyroid is functioning correctly, T_3 and T_4 are produced in the right amounts. Unfortunately, this is not the case for many of us. There are two ways the thyroid can be off-kilter.

Hypothyroidism

Hypothyroidism—*hypo* means "too little"—occurs when the thyroid does not produce enough of either or both T_4 and T_3. Hypothyroidism can cause menorrhagia (heavy periods), more frequent and longer periods, and dysmenorrhoea (painful menstruation).[2] Women with hypothyroidism may also struggle to conceive or have an increased risk of miscarriage when they do get pregnant.[3] Additional symptoms of hypothyroidism include:

- fatigue that feels like bone-crushing exhaustion;
- weight gain without an increase in food intake;
- brain fog and memory problems;
- sensitivity to cold (e.g. you're the only one in the office wearing a jumper);
- lower-than-normal basal body temperature—which you'll notice if you're taking your temperature in the mornings as part of tracking your period (see Chapter 1) or are practising a fertility awareness-based method (FABM) of contraception that uses basal temperature tracking;
- hair loss and/or strawlike hair;
- brittle, slow-growing nails;
- dry skin;
- joint pain; and
- constipation.

Hyperthyroidism

Hyperthyroidism—*hyper* means "over"—occurs when you're generating too much thyroid hormone. With hyperthyroidism, there is the likelihood of delayed puberty, lighter periods, sporadic or infrequent periods, amenorrhoea (absent periods), and subsequent fertility issues.[4] Other symptoms of hyperthyroidism include:

- anxiety, nervousness, and heart palpitations;
- hand tremors;

- difficulty sleeping;
- sensitivity to heat (e.g. you're the only one wearing short sleeves in winter);
- higher-than-normal basal body temperature, which you'll notice if you're taking your temperature in the morning as part of tracking your period or are practising a fertility awareness-based method (FABM) of contraception that uses basal temperature tracking;
- bulging eyes; and
- frequent bowel movements or diarrhoea.

Whether you experience symptoms of hypothyroidism, hyperthyroidism, or a combination of the two, it's time to find the underlying cause of your thyroid imbalance.

CONVENTIONAL MEDICINE'S APPROACH TO THYROID DISORDERS

Over the years, most of the women I've worked with who've had period and fertility problems have had an underlying thyroid condition they were unaware of. They had lots of telltale symptoms (and their own suspicions about what was wrong), but their thyroid tests always came back normal and they were sent on their way. (Perhaps you can relate?)

There are a number of issues at play here. First, their doctors were testing only TSH and total T_4 levels, and sometimes only TSH. While this is standard procedure in Western medical practices, it fails to provide a complete picture of what's actually going on. Thyroid physiology is complex, and the production, conversion, and uptake of thyroid hormone in the body involves several steps. If there is a problem with any of these steps, you may have symptoms, but testing only those two hormones may not reflect that interplay.

Second, the conventional belief is that if TSH is high, then you have hypothyroidism, and if TSH is normal, then you're good to go. Um, no, that is definitely not how it works. In order to get the right data on what your thyroid is up to, you need to get a full thyroid panel. This includes TSH, total T_4 and T_3, free T_4 and T_3, reverse T_3, thyroid peroxidase antibodies (TPO), and thyroglobulin antibodies (TGAB). These last two will help determine if you have an autoimmune thyroid condition.

Third, a range that is considered "normal" varies from lab to lab and is based on a statistical average of people coming in for testing because they are already sick, versus people who are well. But "normal" lab ranges should probably not be determined by people who are already sick, right? Instead, functional or optimal test ranges are much more helpful in determining a thyroid problem; these are narrower than the conventional medicine reference ranges and are based on healthy people who feel great, rather than on sick people.

The idea behind the functional or optimal test range is to assess the risk of a disease before it develops, whereas the conventional range is used to diagnose disease. For instance, the conventional medical TSH range varies by lab but falls somewhere between 0.45 mIU/L and 5.0 mIU/L, whereas the functional reference range is 0.5 mIU/L to 2.0 mIU/L. See the difference? So, you could have a TSH level of 4.0 for years on end, which is considered *way* too high from a *functional medicine* perspective, but because it's within range from a *conventional medicine* perspective, you're unlikely to receive adequate treatment or any treatment, even if you have symptoms. This is why it's so important to be tuned in to your body and pay attention to symptoms that persist, because your body doesn't lie.

OPTIMAL THYROID TEST RANGES

Based on current medical knowledge, these are the optimal test ranges for the thyroid. (Source: Kresser Institute ADAPT Practitioner Training and Certification program.)

TSH: 0.5–2.0 mIU/L

Total T_3: 100–180 ng/dL

Total T_4: 6–12 µg/dL

Free T_3: 2.5–4.0 pg/mL

Free T_4: 1.0–1.5 ng/dL

Reverse T_3: 9–21 ng/dL

*TPO: 0–15 IU/mL

*TGAB: 0–0.9 IU/mL

*To help identify an autoimmune thyroid condition, a TPO antibody test and a thyroglobulin antibody test are required to assess the levels of antibodies present.

SUBCLINICAL HYPOTHYROIDISM

What does this lack of adequate testing and outdated lab ranges lead to? Yup, you guessed it. Millions and millions of women on the planet walking around in a state of what's known as subclinical hypothyroidism for years before being properly diagnosed.

Subclinical hypothyroidism is basically like "hypothyroidism lite," a milder version of full-blown hypothyroidism, where TSH is slightly elevated and free T_4 and/or free T_3 are normal[5]—that's if the doctor even tests T_4 and T_3. Women who have subclinical hypothyroidism exhibit many of the same symptoms as women with full-on hypothyroidism, but the tests come back normal and they're often told that everything is fine and sent on their way.

Listen, when a doctor runs tests and tells you you're fine even when you're clearly stating you don't feel fine—in fact, you feel like sh*t—this is what I call medical gaslighting. Going by the lab numbers alone, the doctor is denying what is real for you and dismissing your experience as if it weren't real. In this case, it's time either to advocate for yourself or to find another doctor, one willing to partner with you to figure out what's really going on "under the hood."

Unfortunately, subclinical hypothyroidism is frequently under-diagnosed and undertreated. To be fair, from a conventional medicine perspective, it is rather controversial and often disputed, which is why doctors rarely assign a diagnosis and recommend an appropriate treatment plan. Remember, the conventional interpretation of such tests is that if a woman's level of TSH, or thyroid-stimulating hormone, is high, then the patient has hypothyroidism; if it's normal, she doesn't—an approach that fails to take any of the other thyroid hormones into account. Naturally, this leaves a huge grey area for a large number of women who have classic hypothyroid symptoms but only slightly elevated levels of TSH and normal levels of the other thyroid hormones based on the ranges recommended in conventional Western medicine.

Countless clients have come to me in desperation after being told their test results were "normal" and that they were fine, even though inadequate thyroid testing was done and/or their test numbers fell within the conventional range but were either at the high or low end (indicating a subclinical thyroid issue). Somewhere between 3 and 8 per cent of people in the United States are affected by subclinical hypothyroidism.[6] So, this is a pretty common problem.

The conventional solution to thyroid disorders is to give women thyroid medication to get the numbers into the healthy range again. You might be one of these women. In fact, if you talk to any woman in her mid-thirties to early forties, she's likely on levothyroxine (a commonly prescribed treatment for hypothyroidism) or knows a woman who is. It's almost become a rite of passage for women in our society to be put on thyroid medication. The problem is that while the women taking this medication may start to feel better, the drug is merely overriding the underlying cause of the thyroid problem without addressing it.

The thyroid doesn't function in isolation. It's very much impacted by autoimmunity and by other endocrine glands and the hormones they make, which is why it's imperative that we search for the reason our thyroids are going bananas.

THE THYROID–MENSTRUAL CYCLE CONNECTION

How can a dysfunctional thyroid cause such a range of menstrual abnormalities and fertility issues? Because of the body-wide hormonal conversation, of course. Let's look at some of the ways the thyroid directly affects your menstrual cycle.

- Thyroid disease (both types) disrupts ovulation,[7] which results in progesterone deficiency. How does this happen? Both hypothyroidism and hyperthyroidism disrupt pituitary hormone production (in particular, the production of prolactin, FSH, and LH), thereby messing with the ovulatory process beginning in the brain.[8] Additionally, hypothyroidism deprives your ovarian follicles of the thyroid hormone they need to develop.[9]
- Hypothyroidism diminishes the body's sensitivity to insulin,[10] which is one reason that thyroid disease is associated with polycystic ovary syndrome and can worsen cases of PCOS.[11] This can further exacerbate oestrogen dominance and progesterone deficiency.
- Hypothyroidism reduces sex hormone-binding globulin (SHBG), which leads to higher oestrogen circulation in the body and, therefore, heavier periods.[12] On the flip side, *hyper*thyroidism increases SHBG, which may lead to lighter periods.[13]
- Hypothyroidism diminishes the body's ability to metabolise oestrogen effectively, which raises oestrogen levels, thus creating an environment that leads to heavier periods.[14]
- There is evidence that hypothyroidism decreases blood-clotting factors, which can cause heavy periods. This is because the role of

clotting factors is to control bleeding. In contrast, *hyper*thyroidism *increases* those clotting factors, which in turn causes *lighter* periods.[15]

- Long and heavy periods caused by hypothyroidism can lead to iron deficiency anaemia, which is very common in premenopausal women. Iron plays a crucial role in ovarian follicle development and hormone production, so an iron deficiency could bring about ovulation and fertility problems.[16]

Generally speaking, a low-functioning thyroid robs the entire body of energy, including the energy needed to keep the reproductive system up and running. Remember, there are thyroid hormone receptors on every cell in the body, so our entire body is dependent on adequate thyroid hormone. Understandably, the body can't put energy into ovulation when it is running on an energy deficit and struggling to keep its engine going.

TRYING TO GET PREGNANT?

Because thyroid function impacts your menstrual cycle, it 100 per cent impacts your fertility. If your thyroid is underactive, your basal body temperature is likely lower than it should be. The rapidly dividing cells of an embryo require a specific temperature range in order for that division to take place (see the temperature ranges under "Get a Full Thyroid Panel or Do Your Own Testing," in the protocol at the end of this chapter). If your body temperature is too low, the embryo may be unable to continue to grow, which will lead to difficulty conceiving and an increased risk of early miscarriage.[17] Many early miscarriages happen because too many women have an undiagnosed thyroid condition. Overt hypothyroidism and hyperthyroidism contribute to pre-eclampsia, preterm delivery, and even stillbirth, which is why you must work with a doctor who will test your thyroid throughout your pregnancy, especially if you have a diagnosed thyroid disorder.[18]

WHAT CAUSES THYROID DISORDERS?

The most common cause of *hypo*thyroidism in the Western world is Hashimoto's thyroiditis, also known as autoimmune thyroiditis; and the most common cause of *hyper*thyroidism is Grave's disease.[19] Like all autoimmune diseases, these thyroid conditions come into play when the immune system is overstimulated or triggered and, through a simple case of mistaken identity, attacks healthy tissue, believing it to be a foreign pathogen. In this case, the unfortunate target of the attack is the thyroid gland. Antibodies are released by the immune system with instructions to destroy cells that resemble the hormone-producing cells in the thyroid, or their receptors. As discussed in Chapter 6, autoimmune disease is rooted in gut health problems. Not surprisingly, lipopolysaccharides (LPS), those obnoxious toxins released from pathogenic bacteria, affect your thyroid in multiple ways. In particular, they attack the thyroid, causing the body to produce antibodies against thyroid cells.[20] LPS also reduces TSH, inhibits the conversion of T_4 to T_3, and interferes with thyroid hormone receptors.[21]

Higher-than-normal levels of oestrogen put a real damper on how your thyroid does business. However, as you now know, hypothyroidism also contributes to elevated oestrogen—quite the hormonal pickle. High oestrogen prevents the thyroid hormone from being able to get into its thyroid receptors.[22] Your thyroid might be working just fine, but you will be feeling symptoms of low thyroid function. Many women with oestrogen dominance are misdiagnosed with hypothyroidism and put on thyroid medication.

Iodine is *the* essential building block of thyroid hormones. No iodine, no thyroid hormones. If we lack this vital mineral, our thyroid can become enlarged—this is known as a goitre—in an attempt to absorb as much iodine as possible. Iodine deficiency used to be considered quite rare in Western culture due to the prevalence of iodised salt in our diets. But recent studies are showing that this deficiency is now back on the rise.[23] However, this isn't a call to supplement: if we consume too much iodine, we can cause hyperthyroidism. Additionally, it appears that iodine supplementation can exacerbate auto-immune thyroiditis, especially in the case of selenium deficiency, so it's critical to work with a skilled practitioner to get the right kind of help for your particular issue.[24]

Unfortunately, increasing amounts of both corticotropin-releasing hormone and cortisol inhibit TSH production.[25] And cortisol slows the conversion of T_4 to T_3. All this will downregulate your thyroid function in a big way.

Persistent organic pollutants (POPs) are industrial chemicals—think dioxin, dichlorodiphenyltrichloroethane (DDT), and polychlorinated biphenyls (PCBs)—that affect your thyroid in multiple ways. They damage the thyroid, reducing T_4 output.[26] They impair the thyroid's ability to absorb iodine,[27] disrupt the hypothalamic–pituitary–thyroid (HPT) axis, and are even linked to thyroid cancer.[28] BPA causes oestrogen dominance[29] and slows down your thyroid by blocking thyroid receptor function[30]—a bit of a double whammy for your thyroid.

The thyroid gland is extremely sensitive to radiation. In fact, 20 to 30 per cent of people who have undergone radiation therapy in the head and neck area have gone on to develop hypothyroidism.[31] Even excess dental X-rays have been shown to increase the risk of thyroid disease.[32] The thyroid is also sensitive to the electromagnetic frequency (EMF) waves generated by all electrical products, but especially mobile phones and laptops—and we're all pretty much attached to them. One study found that an average exposure to mobile phones of just over two hours a day resulted in a higher-than-normal TSH level and lowered T_4.[33]

Both these make your brain think you're in starvation mode. Your brain then sends a signal to your thyroid to slow down hormone production, which slows down your metabolism.[34] Guess what happens next? Because your body is in energy-conservation mode, you actually *retain* body fat.

Birth control pills hijack your thyroid in multiple ways. They not only deplete some of the vital nutrients your thyroid requires, such as selenium and zinc,[35] but they also weaken your gut's ability to absorb those nutrients.[36] On top of interfering with your thyroid hormone levels, the Pill also elevates thyroid-binding globulin (TBG).[37] Once thyroid hormone is bound to TBG, it is not available for use by your cells, so you'll feel like you're in a hypothyroid state. It's no wonder to me that so many of my coaching clients were put on thyroid medication while on the birth control pill, or soon after they came off it.

As you can see, your thyroid has far-reaching effects and if you have a thyroid condition, even if it's subclinical, you'd best believe you're gonna have symptoms. Now you know that a test for just TSH is hardly going to tell you what's up with this endocrine gland, and that more comprehensive testing is in order if you suspect a problem with your thyroid.

WEEK SIX PROTOCOL: SUPPORT YOUR THYROID

So, how do you put all this good information to use and give your thyroid some love? Remember, your thyroid doesn't operate in isolation; it's connected to everything else in the body. This means that by following my recommendations in the previous five weeks of the Fix Your Period programme, you've already taken many of the necessary steps to get your thyroid and your menstrual cycle into amazing shape. And because you've made those changes, your homework this week is to test, girlfriend, test!

Get a Full Thyroid Panel or Do Your Own Testing

It's time to tune in and get in touch with your own personal thyroid status. This week, schedule a full thyroid panel—you can ask your doctor for one or you can order an at-home thyroid panel test kit online—to get a better idea of what's happening with your own body.

Once you have your results, compare them against the "Optimal Thyroid Test Ranges" listed earlier (see page 213). If your test results come back with irregularities, or are out of optimal range, it's time to do more to support your thyroid health. First, ensure you have all the dietary and lifestyle advice from the past weeks on lockdown. Then check out my recommendations for "Additional Thyroid Support" in this chapter. Working with a well-versed doctor or practitioner is important for achieving the best results. You will likely want to retest your thyroid in two to three months to gauge improvements or changes.

If, for whatever reason, you are unable to see your doctor for a thyroid panel or obtain one online, don't despair: your basal body temperature is a great indicator of thyroid function because it is a reflection of your metabolic activity. A thyroid disorder will disrupt your ability to regulate your basal body temperature—a signal that it's time to consult a professional.

If you're not already taking your basal body temperature as part of your cycle-tracking practice, take it for 10 days starting on day 1 of your cycle and up through day 10. Hormonal fluctuations can influence your basal body temperature, so it's best to take it in the follicular phase before ovulation, when there's less fluctuation. If you are not currently getting a period, start taking your temperature at any time.

A normal resting body temperature before ovulation often falls within the range of 36.11 to 36.50 degrees Celsius (97.0 and 97.7 degrees Fahrenheit), according to Toni Weschler, in her book *Taking Charge of Your Fertility*. In my experience over the years, if your temperatures are consistently lower than 36.11, or in the 35s, this could be a sign of low thyroid function. If, however, temperatures are consistently *above* 36.6 degrees, this indicates a possible hyperthyroid state. Of course, keep in mind that one's basal temperature can vary significantly and is not 100 per cent accurate. Still, it should be considered, along with other symptoms, as a first clue that there is a thyroid problem.

If your temperatures are erratic or mixed, both above and below the 36.1 to 36.5 degree range, this is quite often indicative of sub-optimal thyroid function *and* cortisol dysregulation, as the adrenals and thyroid are closely linked. Furthermore, if you are on thyroid medication but seeing lower-than-normal temperatures and/or erratic temperatures, or if you are still feeling symptoms, it might mean you are undermedicated. You'll need to work with your doctor to address this.

If, when you run the thyroid panel or test by tracking your basal body temperature, nothing seems to be off in the numbers and you feel great, that's awesome. However, if the numbers don't seem to be off but you're still showing signs of thyroid imbalance, trust what you feel. Testing is very important, but never discount your feelings. As I've said throughout this book, your body is always talking to you. And I'm in the business of treating a person's symptoms, not her test results. Symptoms may show up before something shows up in your blood work, or they could be indicating something a thyroid panel can't test for, such as the health of your thyroid hormone receptors. Be sure to follow all the diet and lifestyle recommendations from the previous five weeks and then try the suggestions under "Additional Thyroid Support."

IF YOU HAVE HASHIMOTO'S OR GRAVE'S DISEASE

If you have Hashimoto's or Grave's disease, getting off thyroid medication completely or restoring all thyroid function may not be on the cards. Your thyroid may already have endured too much damage, which has decreased its ability to produce and use thyroid hormone correctly. If this is your situation, there is nothing to be ashamed about—the good news is that by following my suggestions in the section "Additional Thyroid Support" (see page 222), you can still see improvement in your periods and quality of life. You may also see a reduction in your other symptoms and even improved thyroid antibody levels. This is important, as it will limit the progression of the disease. However, as you embark on this protocol, I do recommend you work closely with your doctor to test your levels often and adjust your thyroid medication as needed, to keep feeling your best all around.

Additional Thyroid Support

Going gluten-free isn't just good for your gut; it can also support your thyroid. Studies have found that people with coeliac disease are three times more likely to have thyroid disease, which gets better and has even been shown to go into complete remission when gluten is removed from their diets.[38] So, permanently avoiding gluten can help normalise thyroid function. This can be the case even if you don't have coeliac disease.

Selenium, iron, zinc, magnesium, and vitamins A, B_2, B_3, B_{12}, C, and D are all necessary for adequate production and/or conversion of thyroid hormones. Here are the thyroid superstars:

- **Zinc.** This mineral is essential for thyroid function because it helps facilitate the conversion of T_4 to T_3.[39] You can find zinc in beef, shrimp, kidney beans, and spinach. If you're supplementing, the recommended dose is 20 mg to 50 mg of a high-quality zinc such as zinc pincolinate or zinc bisglycinate per day. Make sure to take it with meals to prevent nausea.
- **Selenium.** Your thyroid requires this crucial mineral in order to work properly, and it also reduces thyroid antibodies associated with autoimmune thyroid disease.[40] The best food source of selenium is the Brazil nut (preferably organic). And you need only one or two of these nuts per day to maintain selenium levels. If you plan on getting your selenium in a supplement, do not exceed the recommended dose of 200 mcg per day.
- **Iron.** An iron deficiency signals your thyroid to conserve energy, which leads to lower T_4 and T_3 production.[41] It is best to obtain iron in its "heme" form, which is available only from animal sources such as liver, beef, and lamb. Non-heme iron is found in plant foods and is not as easily absorbed by the body as heme iron.[42] If you choose to supplement, the daily recommended dose is 18 mg.
- **Magnesium.** Deficiency in magnesium is associated with elevated

thyroid antibodies, hypothyroidism, and Hashimoto's disease.[43] Abundant sources of magnesium include dark leafy greens, nuts, seeds, and whole grains. The recommended daily dosage is 350 mg. If you plan on supplementing, take magnesium glycinate or magnesium malate, which are more bioavailable than magnesium citrate and will reduce your chance of experiencing loose stools or diarrhoea.

- **Vitamin A**. Vitamin A increases iodine uptake by the thyroid, lowers TSH, and raises T_3.[44] You'll want to focus on foods that contain retinol, which is the preformed type of vitamin A. Sources of retinol include liver, eggs, butter from grass-fed cows, and cod liver oil (1 teaspoon of cod liver oil a day). Plant sources of vitamin A (carotenoids) while wonderful must be converted to retinol to be used by the body. This conversion is difficult for some people. Unless you're working with a practitioner, I'd suggest sticking to food sources of vitamin A.

- **Vitamin D.** Vitamin D has been associated with helping to prevent Hashimoto's.[45] It can be obtained from some fatty fish, including mackerel, salmon, and tuna; cod liver oil; and, of course, sunlight exposure. Get out in the sun every day between 10 a.m. and 2 p.m. and expose your arms and legs for twenty minutes with sunblock only on your face. If you plan on supplementing, be sure to get your vitamin D levels tested first, to determine your deficiency, and then work with your doctor to supplement with the appropriate dosage. The recommended dose is 2,000 IU per day of vitamin D_3 to maintain current levels of vitamin D if you are not deficient.

Iodine is your thyroid's main squeeze, which means thyroid dysfunction worsens when the body's iodine levels are low. The best sources of dietary iodine are sea vegetables (kelp, kombu, and dulse), ocean fish, eggs, raw dairy, and strawberries. I suggest sticking to food sources of iodine only, but if you supplement with iodine, take no more than 300 mcg in conjunction with selenium.

The thyroid gland is extremely sensitive to radiation and electromagnetic frequency waves, so it's important to limit your exposure.

- At night, switch off your wireless router, put your phone on
  airplane mode, and turn off any Bluetooth devices.
- Keep electronics out of the bedroom. This includes TVs, DVRs,
  mobile phones, fancy alarm clocks, and anything else that emits
  EMFs.
- Use a wired headset instead of wireless earbuds to talk on the
  phone. (Sorry, I know how annoying this one is, but we're talking
  about your brain here.)

Whether it's getting your vitamin D checked and supplementing if
it's low or working on your mobile phone overuse—c'mon, I know
you can do it—whatever strategies you implement from this chapter
will benefit your thyroid. Even if you don't have subclinical or overt
thyroid disease, protecting your thyroid with the right nutrients and
doing your best to avoid thyroid irritants will ensure that your entire
endocrine system, including your menstrual cycle, runs smoothly.

PART III

LIVING LIKE A MENSTRUATION MAVEN

10

AFTER THE SIX WEEKS

Congratulations on completing the Fix Your Period programme! Your commitment to your health and to the hormone repair process is to be celebrated. So, celebrate! Give yourself kudos for all the positive changes you've made over the past several weeks and the progress you've made on your health journey. Rehabbing your hormones is not for wusses. As one of my amazing teachers, Dr Sara Gottfried, MD, says, "It's the path of the warrior princess." And by now, I hope you see that it's a better path, one that is more aligned with who you are at your deepest level and that will lead you to better health and, more important, a better period.

Make sure to acknowledge your new relationship with your body, too. Are you listening to her, trusting her, loving her more, and truly honouring her needs? Hell yeah, you are!

TAKE AN INVENTORY OF WHERE YOU ARE NOW

Now that we're at the end of the programme, let's take an honest, unflinching inventory of where you are. What were your symptoms when you started? Are you still experiencing them now? If they haven't disappeared completely, have they lessened? It's easy for us to notice only the symptoms we're still dealing with and not the ones we've resolved or improved. So, let's tune in to what was hugely problematic for you at the start and see how that's shifted.

What Has Changed?

What has changed since you began six weeks ago? Are you:

- Experiencing lighter periods?
- Using fewer tampons and pads?
- Ovulating or getting a period for the first time in a while?
- Having less intense cramps?
- Experiencing two migraines this month instead of five?
- Seeing clearer skin and stronger, healthier hair and nails?
- Experiencing better digestion?
- Experiencing more energy, vitality, and mental clarity?

What else? Be specific. Taking an inventory of how much has changed, even if *nothing* has changed, is a powerful way to track your progress and identify areas that need more attention going forwards.

If some of the diet and lifestyle changes in the six-week programme have been more challenging to implement than others, don't sweat it. Change ain't easy. But bit by bit, week by week, if you keep adding the hormone-healthy practices I've outlined, your health should continue to improve.

MOVING FORWARD

Your period is like a crystal ball for your hormonal health, so continue to pay attention to it moving forwards. Even if you haven't yet seen all the changes you hoped for, keep up the great work. Continue to fill your plate with a rainbow of foods to prevent blood sugar spikes and crashes; maintain a healthy gut; support efficient detoxification;

manage your stress like a boss; and pay attention to what your thyroid is telling you—all these steps are as essential now as they were six weeks ago. Sustain what you've been doing, taking care to make your way through *all* the recommendations in each chapter—go back and check. Achieving hormone balance is about building a strong foundation, and these recommendations are your foundation for continued change. And change can take time. Hey, Rome wasn't built in a day. It may take *two to three months* of consistently following the recommendations in the programme for you to see the desired results.

Additional Steps

If you have oestrogen dominance (PMS symptoms, heavy or long periods, anovulation, breast pain or tenderness, a short luteal phase, and spotting or bleeding between periods), PCOS, endometriosis, adenomyosis or hypothalamic amenorrhoea, I can recommend a few additional steps to boost your healing. Check out the advanced protocol for each of these conditions later in this chapter. I've also outlined some general period-supportive practices that anyone can do, no matter your period problem.

Wherever you are on your health journey, I encourage you to consider working with a qualified functional medicine or naturopathic doctor for more one-on-one help. These practitioners are specially trained to identify and treat the root cause of your symptoms, no matter how complex your case. If you are unable to work with a doctor, you might want to seek out a certified women's health coach, nutritional therapist, or holistic nutrition consultant.

Now, let's find your new normal diet.

HOW TO END THE ELIMINATION DIET

Starting in week three and throughout the rest of the programme, you removed inflammatory foods from your diet. Now it's time to see which foods are the triggers for your specific symptoms or conditions by adding them back in one at a time. But before you begin reintroducing foods, I encourage you to assess how you're feeling after four weeks without inflammatory foods. What symptoms have changed or improved? Have you developed any new symptoms? Did you notice you had special cravings at certain times of the protocol? Any changes in your mood, energy, bloating, or bowel movements?

Reintroduce Inflammatory or Problematic Foods

After following an elimination protocol, the tendency can be to add everything back in too quickly. This is a mistake, as it leaves you without the desired conclusions about what does and doesn't work for your body in this season of life. So, to make sure you get the most out of the work you've put in, add foods back in strategically.

BE STRATEGIC

I suggest you begin by reintroducing the foods that are least problematic for many people and work towards adding those that tend to be highly problematic. These are (from least to most problematic):

- caffeine;
- pulses (if you removed them);
- eggs;
- dairy (if you have heavy, painful periods or acne, give yourself sixty days before reintroducing dairy);
- grains (bring them back one type at a time);
- corn (make sure it's organic);
- soy (make sure it's organic); and
- sugar and alcohol.

You may want to bring sugar and alcohol back into your diet, but the hormonal consequences of ingesting these in even small amounts might not be worth it—especially if you're now feeling good. Consider the fact that alcohol and sugar place a high burden on your blood sugar and detox pathways, creating a lot of hormonal vulnerability.

No, you don't have to swear off all sugar for life, but you'll experience the greatest positive changes if you let it creep into your diet only on occasion. Trust how your body reacts when you eat it—you'll feel the difference.

POSSIBLE OUTCOMES

When you reintroduce a food, look for one of three possible outcomes:

- You feel absolutely fine immediately afterwards and in the coming days. Conclusion: this food is okay to add back into your diet.
- You feel an immediate negative reaction. Conclusion: this food is currently problematic for your system; better to keep it out of your diet a while longer and reintroduce it again in twenty-eight days (more on how to do this later in this chapter).
- You feel fine upon eating the food, but within twelve to seventy-two hours, you notice a reaction or symptoms. Conclusion: this food is not supportive at the moment but may be okay to eat on occasion after further gut healing.

SYMPTOMS TO WATCH OUT FOR

Reactions or symptoms to look for as you reintroduce foods (these can be immediate or delayed) include:

- changes in energy levels, fatigue, or low mood;
- interrupted sleep;
- runny nose, nasal congestion, sneezing, or quick onset of sinus infections;
- sore throat;
- mouth sores or an itchy mouth;
- joint pain;
- acne breakouts, rashes, itchy skin, and hives;
- stomach cramps, bloating, acid reflux or other digestive problems, including changes in bowel movement frequency or consistency;
- weight gain or water retention; and/or
- swollen hands and feet.

TIP: It's helpful to keep a food journal while reintroducing foods into your diet. Keeping track of your symptoms will be your way of knowing if your body is saying, "Hey, this food feels great," or "Hmm, I do my best when I don't eat that." The bottom line? Pay attention to your symptoms either in a food diary or using a food journal app. There are plenty of free ones available.

Now that you are clear on where to start and what to look for, let's talk timing.

THE 1–2–3–4 TECHNIQUE FOR FOOD REINTRODUCTION

Some foods may give you a delayed reaction, so if you don't want to be confused as to which food is causing which reaction, reintroduce one food at a time, consuming one serving of it one to two times a day, for three days, before eliminating that food again for four days. This is what I call the 1–2–3–4 Technique:

1 food at a time
2 times per day
For 3 days
Then eliminate that food again for 4 days

If you begin to experience negative reactions to a particular food, you don't need to continue the reintroduction process. You'll already know that that food isn't right for you in this moment and that it's time to remove it, per the instructions below.

After the three days have passed, depending on your symptoms or lack thereof, you'll have a few options:

- **IF THE REINTRODUCTION CAUSED ZERO SYMPTOMS,** remove it again for four days to make sure there are no delayed reactions. If you still have zero symptoms after those four days, you're in the clear and can include this food in your diet as you wish. Now move on to reintroduce the next food on the list.

- **IF THE REINTRODUCTION CAUSED SYMPTOMS OF ANY KIND,** eliminate this food for another twenty-eight days, to allow for further healing. (Important: You don't have to wait the entire twenty-eight days to reintroduce the next food on the list; you just need to wait seven days. After those seven days, your inflammatory response will have died down enough for you to move ahead with the next food on your list.) After twenty-eight days, try reintroducing the original offending food again, to see if your response has changed. If it has and you seem to tolerate the food well, continue the reintroduction process over the course of three days and continue to observe your symptoms. If you still experience symptoms, this food is likely causing inflammation in your body, and I suggest working with a trained medical professional to explore this further.

IF YOUR HEAD IS SPINNING AS YOU READ THIS, HERE'S HOW THIS PROCESS SHOULD LOOK: Let's say you introduced caffeine and successfully detected that it was an acceptable food for you by introducing it for three days, seeing no symptoms, waiting four more days, and still experiencing zero symptoms. You then continued on to beans, at which point you noticed painful bloating, stomach cramps, and smelly wind each time you ate them. You would then eliminate beans from your diet again and wait seven days before reintroducing eggs. You will not reintroduce beans again until twenty-eight days later. Once you reintroduce eggs, pay attention to your symptoms. If you do well eating them, move on to the next food group on the list until you feel confident about your body's response to each food.

I know. This whole operation is not exactly easy-peasy, but after the intentional effort you've put into the programme over the last six weeks, I trust that you'll want to close out the elimination diet correctly. If you start to feel impatient and just want it done with already, take a deep breath and remember your original desire when you bought (or borrowed) this book. Remembering your unpleasant symptoms and your need to find freedom from period drama will give you the motivation to keep going. Do your best, try not to get frustrated, and remember 1–2–3–4.

Identifying which foods cause an inflammatory response in your body is only one step on the road to fixing your period, but it's an eye-opening one, allowing you to see the rapid rate at which your body can change and heal when extra stressors are removed.

That being said, there is a common misconception that simply eliminating foods that aren't working for you is enough to reboot your health in the long term. Yes, it is a revolutionary first step, but it can be dangerous to overly embrace or become obsessed with the elimination of more and more food groups. After all, eliminating everything for life is not the answer.

Reacting poorly to more than two foods in the reintroduction phase is a warning sign of some deeper things happening, such as an inability to break foods down properly, malabsorption of nutrients, leaky gut, or even autoimmune disease. Remember: your ultimate goal is to be able to include as many nutrient-dense and hormone-supportive foods in your diet as possible, so don't get stuck in step one and call it done. If you find you're reacting to more than two food groups on the list, working with a skilled practitioner to determine the right next step for your gut healing can be extremely beneficial.

GENERAL PERIOD-SUPPORTIVE PRACTICES ANYONE CAN DO

SEED CYCLING: The strategic consumption of flax, pumpkin, sesame, and sunflower seeds at different times of the month to balance hormones, seed cycling is an excellent addition to anyone's hormone-supportive lifestyle, especially if you're dealing with amenorrhoea, irregular cycles, PMS symptoms, cramps, a short luteal phase, or other symptoms of imbalanced oestrogen and progesterone. Take 1 tablespoon each of pumpkin seeds and ground flaxseed from day 1 until you ovulate, and then switch to 1 tablespoon each of sesame and sunflower seeds from the day after ovulation until your next period. If you're not ovulating, you'd switch seeds at day 14 and then again at day 28. For more detailed instructions on adding seed cycling to your routine, go to fixyourperiod.com to get my Seed Cycling Protocol.

CASTOR-OIL PACKS: These sound scary, but they work wonders for period pain, improving scar tissue and bringing blood flow to the pelvic region, which can reduce brown or very dark blood. Purchase a castor-oil pack kit and apply the pack to your lower belly with a heating pad for thirty to forty-five minutes one to three times a week.

> **IMPORTANT:** I do not recommend *drinking* castor oil. Also, do not use castor oil packs during your period or if you are pregnant or breastfeeding. If you are trying to conceive, do not use them after ovulation. Visit fixyourperiod.com to get my **Castor Oil Pack Guide.**

CBD OIL: Cannabis has been used for menstrual pain for centuries.[1] According to Jenny Sansouci, author of *The Rebel's Apothecary*, "We all have a system in our body called the endocannabinoid system, which plays a role in regulating pain and inflammation. Compounds in the cannabis plant called cannabinoids (this includes CBD and THC) directly interact with receptors in the endocannabinoid system to help us maintain homeostasis (balance) in the body." As it turns out, we have an abundance of these cannabinoid receptors in our reproductive organs and tissues, including our uterus and ovaries, which points to why so many women find relief from period pain with cannabis products.[2] Visit fixyourperiod.com to get my CBD for Your Period Guide.

ADVANCED PROTOCOLS FOR SPECIFIC PROBLEMS

Advanced Protocol: Oestrogen Dominance

If you've gone through the six-week programme and haven't seen much improvement in your symptoms, don't forget, you may just need more time. Remember, it probably took a long time for these imbalances to develop, so I suggest giving yourself one to two months of healing time for every year you've experienced symptoms.

The gut, liver, and adrenals create a perfect hat-trick. If any combination of the three has diminished function, it can throw off your oestrogen and progesterone levels. So, be sure to revisit Chapters 6, 7, and 8 to review the diet and supplement suggestions in each.

In the meanwhile, there are some advanced steps you can take to reduce your oestrogenic load and/or increase progesterone.

STEP 1: TEST, DON'T GUESS

Understanding precisely what's happening to you internally will help you avoid cherry-picking solutions and wasting money on things that might not be tailor-made for your specific issue. I recommend getting the following two tests done. These will detect actual hormone levels, tell you how the liver is processing your hormones, and identify any genetic reasons for your period/fertility issues.

DUTCH. For advanced help, get the DUTCH test done. In the UK, this would not normally be done on the NHS and you would need to seek out a private clinic and pay for this test to be carried out (see appendix B), and work with a practitioner to interpret the results. This test will show how much of each oestrogen metabolite, 2-OH, 4-OH, and 16-OH, your liver is producing and provide detailed information on what your other hormones are getting up to. Depending on your test results, your practitioner may recommend a specific diet or supplement regimen.

GENETIC TESTING. Testing *MTHFR*, *COMT*, and other genes can reveal additional ways to resolve stubborn symptoms and issues with your detoxification pathways. I recommend Nutrition Genome or StrateGene (there are financial costs attached to these tests).

STEP 2: REBALANCE YOUR GUT MICROBIOME

As discussed in Chapter 6, our microbiome and estrobolome play a massive role in how we produce and use oestrogen. That's why it's important we know what's going on down there. Work with a naturopathic or functional medicine doctor to properly test for SIBO, *H. pylori*, parasites, yeast overgrowth, or other gut infections slipping under the radar. A great place to start is with the Comprehensive Stool Analysis or the Comprehensive Stool Analysis with Parasitology, by Doctor's Data. These tests will give you a broad overview of what's happening with your microbiota, including details on pathogenic bacteria, yeasts, and, with the second test I mentioned, parasites.

STEP 3: NOURISH YOUR ADRENALS TO SUPPORT PROGESTERONE PRODUCTION

If, while reading Chapter 8, you were like, "Wow, all this talk about stress applies to me!" then repairing your adrenals should be a high priority for you; improving their function will increase your ability to ovulate consistently and produce progesterone. Managing your stress is a lot about effecting and managing behaviour change, and that's sometimes tough to do, even for the most stress-resilient of us. I therefore suggest you enlist the support and guidance of a certified health or life coach, who can work with you to develop and implement the best step-by-step approach to getting you in a state of flow rather than feeling like you're constantly swimming upstream. But be patient with yourself: digging out of ingrained behavioural patterns and years of fight-or-flight is no picnic. In the meantime, there are a few supplements that can be helpful in restoring a healthy stress response and boosting progesterone:

PHOSPHATIDYLSERINE. (I know. How the heck do you pronounce *that* one?) This supplement dampens the effect of external stress on the HPA axis and lowers cortisol production, which can improve your response to stress and anxiety and even your memory.[3] The recommended dose for phosphatidylserine is 400 mg a day.

B-COMPLEX WITH AT LEAST 100 MG B$_5$. The B vitamins play an important synergistic role in helping us combat the effects of stress.[4] And because every woman on the planet experiences stress, every woman on the planet probably should be taking a B-complex vitamin daily, as chronically high levels of cortisol deplete vitamins B$_1$, B$_5$, B$_6$, and B$_{12}$. Apart from their stress-reduction role, B vitamins are extremely energising and may help improve your cortisol rhythm.[5] They are best taken in the morning with food to help boost mood and energy for the day.

VITAMIN C. The adrenals can boast one of the highest concentrations of ascorbic acid in any tissue in the body. A potent antioxidant, vitamin C, as it is more commonly known, protects the function of your adrenals and reduces cortisol and inflammatory cytokine production.[6] It also has been shown to increase progesterone levels.[7] The recommended dose is 250 mg to 500 mg of vitamin C twice daily. Breaking up the dose prevents diarrhoea, which can happen with higher doses. I also suggest taking it after ovulation (i.e. only in the second half of the cycle), as it can dry up fertile-quality cervical fluid.

ASHWAGANDHA. Commonly used in Ayurvedic medicine, this popular herb has been around for thousands of years. It is not only an effective anti-anxiety remedy,[8] but can also treat fatigue and sleep disorders and boost endurance.[9] It has even helped a few of my super-stressed clients with amenorrhoea get their periods back. Recommended dosage is 250 mg to 300 mg a day in the morning.

Advanced Protocol: Polycystic Ovary Syndrome

If you have been diagnosed with PCOS, or you have the hallmark symptoms of PCOS—high androgens, chronic anovulation, long menstrual cycles, hair loss on your head, excess body hair growth, acne, insulin dysregulation, and/or weight gain—you'll benefit from the recommendations listed under "Advanced Protocol: Oestrogen Dominance," so please start there. In addition to proper testing, addressing your gut health more completely, and supporting your adrenals, you can do the following to see decreased PCOS symptoms and increased fertility:

STEP 1: TRY A MORE SPECIALISED DIET

When it comes to the way we eat, there is no one-size-fits-all way; there is only the right way for you. If you're still struggling with symptoms or feeling unsatisfied with the foods you're eating, you may benefit from a more specialised diet with a different balance of carbs, protein, fat, and nutrients. I recommend you work one-on-one with a qualified professional to find the best fit for you. However, the following two specialised diets can be very helpful when done correctly.

PALEO. You may think of this diet as "trendy," but it's been studied for more than twenty-five years and has many benefits, including improved gut health[10]—and we know how important that is for your hormones! There is a misconception that Paleo means eating only meat, but this is not the case. There are slightly different opinions about what the Paleo diet should look like, each of which varies on the types of acceptable vegetables and fruits, and whether grains, potatoes, and dairy are allowed. But for the most part, the Paleo diet emphasizes grass-fed (pastured) wild meats, wild-caught fish, lots of organic vegetables, some seasonal fruit (like berries), healthy fats, nuts, seeds, and fermented foods, but no processed foods, sugars, alcohol, or legumes. Chris Kresser's book *The Paleo Cure* is a great place to start.

KETOGENIC. While there are some similarities between the keto diet and the Paleo diet, they are actually quite different. For instance, the Paleo diet is based on a list of foods our ancestors would have theoretically eaten, whereas the keto diet is simply a state of metabolism achieved by lowering your carbohydrate intake. When your body doesn't have carbohydrates to run on, it uses fat for fuel. When fat is broken down in the liver, ketones, beneficial to the brain and GI tract, are produced. When large amounts of ketones are made, the body enters a ketogenic state— hence the diet's name. On a ketogenic diet, you eat meat, fish, eggs, vegetables, nuts, whole-fat dairy, and berries (the last, in moderation). You avoid all other fruit, processed carbohydrates and sugar, grains, starch, and alcohol. Leanne Vogel's *Keto for Women* is an excellent resource.

STEP 2: SUPPLEMENT WITH INOSITOL, CHROMIUM, ZINC, AND VITAMIN D

INOSITOL. This substance is found in a number of foods and in our bodies, and helps improve insulin sensitivity. Women with PCOS tend to be deficient in inositol, a deficiency linked to insulin resistance and subsequent anovulation and irregular cycles.[11] Two types of inositol are recommended for women with PCOS, D-chiro-inositol and myoinositol; both work very well together.[12] The recommended dosage of these two supplements is in a forty-to-one ratio, which is the ratio found in the body naturally, so 1,000 mg twice a day of myoinositol plus 25 mg twice a day of D-chiro-inositol.

CHROMIUM. Chromium is a mineral that promotes proper insulin utilisation and helps with blood glucose management.[13] Chromium can be found in a wide range of foods such as broccoli, sweet potatoes, grass-fed beef, eggs, and raw onion. If you are not getting enough of these foods or continue to experience blood sugar issues, take 200 mcg of chromium picolinate a day.

ZINC. Zinc has been shown to help reduce hair loss and hirsutism (unwanted male-pattern hair growth) in women with PCOS,[14] as well as improve blood sugar and insulin markers.[15] The recommended dose is 20 mg to 50 mg of a high-quality zinc supplement (zinc picolinate or zinc bisglycinate) daily, with food. It can cause nausea if taken on an empty stomach.

VITAMIN D. I often refer to vitamin D as the "period vitamin" because it plays such an important role in follicle development, follicle sensitivity to FSH, and progesterone production.[16] The majority of women diagnosed with PCOS are deficient in this critical vitamin.[17] Before supplementing, get your vitamin D levels tested to determine if you have a deficiency. To start building up your vitamin D levels, go out in the sunshine every day and expose your arms and legs for twenty minutes between 10 a.m. and 2 p.m. (with sunblock on your face only), and/or supplement per your doctor's instructions. If you don't have access to testing, a safe dose of vitamin D to maintain current levels is 2,000 IU a day.

Advanced Protocol: Endometriosis and Adenomyosis

You'll benefit from the recommendations listed under "Advanced Protocol: Oestrogen Dominance," so please start there. In addition, I suggest the following:

STEP 1: GIVE YOUR IMMUNE SYSTEM A BREAK WITH THE AUTOIMMUNE PROTOCOL

The causes of endometriosis and adenomyosis are yet to be determined, but the two share a number of features, including a dysregulated immune system. The autoimmune protocol (AIP) is a therapeutic diet aimed at restoring proper immune system function. Dr Sarah Ballantyne (thepaleomom.com) and Mickey Trescott (autoimmunewellness .com), two leaders in the AIP community, have excellent resources on their websites for how to follow this diet.

STEP 2: TAKE SUPPLEMENTS TO REDUCE INFLAMMATION AND PAIN

CURCUMIN. Curcumin, the powerful anti-inflammatory antioxidant present in turmeric, a spice with a long history of medicinal use, can really make a big difference for someone with endometriosis. Oestradiol levels in the endometriotic cells are higher than in the regular endometrial tissue lining your uterus. Curcumin has been shown to reduce the oestradiol levels in those cells and subsequently reduce the number and size, and slow the growth, of endometriotic cells.[18] Curcumin is also a major pain reducer for women with endometriosis and adenomyosis. Take the recommended daily dose of curcumin (500 mg to 1,000 mg) with a meal that contains fat, for improved absorption.

N-ACETYL CYSTEINE (NAC). I mention this supplement in Chapter 7; it is the precursor to one of the body's most potent antioxidants, glutathione. NAC has also been shown to support the reduction of endometriotic cysts (endometriosis located on the ovaries) and support fertility in women with endometriosis.[19] Anecdotally, I've seen it improve pain in women with adenomyosis. The recommended dose is 600 mg daily.

FISH OIL. Omega-3 fish oil has some next-level anti-inflammatory powers, and preliminary evidence suggests that it can reduce the size of endometriotic lesions, and reduce pain and inflammation associated with endometriosis.[20] It's also great for period pain not associated with endometriosis and adenomyosis. The recommended dose is 1,000 mg to 2,000 mg a day.

Advanced Protocol: Hypothalamic Amenorrhoea

STEP 1: FOLLOW THE EAT-MORE DIET

Yes, I made that up, but basically, it's the diet you may need to be on if you're experiencing hypothalamic amenorrhoea. So many instances of amenorrhoea or missing periods can be linked to decreased food intake, rapid weight loss, high stress, and increased exercise intensity. So, if you've been diagnosed with HA or suspect you have it based on what I've described in this book, I encourage you to increase your intake of carbs, protein, and fat and, simultaneously, your caloric intake to at least 2,500 calories a day. This might mean fewer salads and a higher intake of more calorie-dense foods, which are necessary for the return of your menstrual cycle. If you've lost your period to the Paleo, keto, or any low-carb diet, this applies to you, too. I highly recommend *No Period. Now What?*, by Dr Nicola Rinaldi, for in-depth information on next steps if you have this condition.

STEP 2: GET TESTED

In some cases of HA that I have seen, underlying gut health issues, such as parasites, SIBO, or other hidden infections, are throwing off thyroid production, cortisol levels, and nutrient absorption. Get your hormones tested with DUTCH (appendix B) and work with a doctor who can order a functional stool test, such as the Comprehensive Stool Analysis or the Comprehensive Stool Analysis with Parasitology, by Doctor's Data, to uncover the hidden stressors keeping your period at bay. (See additional hormone testing recommendations in appendix B.)

STEP 3: DON'T UNDERESTIMATE THE POWER OF MENTAL AND EMOTIONAL STRESS

If you haven't had a period for three months or more, it's time to work with a certified health or life coach to explore unaddressed stress and mind-set issues that may be creating a sense of scarcity in your body. Remember, getting a period and ovulating can happen only when our survival is not in question and our bodies feel safe to perform those functions. Addressing any unresolved trauma and underlying limiting beliefs (beliefs that negatively impact different aspects of your life and create feelings of not-enoughness, fear, dissatisfaction, and resentment), can create huge shifts in your emotional health and bring your period back.

STEP 4: USE SUPPLEMENTS

HIGH-QUALITY MULTIVITAMIN OR PRENATAL VITAMIN. While increasing your calories, supplement with a high-quality multivitamin or pre-natal vitamin to help address any nutrient deficiencies that could be affecting the return of your period.

RHODIOLA. This adaptogen (i.e. a herb that deals with stress) has been used for centuries to combat fatigue and memory loss, increase productivity, and mitigate the general effects of stress.[21] What's even cooler is that rhodiola has been shown to be effective for lack of ovulation and irregular or infrequent periods[22] due to its positive effect on both cortisol output and the thyroid. The recommended dosage is 200 mg *Rhodiola rosea* one to two times a day.

STEP 5: TAPER YOUR EXERCISE

If you have amenorrhoea you should *reduce* high-intensity exercise, including CrossFit, running, and spinning. Your body interprets this exercise as a stressor. Oestrogen at normal levels is a stress buffer, but because your oestrogen levels are low, your body doesn't have the oestrogen reserves to counter the impact of the exercise.[23] When you exercise intensely, you experience a heightened stress response, which makes it harder to bring your period back or regulate your cycle. Instead, try low-intensity exercises such as restorative and yin yoga (no Bikram yoga, please), Pilates, walking, Barre and ballet, tai chi, swimming, and functional movements (exercises that mimic real-life movements) such as lunges, knee-ups, and step-ups.

HARNESS THE POWER OF YOUR CYCLE

In the beginning of 2019, the US women's football team was in its final phase of preparations for the upcoming World Cup in France. At their training facility in Santa Barbara, California, players were put through a rigorous fitness regimen designed by Dawn Scott, the national team's fitness coach. Scott had been the team's fitness coach for nine years in the run-up to the 2019 World Cup, but this year she decided to do something different. In addition to her team of strength coaches and nutritionists, she added a new specialist: "period consultant" Dr Georgie Bruinvels.

Bruinvels, a specialist in optimising the performance of female athletes, had done extensive research into how each phase of the menstrual cycle impacts a woman's athletic performance. By tracking each team member's period, Scott and Bruinvels were able to gain a comprehensive understanding of her cycle and design strategies to maximise her performance during each phase. These strategies included adjustments to the sleeping schedules, diets, lifestyle, and training for each player. "It empowered them to be proactive," said Bruinvels. "There's no evidence that someone can't perform to their best at any time in their cycle if they are proactive about taking steps."

The American team went on to win the 2019 World Cup, with Rose Lavelle scoring the winning goal in the finals. Rose got her period the next day.[1]

As the US team's story illustrates, learning about and embracing your internal cyclical nature is one of the most powerful and effective ways to maximise your true potential in all areas of life. That's right. Our periods don't have to hold us back, even when we assume they will.

We women work hard to stay on top of everything we do, and we expect to have the same energy level every single day of every single month. However, the cyclical nature of our bodies makes that impossible.

Your hormones, particularly oestrogen, progesterone, and testosterone, are meant to ebb and flow throughout the four phases of your menstrual cycle. As it cycles through the bleeding, follicular, ovulatory, and luteal phases, your body changes nearly every week—heck, sometimes every day. Just as each season brings its own distinct characteristics, such as the cold quiet of winter or the light-filled fecundity of spring, the hormonal shifts occurring in each phase of your cycle create different physical responses and emotions.

The hormonal changes occurring on an almost weekly basis throughout your cycle impact:

- your mood (whether you feel happy, sad, anxious, or calm);
- your sleeping habits;
- how you react to situations and people;
- the decisions you make;
- how social or introverted you are;
- your motivation and energy level;
- the nutrients you need most;
- the type of exercise that will best support you; and
- your libido.

When Dawn Scott and Dr Bruinvels embarked on their plan to optimise their players' training based on their cycles, before they could do anything, they first needed to understand the symptoms each player was exhibiting during each phase. Same goes for you. By recognising these changes and living in sync with them, you can ensure that you're always performing at your best. Remember, there is no one-size-fits-all approach to this. It's your own unique cycle, and you will need to learn to observe it, understand it, and work with it.

Working against your natural cycle results in frustration and burnout. Once you start to tune in to the nuances of the four phases of your cycle, begin noticing your body's messages, and work with your innate female wisdom, you'll see profound shifts in your health and life. For example, during your cycle's less active phases, you'll know to honour your body's need for rest and relaxation. During your cycle's more active phases, you can take advantage of your increased energy to get more done.

To do this, begin to pay attention to your symptoms during each phase—how you feel physically and emotionally. Notice what feels off or not right. For a refresher on these symptoms, refer back to "Basic Cycle Tracking" at the end of Chapter 1. Add these symptoms to your paper chart or your period-tracking app. Next, start implementing some of the suggested ways to take advantage of the natural tendencies and changes associated with each phase of your cycle outlined in this chapter. Over the coming weeks and months, pay attention to whether adjustments to your diet, exercise routine, social calendar, and work engagements improve or even resolve your symptoms.

THE MAGIC OF THE MOON

According to astrologer Jennifer Racioppi, "The menstrual cycle and the moon cycle are exact mirrors of each other." The four phases of the moon's approximately 29-day cycle (new, waxing, full, and waning) synchronise perfectly with our four biological phases (bleeding, follicular, ovulatory, luteal). It's as if the cycle of the moon were meant for us! Hey, a girl can hope, right?

Aligning with the Moon's Phases

If you have hypothalamic amenorrhoea or you don't have a period for whatever reason (you're pregnant, breastfeeding, in perimenopause, or in menopause or have had a hysterectomy), harnessing these external moon phases will help you recreate the phases you have lost if your period is missing in action. Living in accordance with the moon cycles will provide a framework for you to live as if you're still cycling menstrually. In my experience with clients, this practice may even encourage your period to return if you have hypothalamic or post-birth control amenorrhoea. Similarly, if you have an extremely irregular cycle (e.g. you get a period every two to three months), aligning your energetic patterns with the phases of the moon during the times you don't have a period can be very helpful.

HERE'S HOW

Add the moon cycles to your calendar—Google Calendar allows you to do this—download a moon calendar app, or purchase a paper moon calendar, so you know when the different phases of the moon occur.

Each moon phase indicates the start of a new biological phase and a new set of lifestyle guidelines to follow for that phase. Start day 1 of the "cycle" on the day of the new moon, which is the beginning of the moon cycle. The "follicular" phase would be the waxing phase between the new moon and full moon. "Ovulation" would be at the full moon, and then the "luteal" phase would be the waning phase or the time in between the full moon and new moon. Even though your period is absent, act as if you are in each phase by following the same guidelines for food, self-care, and activities as outlined for the four phases of a regular cycle. At the next new moon, start the process over again.

Phase 1: The Bleeding Phase (Menstruation)—
Winter and New Moon

THEMES: rest and relaxation, quiet time, shedding, trust, intuition

This phase is characterised by a decline in oestrogen and pro-gesterone, so it's little wonder that many women feel fatigued, with-drawn, and introspective and want to rest or retreat. I've found that all those disruptive symptoms such as bloating, cramping, lower-back pain, and headaches or migraines are often a message from your body to slow down or just stop. This is a time to focus on nurturing yourself.

MAKE THIS PHASE WORK FOR YOU

Food

Your focus during this phase should be on replacing the minerals (especially iron) you lose while bleeding, decreasing inflammation—menstruation is an inflammatory process—and supporting your energy levels by getting plenty of B_{12}. Red meat, salmon, sardines, and bone broth with added spring onions, seaweed, and mushrooms will replenish iron, zinc, and other minerals. Antioxidant-rich fruits and veggies such as berries and leafy greens will quench inflammation, and don't forget those vitamin C–rich foods to help absorb iron.

Comforting chillis, soups, stews, or stir-fries containing warming spices such as turmeric, cayenne, and cinnamon make for great meals during this phase, as they help to reduce inflammation and encourage blood flow. Hydration is also crucial during this phase, particularly if you struggle with diarrhoea, so I recommend you ramp up your intake of cucumbers, celery, watermelon, cantaloupe, and other water-rich foods. Tempting though a sugar fix may be, avoid it to keep your moods stable and to diminish inflammation; the same goes for cold smoothies and ice water, as they may intensify cramps.

Lifestyle and Career

This is the winter season, so it's time to slooowww down. Your period's arrival is your body's way of forcing you to relax—although plenty of us don't get the memo. After all, we've been programmed to believe we have to have the same energy level all month long and that we can be everything to everyone while we're at it. Not so. During this phase, hit the Pause button.

Clear your calendar of big social events, dating, and work activities. Instead, support your emotional well-being by spending some quality "me" time: binge on Netflix, attend to a hobby or other activity you enjoy, write in your journal. Focus on your needs, including taking note of the things in your life that require your attention along with setting intentions and goals for the month ahead. Retail therapy may seem like a good idea—I know the power that a new lipstick has to distract from period-related aches and fatigue and to lift a mood—but the high it brings is fleeting. Instead, make activities that restore energy a priority.

Exercise

"Gentle" is the name of the game for most of us during this phase. Exercise should be limited to moderate movement and stretching such as yoga, Pilates, and walking, especially if you have period pain and other less-than-desirable period symptoms. Unless you're an athlete who's required to perform during your period, I suggest avoiding extremely strenuous exercise; no CrossFit, boot camps, spinning, or running. If you're an athlete or you work out often, consider focusing on high-intensity interval training (HIIT) and strength training.

Sex

Some women experience low desire at this time, while others want sex because of the increased blood flow to the pelvic region or the slight rise in testosterone that may happen during this phase. Regardless of how you feel, it's A-okay. That being said, physical touch and orgasms trigger the production of oxytocin, the hormone of love and bonding, which also happens to reduce physical pain. Finding a way to be intimate that feels good to you during this phase brings multiple benefits. Penetrative sex isn't the only way to go. You may feel too sensitive down there even to consider it. Instead, get an oxytocin boost from gentle touching and other signs of affection, like a little make-out session.

If penetrative sex is on the agenda, keep in mind that blood is not the greatest lubricant. Use lots of lube to avoid sex that feels uncomfortable or hurts. Menstrual blood raises the pH in the vagina, making it more alkaline and less able to ward off bacterial overgrowth. Coupled with decreased oestrogen during this time, the likelihood of vaginal infections *increases*, so your partner might want to ejaculate outside your vagina.[2]

Phase 2: The Follicular Phase—Spring and Waxing Moon

THEMES: renewal, creativity, and new beginnings and connections

This is the non-bleeding part of your follicular phase, when your body starts the fertility process all over again. Oestrogen and testosterone levels start to rise, boosting your energy, mood, and brain skills. Rising oestrogen makes you feel more extroverted and suppresses your appetite. More oestrogen also means more dopamine and serotonin, those lovely feel-good neurotransmitters, while testosterone stokes your libido. You'll start to feel more confident, outgoing, and willing to take more risks. You're gonna start feeling like a whole new woman who can take on the world—so, get to it! Start new projects, take on a new challenge, embrace a new relationship. Self-care during this phase will focus on providing all the nutrients and emotional support you need to keep your energy levels high and your mood upbeat.

MAKE THIS PHASE WORK FOR YOU

Food

Your appetite and nutrient needs will likely fluctuate during this phase. Higher oestrogen levels mean increased sensitivity to insulin, and because oestrogen also regulates the hunger and satiety mechanisms (leptin sensitivity) in the brain, your appetite may decrease or you may notice that you feel fuller on less food. In the first part of this phase until about a few days before ovulation, you might find you crave lower-carb meals. Eat light, fresh, vibrantly coloured foods such as salads with a base of greens such as rocket and baby kale, lean protein, and a variety of veggies and other healthy toppings. Increase healthy fats such as avocado, olive oil, butter, nuts, and seeds (in particular pumpkin and flax) to support oestrogen production.

As you approach ovulation, you'll notice your appetite increasing. Time to up your carb intake; the mere act of ovulation requires a lot of energy. Complex carbs such as gluten-free whole grains, sweet and regular potatoes, and squashes are excellent choices that support ovulation. To prevent ovulatory bloating, add more microbiome-friendly foods to your plate, such as sauerkraut, kimchi, and coconut kefir.

Lifestyle and Career

The follicular phase of the cycle correlates with spring. This is a time for renewal, for beginning new things and making social connections. Brainstorming, problem solving, and creativity will be major strengths during this phase, so initiate new projects, make big decisions, and take on mentally challenging assignments. With clear thoughts and soaring social skills, make your voice heard by speaking up in meetings and taking charge on projects. Put yourself out there and engage with others. Join a new social or networking group and schedule time with friends. You're flying high in this phase, but make sure not to overdo it by saying yes to everything, or you'll burn yourself out. Be your bold self in ways that support your long-term health and goals.

Exercise

Now is a good time to try a new workout or a different type of exercise, especially something more demanding. Your energy and strength will rise to peak levels because of increasing oestrogen and testosterone, so push yourself with more challenging workouts or physical activities, especially as you get closer to ovulation. Research shows that muscle is built faster and repairs better in this phase, so if you're strength-training, prioritise anaerobic exercises (short exertion, high intensity) such as weight training and high-intensity interval training (HIIT) workouts.[3]

Sex

You guessed it: this phase is a great time to try new positions, toys, and locations. Earlier in the follicular phase might be a drier time of the month, especially right after your period. So, make time for fore-play and use lots of lube, if necessary.

Phase 3: The Ovulatory Phase—Summer and Full Moon

THEMES: fertility, energy, irresistibility, seduction

Ovulation is the culmination of all the hard work your body has been doing over the last couple of weeks. This is the shortest phase of your cycle, but it is the most action-packed because of all the hormonal activity happening. You'll look more attractive and feel more confident (thanks, oestrogen!), so it will be easier to verbalise your thoughts and feelings. Plus, your sex drive will be at its peak![4]

A lot of oestrogen also means a lot of dopamine. More of this feel-good neurotransmitter can improve your focus, concentration, and motivation, making goals easier to achieve. For women who tend to have more dopamine roaming around their bodies, ovulation can push them into the dopamine red zone. Yup, too much of a good thing may make you irritable, snappy, and quick to anger.[5] So, if you experience these feelings at ovulation, now you know why. Overall, though, you are in full-on Superwoman mode, with your energy cranking even higher than in the follicular phase. To get the most out of this phase, you'll want nutrient-dense, power-packed foods, lots of physical activity (including sex), and opportunities to use your brainpower.

MAKE THIS PHASE WORK FOR YOU

Food

Your ovaries have been running a marathon, and during this phase you'll want to give them the sustenance they need to cross the finish line. Eat those carbs (sweet potatoes, rice, quinoa, and starchy vegetables) and heartier breakfasts (free-range eggs, veggies, and avocado) to give your body the energy it needs to ovulate. Rich in vitamins and nutrients, bone broth is an ideal food during this phase (but remember, if you have histamine problems, bone broth might not be a good idea).

Oestrogen peaks during this phase, so you'll want to support phases one and two of your liver's oestrogen detoxification (see Chapter 7) with one to two servings a day of steamed or sautéed cruciferous veggies such as broccoli, cauliflower, cabbage, and kale.

Lifestyle and Career

In the summer phase of the cycle, you're saying yes to all the BBQs and beach invites because life is so damn good. Oestrogen affects the hippocampus, where you store memories, so you are much better at recalling important information at this time of the month.[6] Now is the time for job interviews, public speaking, trivia night, and winning arguments (haha). You will feel most charismatic and energetic at this time of the month, with lots of motivation to get things done—thanks, testosterone—so, I highly recommend scheduling bigger tasks or anything that will require a lot of energy and output.

You'll also find it easy to verbalize your thoughts and feelings during this phase, and you're more receptive to others' opinions and feelings.[7] Use these heightened social skills to connect with your friends, family, and community. Now is the time to ask for a rise, go to networking events, and have important business or personal conversations. This is even a good time to say yes to those appointments you've put off. Your pain threshold is at its highest when oestrogen is high, so consider making your dental, gynaecology, or waxing appointments during your ovulatory phase.[8]

Exercise

Keep enjoying lots of physical activity and high-impact workouts, such as max weight lifting, running, plyometrics (jump training), and spinning. Caveat: when oestrogen peaks, you're at a higher risk for an anterior cruciate ligament (ACL) injury, as oestrogen increases joint laxity.[9] So, be sure to warm up properly if you're playing sports where you might be making sharp direction changes, as in football or netball, or hockey, and use a foam roller afterwards to decrease muscle tightness and reduce risk of injury.

And remember, if you have amenorrhoea or extremely irregular periods, you should *reduce* high-intensity exercise. Stick to low-intensity options until you get your period back and it arrives consistently for at least three months in a row.

Sex

You are naturally very lubricated at this time, and your sex drive is often the highest it will be in your cycle, so you may find yourself wanting more passionate and intense sex during this phase, without needing as much foreplay. Own it!

Phase 4: The Luteal Phase—Autumn and Waning Moon

THEMES: slowness, sensitivity, self-care, attention to detail

The first 2 to 3 days of this phase will feel a lot like the ovulatory phase. This changes when oestrogen and testosterone decline and your body starts producing progesterone, a natural sleep aid and anti-anxiety hormone. You'll either notice a subtle energy shift similar to the one that happens when summer turns to autumn: you'll feel quieter, more withdrawn, and less social and find yourself buckling down; or, if you're sensitive to that post-ovulation oestrogen drop, you'll feel like you've crashed into autumn. Like, "Where did all those positive summer vibes go?"

In the second half of the luteal phase, you might feel PMS symptoms—cravings for carbohydrate-heavy comfort foods, anxiety and moodiness, or PMDD symptoms. These symptoms are not all in your head, but they aren't something you should suffer through, either. After the go-go days of the follicular and ovulatory phases, during this phase it's time to turn your focus to rest, recovery, and restorative self-care.

MAKE THIS PHASE WORK FOR YOU

Food

Progesterone dominates in this phase, and it brings with it a higher chance of blood sugar crashes. As described in Chapter 5, our bodies are more prone to blood sugar and insulin imbalances in the second half of our cycle, and these can worsen PMS or PMDD symptoms. For that reason, you'll want to stick to higher-protein, higher-fat, lower-carbohydrate meals to avoid blood sugar spikes and crashes. Roasted veggies such as sweet potatoes, carrots, beetroot, parsnips, turnips, and onions (for fibre and complex carbs) will support your mood and help you avoid caving in to the cravings. Focus on high-protein/high-fat snacks like power balls, avocado wrapped in sliced turkey, nuts, and seeds (particularly sesame and sunflower seeds).

To satisfy cravings for chocolate, go for super dark (70 per cent cacao or above). High in antioxidants and rich in magnesium, this is a much better option than sugar-filled milk chocolate.

Lifestyle and Career

Now we're in the autumn phase of the cycle. Summer is over, and you begin easing back into a routine. As you progress through this phase, think of ways to limit overstimulation. Consider working from home, if that's an option, or scheduling social events for other times in the month. Progesterone brings focus, rationality, and attention to detail. This makes it a great time for you to do your bookkeeping or close out a project at home or at work.[10] You might also find you have a strong desire during this phase to clean and organise your home and take care of your to-do lists as you prepare for menstruation.

As Dr Christiane Northrup says in her book *Women's Bodies, Women's Wisdom*, "Premenstrually, the veil between the worlds of the seen and unseen is much thinner." This is the time in your cycle when the decks are cleared (you no longer have the happy oestrogen blinders on), and you begin examining what's working and not working in your life. How's your job going? What about your relationship, or even certain friendships? If you find yourself experiencing heightened emotions—flashes of anger, impatience, and irritation with what feels like everything—that you don't necessarily experience in the first half of your cycle, take a minute to reflect on the deeper reasons for your feelings.

Go easy on yourself. If necessary, practise lots of soothing self-indulgence throughout this phase, but especially in the latter part, to counter irritability or that down-in-the-dumps feeling. Get one-on-one time with a close friend, take an extra hour of sleep, meditate each morning, ask your family to help with household chores—anything that helps you feel taken care of.

Exercise

In the first week of the luteal phase, you may want to keep up the strenuous activity you were doing around ovulation. This is a good time to focus on moderate-intensity cardio exercises like dance classes, running, kickboxing, and spin. You might find you have more endurance in this phase, so consider doing longer workout sessions.

As you get closer to your period, tune in to your energy levels and slowly taper down your exercise or include more recovery days, if that's what your body is telling you it needs. Swap out higher-intensity workouts for swimming, hiking, hot yoga, a Barre or Pilates class, or a walk after dinner.

Sex

During this second half of your cycle, oxytocin, the hormone of love and bonding, is lower than in the first half.[11] It falls after ovulation and is very low in the late luteal phase. This makes a lot of women feel they need to be alone and avoid excess stimulation. Sex may not be a priority at this time. Instead, you may prefer lots of hugs and other kinds of intimacy. Or, the desire to spend more time alone may translate into a preference for self-pleasure, instead of engaging with someone else sexually. If you do engage in sex, foreplay is important in this phase because it might take you longer to warm up.

Working with Your Cycle Made Easy

To harness the power of your cycle, look at your calendar and pin-point the first day of your period. This is the kickoff point for everything that is to follow. If you track your cycle using a period-tracking app, then you're already ahead of the game.

Next, I suggest colour-coding each week based on the phase of your cycle. For instance, the first week can be red in honour of your period. The second week can be orange; you're getting your energy back and starting to jump into new things. The third week can be green, to represent the high-energy vibe of the ovulation phase. And the fourth week can be purple, to signify the time when you're winding down. Or choose whatever colours you like.

Finally, start mapping out your month based on your strengths in each phase of your cycle. Add reminder notes about food and lifestyle recommendations so that you can make time for a yin yoga class during your bleeding phase, do some serious networking when you're ovulating, and Marie Kondo your closets in your luteal phase. Over time, making these adjustments will become second nature.

Of course, we can't schedule everything around our cycles. Big meetings, deadlines, important life events, and social activities are going to happen during every phase. But here's where knowledge is power. Now that you know what your hormones are doing and how you'll likely be feeling physically, mentally, and emotionally, you can plan to give yourself the support you'll need to function at your best no matter what phase of your cycle you're in. This may mean allocating extra time to prepare for a presentation when you know your motivation will be low, or doing a high-intensity workout to burn off some energy before buckling down for a long work session. After all, if the US women's football team can do it, so can you! Do what you can to live more in alignment with your cycle and you will reap the benefits.

Mapping your menstrual cycle and aligning your life with its phases allows you to anticipate how you'll feel and, subsequently, make a plan for how best to support your body each month. By paying attention to what you're experiencing during each phase of your cycle—what you most want to eat, your mood, the types of exercise that satisfy you, the intimacy you're craving (or not)—and working with your cycle instead of fighting against it, you'll promote healthy hormone balance and harness your innate lady superpowers so you can slay life.

BETTER BIRTH CONTROL

Your menstrual cycle and your fertility are not mutually exclusive entities. Everything you've been doing as part of the Fix Your Period programme, from balancing your blood sugar to loving your liver and supporting your thyroid, will help improve or even resolve your period problems and support your fertility at the same time.

This is a good thing, I promise. A naturally fertile body is exactly what you've been aiming for throughout this book. And while it's easy to dismiss or even fear improving your fertility, being fertile isn't just about whether you want to become pregnant. When you ovulate on a regular basis, your body produces extremely beneficial hormones that it would otherwise not produce if you were suppressing your cycle on some form of hormonal birth control.

Over these past six weeks, I've empowered you to take ownership of your hormones. Now I want to help you do the same for your birth control. I believe that all women should be taught to partner with their bodies to better understand their fertility, rather than live in perpetual fear and distrust of this fundamental aspect of their health. (Pretty sure you've probably figured that out by now, though!)

Holly Grigg-Spall's groundbreaking book, *Sweetening the Pill*, sounded the alarm and woke us all up to the fact that something was not quite right with the Pill. As she writes, "The choice to take the pill is fiercely protected and yet that choice is rarely autonomous and informed."[1] Like Holly, I fully believe women should be able to choose the birth control they want to use, but that decision should be based on fully informed consent—meaning, a medical doctor should explain *all* the potential benefits and risks and the alternatives. That has not been the case for most women I've worked with over the years. When you are not offered all the birth control options available or are not aware of the risks to your health of each of these options, you are not 100 per cent informed. It's time to change that.

SAY GOOD-BYE TO HORMONAL BIRTH CONTROL

Even though it's been around since 1960, the Pill is still the most popular form of reversible contraception in the United States today, with 16 per cent of all women between the ages of fifteen and forty-four using it, and 25.9 per cent of those currently on some form of contraception using it.[2] It is currently prescribed to 3.5 million British women, 25 per cent of all women between sixteen and forty-nine. But while the Pill is an effective form of birth control, there is a laundry list of potential side effects associated with it, including migraines, lowered sex drive, vaginal dryness, abnormal uterine bleeding and spotting, thyroid dysfunction, blood clots and deep vein thrombosis, nutrient deficiencies and mood swings, anxiety and depression, and the list goes on.[3]

Why is it still so popular, then? Because it fits into the cultural narrative that convenience is everything. Popping a little pill every morning is a pretty easy way to prevent pregnancy, right? This is not dissimilar to our use of blood pressure or cholesterol drugs. It takes a significant amount of work to figure out the underlying cause, and often the treatment requires substantial long-term changes in lifestyle. A pill that will produce the same desired results is therefore much more enticing.

The fact is no woman's body is capable of functioning at its best on the Pill because the synthetic hormones in it disrupt the conversation between the hypothalamus, pituitary, and ovaries, which prevents ovulation. Other hormonal methods work along the same lines, either by stopping ovulation or making implantation of a fertilised egg very difficult or even impossible.

These types of birth control come in the form of combination pills (oestrogen and progestin), progestin-only pills (known as the mini pill), hormonal intrauterine devices (IUDs), implants, injections, skin patches and vaginal rings.

But we simply can't ignore our biology and suppress our natural cycles (sometimes for years on end) without at least a few consequences. There has to be a better way. This is why I do the work I do—because the one-size-fits-all approach does not work for women's biology.

Even though I could have been the poster child for birth control pill side effects, getting off the Pill was no small feat. I was absolutely terrified of no longer having a reliable form of birth control, or the crutch that saved me from my period problems when I was a teenager. It took me a few months to work up the nerve just to stop taking it, but working with my acupuncturist to understand my cycle and address my symptoms holistically helped me make the decision.

When my period finally came back (and came on strong), to my surprise, it was manageable. A period that was no big deal sans birth control? Who would have thought it? But there I was, getting my period after months of acupuncture and diet and lifestyle changes and I was a functioning human who could go to work and live her life. This was a revelation after my multi-year journey involving countless doctors and specialists, endless testing, and multiple unnecessary procedures.

If you're in a similar position, please know that I see you, I hear you, and I totally get it. Even if you're convinced that your hormonal birth control is no longer serving you, and you've spent the last six weeks working through the programme, it can be downright difficult to say sayonara to something you've depended on for pregnancy prevention or symptom reduction. The physiological upheaval that happens when you come off the Pill can be no joke, but by going through the Fix Your Period programme, you'll soften the blow to your body when you do decide to quit it for good.

Ultimately, you're the only one who can decide when it's right to ditch your birth control method for something that won't interfere with your body's natural hormones. I trust that you will know when that time comes.

NON-HORMONAL BIRTH CONTROL 101

You know that feeling you get when you're trying to choose a paint colour at a DIY shop? The total bewilderment as you stare at the 437 different shades of yellow? Most of them would probably work in your bedroom, but each has its own unique yet subtle qualities, making it impossible to choose just one. And when you finally get over that hurdle, you then have to decide on the brand of paint, along with whether you want an eggshell, semigloss, or flat finish. Decisions, decisions. Well, I liken trying to navigate the vast array of birth control options, methods, and brands, and determining which one (if any) is for you, to the task of choosing a paint colour. A daunting mission to say the least.

There's a reason I call this section "Non-hormonal Birth Control 101." While it's not necessary to get a master's degree in this subject, it is important to educate yourself about the various birth control options available, so that you can make an informed decision about which one is right for you.

Regardless of where you are on the birth control spectrum, the non-hormonal options I outline in this chapter vary in their effectiveness. This is by no means a comprehensive list; nor is it a how-to guide to any of these methods. Once you make a decision about the birth control method(s) you'd like to use, and before you rely on any of them for birth control, please make an appointment with your doctor or work with a trained fertility awareness educator. If you're trying to avoid pregnancy, you definitely don't want to take any chances.

"Perfect" Use Versus "Typical" Use

When it comes to birth control, there are two types of effectiveness: perfect use and typical use. Perfect use is when you use the birth control method exactly as indicated by your healthcare provider every time. Typical use means that you don't follow the exact recommendations for how to use that form of birth control. Examples of typical use include skipping pills, putting a condom on incorrectly, or positioning a cervical cap or diaphragm incorrectly or removing it too soon after intercourse. The following sections include pregnancy statistics for both perfect and typical use.

Non-Barrier Methods of Non-hormonal Birth Control

FERTILITY AWARENESS METHOD (FAM), OR NATURAL FAMILY PLANNING (NFP)

No drugs, no devices, and very inexpensive—what more could you want? The fertility awareness method, also known as natural family planning, is a type of birth control method in which you track the signs of fertility to determine your fertile window during each cycle. These signs include:[*]

- your cervical fluid, which changes significantly throughout your cycle;
- your basal body temperature (i.e. your temperature upon waking); and
- your cervical position and firmness, which changes, along with whether it is open or closed, depending on where you are in your cycle.

By the way, this is exactly what you are doing when you track your cycle (see "Advanced Cycle Tracking" in Chapter 1); you just interact with the data differently when using them as a method of birth control.

A number of fertility awareness methods use one or more of the signs of fertility just mentioned, but I recommend the sympto-thermal method, which is most effective and measures all three signs—cervical fluid patterns, cervical position (*sympto*), and basal body temperature (*thermal*)—throughout your cycle to determine your fertile window. Tracking these signs and symptoms gives you an accurate indication of your fertility status and facilitates the informed decisions you need to make about how to avoid pregnancy.

Believe it or not, you're fertile for only 6 days per cycle. This is because ovulation happens on a single day of your cycle, while sperm can survive in your body for up to 5 days during your fertile window.[5] For clarity, once you ovulate, your egg survives for a maximum of twenty-four hours. You may release more than one egg within that twenty-four-hour window (which could produce fraternal twins if you were to get pregnant), but once you ovulate, a series of hormonal changes—progesterone rises and suppresses LH from surging again—prevents ovulation from happening again for the rest of your cycle. In other words, outside that window it is physically impossible to ovulate again in your cycle.

All fertility awareness methods add an additional buffer period to allow you to confirm ovulation and ensure that your fertile window has ended, which is why your fertile window can be longer than 6 days, depending on the method you use. Once you identify the days on which you're fertile, either abstain from intercourse or use a barrier method to prevent pregnancy. After you confirm that ovulation has occurred, you can have unprotected sex without risk of pregnancy for the rest of your cycle. However, just like the Pill, this method does not protect against STIs, so a barrier method is advised.

ARE FAM AND NFP THE SAME?

Although the terms *fertility awareness method* and *natural family planning* are often used interchangeably, there are historical differences between the two. Natural family planning is often associated with religion. In fact, it is the only method of family planning approved by the Roman Catholic Church and other religious institutions because it encourages abstaining from intercourse during fertile days to avoid pregnancy. The fertility awareness method has no ties with religious institutions. FAM users can freely use barrier methods on fertile days if they decide to do so, or engage in non-penetrative sex or outercourse.

FAM is by far the healthiest of all the birth control options because it allows you to be in control of your fertility, which can be hugely empowering. All it requires is a basal thermometer and a fertility-tracking app (more on those later in the chapter) or paper chart to record your cycle information. While there is information in this book on how to track your cycle (see "Advanced Cycle Tracking" in Chapter 1 on page 26), I always recommend seeking the help of a trained fertility awareness educator to fully understand and use the method effectively. Please keep in mind that you must use a backup form of birth control until you feel comfortable and confident using FAM as your main birth control method.

Effectiveness

Of 100 couples who use the sympto-thermal method correctly for one year, 0.4 (fewer than 1) will have a pregnancy. That is a 99.6 per cent effectiveness rate with perfect use, making the sympto-thermal fertility awareness method just as effective as all hormonal birth control methods.[6] With typical use, however (see "'Perfect' Use Versus 'Typical' Use" on page 263), the number drops down to 1.8, meaning that fewer than 2 out of every 100 couples will have a pregnancy.[7]

What Else You Should Know

The most common question I get is "Isn't this just the rhythm method?" No. The rhythm, or calendar, method is an outdated and ineffective form of birth control based entirely on determining your fertile window from previous menstrual cycles. Even if your cycles are pretty regular and predictable, at some point there will be an early or late ovulation, which can throw off your fertile window and end in an accidental pregnancy. A quick search online brings up many reputable sites that use *FAM/NFP* and *the rhythm method* interchangeably. It is unfortunate that FAM is often lumped together with the rhythm method because it scares women away from learning what I believe to be the most important information they'll ever learn about their bodies.

The sympto-thermal method is effective because you are measuring your own fertility signs and symptoms every day, and determining the exact days you're fertile every single cycle. During the "you could get pregnant" window, you can either avoid sex or use a barrier method or the withdrawal method.

Added bonus: the sympto-thermal method of FAM can indicate other issues as well. Taking your basal temperature can help detect an underactive thyroid (see the Chapter 9 protocol on page 219) and can tell you whether you're ovulating; if your luteal phase is too short; and if your follicular phase is too short or too long. Charting your cervical fluid can help you become aware of abnormalities that may occur due to yeast or bacterial infections or sexually transmitted infections (STIs). I mean, look at all the bonuses that come with this method of birth control.

NATURAL CYCLES APP

Birth control has gone digital. This form of birth control is similar to FAM in that it uses your basal body temperature. Developed by Elina Berglund, a former physicist who wanted to create a birth control option that didn't have side effects, Natural Cycles was the first app ever to be approved for contraception. (It was approved for use in the European Union in 2017 and shortly thereafter in the United States by the FDA.)

You simply take your basal temperature each morning, using either the thermometer included in your Natural Cycles yearly subscription or one you purchase on your own, and input it into the app. Using an algorithm based on the cycles of more than fifteen thousand women, the app takes your data and tells you whether you are fertile: a red signal in the app means you are potentially fertile and need to abstain or use protection, while a green signal in the app means you are infertile on that day and can have unprotected sex.

Effectiveness
Natural Cycles boasts a 98 per cent effectiveness rate with perfect use, and a 93 per cent effectiveness rate with typical use (see "'Perfect' Use Versus 'Typical' Use" on page 263).

What Else You Should Know
Similar to practising FAM, Natural Cycles tells you only when you are fertile or infertile. For it to be effective during your fertile window, abstain from intercourse (penis-in-vagina sex), try alternatives such as oral sex, or use another form of birth control such as withdrawal or a barrier method.

It's important to remember to take your temperature every morning at roughly the same time, so the app can learn your unique cycle and you can achieve more "green" days.

WITHDRAWAL METHOD
The withdrawal method, or coitus interruptus, is more commonly known as the "pull-out method" or "pull and pray" (haha). This method is simply the penis being withdrawn from the vagina before ejaculation occurs. This means that your male partner must know when to withdraw so that ejaculation happens outside the vagina. Most women I talk to are terrified of this method, while others tell me it's the only one they use. Whether you choose to use this method has a lot to do with your partner's ability to pull out in time and how risk averse you are when it comes to potentially getting pregnant.

Effectiveness

The withdrawal method can be surprisingly effective. I know, shocking, right? But it's true: when used correctly, it can be up to 96 per cent effective. However, if it is used incorrectly, it is only 78 per cent effective.[8] In order to practise the withdrawal method properly, the man must pull out before ejaculation. If you both decide to go for round two, he must use a barrier method or thoroughly wash his hands and penis and urinate to clear any remaining sperm from his urethra.

What Else You Should Know

While some evidence suggests that pre-ejaculate secretions do not contain live sperm[9], there are studies that have found sperm in the pre-ejaculate fluid in a minority of their participants, which means that sperm seem to be able to get into the pre-ejaculate fluid of some men.[10] Since the research doesn't give us a definitive answer, it would be wise to use this method with caution.

COPPER T IUD (INTRAUTERINE DEVICE), AKA THE COPPER IUD

An IUD is a small T-shaped device that your gynaecologist inserts into your uterus through the cervix. (Once it's been inserted, you shouldn't feel it.) At the base of the IUD is a nylon string that hangs down through the cervix so that when it comes time to remove the IUD, your doctor can pull it out. This IUD does not contain synthetic hormones. Instead, it releases copper ions, which create an inflammatory response that impairs sperm motility, thus preventing egg fertilisation.[11] This inflammatory response in the uterus can also impair implantation. This means that sometimes the copper IUD is effective post-fertilisation, and this is why it can be used as emergency contraception after unprotected sex, to prevent implantation of a fertilised egg.

Effectiveness

The copper IUD is 99.2 per cent effective for up to ten years.[12]

What Else You Should Know

IUDs are a long-lasting and very effective form of birth control and, on the whole, have some of the highest satisfaction and continuation rates among users. However, there can be quite a few side effects, both while you have it in and after it is removed.

A significant number of women have reported tremendously long and painful periods along with very heavy bleeding when using the copper IUD. If you already have painful and/or heavy periods, this might not be the best form of birth control for you.

There is also an increased chance of bacterial vaginosis because of the disruption of the vaginal microbiome, and a slightly increased risk of pelvic inflammatory disease.[13]

I've received reports anecdotally of copper excess or copper toxicity symptoms in women using the copper IUD, including heart palpitations, panic attacks, anxiety, depressive episodes, and even suicidal thoughts. If you have an allergy to copper or a condition such as Wilson's disease (in which the body doesn't effectively eliminate copper), then you should not use the copper IUD. On the other hand, I have worked with many women who don't experience side effects at all and are extremely happy with their copper IUD.

TUBAL LIGATION

Tubal ligation is a surgical procedure that permanently closes or blocks the fallopian tubes. When the fallopian tubes are blocked, sperm can't meet an egg and cause a pregnancy. This procedure may also be referred to as "getting your tubes tied" or "female sterilisation."

Effectiveness

Tubal ligation is more than 99 per cent effective at preventing pregnancy due to its being permanent.[14] Fewer than one out of a hundred women who are sterilised will get pregnant each year. After you've had this procedure, and once your doctor gives you the green light, it is safe for you to have sex without any other form of birth control.

What Else You Should Know

Tubal ligation is considered a permanent form of birth control, so you must be absolutely certain that it's right for you. If you later decide you want to get pregnant, IVF (in vitro fertilisation) will be your best option, but there are no guarantees.

Studies have found that tubal ligation does not affect the structure of ovarian tissue, and thus, ovarian function. However, evidence suggests that women who've had their tubes tied experience menstrual irregularities such as heavier periods, more period pain, and more frequent periods.[15]

VASECTOMY

A vasectomy is a relatively simple procedure undergone by men, most often performed by a urologist, in which the small tubes in the scrotum that carry sperm are cut or blocked off so sperm can't leave the body. This procedure is very quick, and the patient can go home the same day.

Effectiveness

A vasectomy is considered permanent. It is very effective at preventing pregnancy, with a failure rate of less than 1 per cent.[16] It is not considered effective right after surgery, and a backup form of birth control should be used until a doctor has confirmed it is safe to have unprotected sex. This is a far less invasive procedure than tubal ligation, which means there is a lower risk of infection and other complications, and it generally takes less time to heal from the procedure.[17]

What Else You Should Know

Vasectomies don't change how ejaculating feels. Semen will still look and feel the same after the procedure. It just won't contain sperm or be able to get you pregnant. In my opinion, vasectomy is a pretty underused method of birth control, with three times as many couples in the United States, for instance, choosing tubal ligation over vasectomy.[18]

Barrier Methods of Nonhormonal Birth Control

MALE CONDOM

Ah, condoms, the old faithful birth control method. In case you weren't paying attention in Sex Ed, a condom is a thin sheath made of latex, polyurethane, animal membrane, silicone, or other material that is placed over the erect penis right before intercourse.

Effectiveness

When used correctly, condoms are 98 per cent effective, but that figure drops significantly, to 82 per cent, if the condom is used incorrectly.[19] This includes putting it on or removing it incorrectly or using oil-based lubricants such as coconut oil and petroleum jelly, which cause condoms to break. Don't believe me? Take a condom out of the wrapper and rub some coconut oil on it for a few minutes. It will disintegrate right before your eyes.

What Else You Should Know

When choosing condoms, look for brands that don't contain spermicide. As you know from Chapter 7, you don't want harsh chemicals up in your business. This goes for nonoxynol-9 and other spermicides that can cause an array of symptoms such as vaginal irritation and disruption of the vaginal microbiome (which can lead to vaginal infections).

Ensure that your partner is wearing the appropriate-sized condom. This will provide even more insurance during sex and no worries of it sliding off or breaking. (Check out luckybloke.com for an easy guide to getting the right condom fit.)

DIAPHRAGM

A diaphragm is a silicone dome that you place over the cervix before sex. It works by physically blocking sperm from entering the uterus, in combination with the spermicide you apply before inserting it, to catch any sperm that might escape around the edge of the diaphragm. Every time I think of diaphragms, I am reminded of the *Sex and the*

City episode in which Carrie needs Samantha's help to retrieve her stuck diaphragm. (It was 1999, and diaphragms were still popular back then.) Most young women today have no idea how a diaphragm works, much less where to get one. Diaphragm use has dropped precipitously in the last three decades, replaced by other, easier methods such as the IUD and implant.

Effectiveness

Diaphragms are not the most effective type of birth control. If used correctly, a diaphragm prevents pregnancy 94 per cent of the time; with typical use, that figure drops to 88 per cent.[20] A diaphragm should always be used with spermicide and can also be used with a condom or the withdrawal method to increase effectiveness. I recommend the non-toxic spermicide ContraGel.

What Else You Should Know

While the diaphragm is inexpensive and has no adverse effects on your health, it does need to be fitted by a doctor, or a sexual health practitioner, can be difficult to insert, can move around during sex, and must be used with spermicide to achieve maximum effectiveness. Also, it can't be used during your period; it has to be inserted anywhere from two hours to right before the fun begins, which is kind of a mood killer; and it has to stay put for eight hours after sex. There is also an increased risk of toxic shock syndrome with this method of birth control.

There is a relatively new diaphragm kid on the block called Caya. It is anatomically designed to fit most women and does not require a pelvic exam or fitting, as with the traditional diaphragms.

CERVICAL CAP

The cervical cap is basically the diaphragm's little sister. It is smaller, made of silicone, and like the diaphragm, it slips into place over the cervix and must also be used with spermicide. It comes in three sizes and must be prescribed and fitted by a doctor, or a sexual healthcare professional.

Effectiveness

The cap prevents pregnancy 92 per cent of the time with typical use, but with perfect use, it is up to 98 per cent effective.[21]

What Else You Should Know

You'll need to use spermicide with a cervical cap for it to be most effective. If you're allergic to silicone, consider another method. As with the diaphragm, there is an increased risk of toxic shock syndrome.

BIRTH CONTROL SPONGE

This birth control option is made of plastic foam and contains spermicide. Like the diaphragm and cervical cap, it is inserted into the vagina before sex, where it physically blocks the cervix while the spermicide kills the sperm. It's sold at pharmacies and online and is intended for one-time use only.

Effectiveness

With perfect use, the sponge has a 91 per cent effectiveness rate in women who have never given birth; women who don't use it as directed experience 88 per cent efficacy. This drops significantly for women who have given birth: to 80 per cent for those who use it correctly and 76 per cent for those who don't.[22]

What Else You Should Know

It can be inserted up to twenty-four hours before sex. If the sponge is left in for longer than twenty-four hours, there is an increased risk of toxic shock syndrome and yeast infections. Also, you may experience vaginal irritation from the spermicide.

FERTILITY TRACKING DEVICES AND APPS

Femtech is the term used to describe technologies aimed at managing and improving all areas of female health. From periods and pelvic floors, to fertility and pregnancy, there is no shortage of innovative products that are changing the way women manage their health and lives. As a bit of a women's health tech junkie, I've tried dozens of apps and devices and can't get enough of all the innovation happening in this space.

To say that women's health has been ignored for most of history is an understatement. I mean, including women in clinical trials for new medical treatments wasn't even required in the United States until 1993.[23] Innovation in the birth control arena has been stagnant since 1960, when the Pill came on the market, and then there was that time when Apple forgot to include period tracking in its revamped HealthKit app in 2014.

All this is to say that I am more than thrilled to see the emergence of so much innovation in the women's health space in such a short span of time. Period- and fertility-tracking apps and devices, period underwear, smart sex toys, pregnancy-tracking apps, and tampon delivery services are just a few of what you'll find. Like the Pill when it first came to market, this technology gives women more control over their bodies and fertility. However, unlike the Pill, which shuts off our cycles, this technology provides important data and valuable insights into our unique menstrual cycles in a safe, accessible, nonhormonal way.

Depending on your needs, I recommend you look into any of these devices, including the Daysy Fertility Monitor, the Ava Fertility Bracelet, iFertracker, the Mira Fertility Tracker, OvuSense, and Tempdrop, all of which are available online. I have used almost all of these but have the most experience with Daysy and Ava.

Daysy Fertility Monitor

A device I have used and loved is the Daysy Fertility Monitor. While this device is not labelled as a contraceptive method, I (and many of my clients) have used it for that purpose with great success. When you take your basal body temperature each morning, the Daysy device uses an algorithm based on the menstrual cycles of more than five hundred thousand users to determine whether you are fertile, giving you a green light if you're infertile, a red light if you're fertile, and a yellow light for caution days or for when it is still learning your cycle. Daysy also comes with an app, which you can wirelessly sync to the device to see your data via the calendar and temperature chart.[24]

Ava Fertility Bracelet

Another device I've used, and can highly recommend, is the Ava Fertility Bracelet, which I've christened the Fitbit for your menstrual cycle and fertility. You wear it around your wrist while you sleep, and it measures your body temperature, breathing rate, and heart rate variability, among other parameters. All these measurements, which change depending on which menstrual cycle phase you're in (follicular or luteal), can help Ava predict your fertile phase in each cycle. Each time you sync to the Ava app, you'll get a notification about how fertile you are that day.[25]

And there you have it! There are probably more options for nonhormonal birth control than you may have realised. And with femtech, there is more innovation in the birth control space now than in the past twenty-five years. This will lead to even more birth control and fertility tracking solutions in the future.

Conclusion

PERIOD POWER

How does it feel to be in the driver's seat, getting more and more familiar with your body, expanding your period literacy each and every day, and playing an active role in solving your period-related issues? Pretty damn good, right? Over the course of the six-week Fix Your Period programme, you've gained some serious ground on your period health journey. Just think about how much you and your body have learned!

You're feeling better than you ever have before and have the know-how to continue to make progress and live in harmony with your cycle. And I'm not just talking about the diet, supplement, and lifestyle recommendations, though those are definitely part of it. No, what I mean is that you are listening to your body and understanding what she's telling you.

And what an incredible body it is! You are an impossible assembly of trillions of cells all working towards one singular goal, to make you your *best* you. Your body is by far the most extraordinary thing in our known universe and now you've gained a greater appreciation for her true majesty and brilliance. Trust her and listen to her and remember that she is always only trying to do what's best for you.

And, speaking of you: there is no other person who has ever existed that is exactly like yourself. Now you know that only *you* are the expert of you and that no matter what anyone says, you do not have to just "deal" with your period-related problems. Not when there are natural, science-backed ways to rescue your hormones and create trouble-free periods.

Fixing your period isn't just one and done, though. It's a long-term commitment, and it's not always easy. The dialogue you have started with your body is a conversation that will continue for the rest of your life. You'll have numerous chats with it about your menstrual cycle, perhaps a conversation or two about having a baby, and you'll talk in depth about perimenopause and menopause when the time comes. Just keep listening. And as you take your next steps I want you to keep in mind:

THERE IS NO SUCH THING AS A PERFECT PERIOD. Continually striving for *the* perfect period will only use up your precious bandwidth and lead to continued frustration with your body. So, aim for *your* perfect period. Define what that looks like to *you* (less cramping, more regularity) and focus on making that happen.

YOU NEED TO DO YOU. Your body is unique, and so is the fix for your period problem. There is no one-size-fits-all solution. This means embracing trial and error and getting comfortable with disappointment. Not every intervention is going to provide the results you're looking for. And what does work for you may not work for your sister or your BFF. Still, now you know there are lots of options available to you. Use this book, my online resources, and the resources suggested in the appendices to help you along. Remember: you are not alone. Besides, it's good to ask for help and support. If you determine you need more specialised treatment, I encourage you to partner with a functional medicine provider who is committed to helping resolve the root cause of your period issues and who can order the right tests and interpret them with you. Hang in there, and be willing to adjust your approach, and you *will* see results.

IT'S OKAY TO MESS UP. Life happens. Your food and self-care aren't always going to be stellar, and that is totally fine. Don't beat yourself up; just practise self-forgiveness and move forwards. Acknowledge where you went wrong and troubleshoot how to prevent it from happening again. After reading this book, you now have a blueprint for what works for you, which means you can alter your course with relative ease. Do you need extra help or support from your family or a friend? An app or tech support to keep it simple? Do your best to figure out the root cause of the problem and try some solutions. You're worth the effort!

IT'S IMPORTANT TO BE ACCOUNTABLE. In a journal, keep track of the changes you're making and the results you experience. Pick a regular daily, weekly, or monthly check-in date and time—based on your menstrual cycle or the moon cycle. How are your symptoms changing? What's working for you? What isn't? What do you need to keep doing or try next? These check-ins aren't a report card, but rather, an opportunity to appreciate the amazing complexity of your body and keep yourself accountable in order to continue making positive changes for your health. Your goal is to continue to cultivate the new habits that support your Fix Your Period mission. You can't achieve your goals without a clear idea of how to go about making them a reality. So, use your journal to remind you of those goals, set new ones, and map out next steps. Remember, you are the designer of your own life.

THINGS CHANGE. Yup, they do. The march of time will impact your hormones and what you need to do to keep feeling your best. So will pregnancy, injury, or any intense lifestyle change. Maintaining hormone balance at age twenty-five will look quite different from how it looks at age forty-five. That's why it's important to listen to your body, pay attention to her signals, and adjust and experiment as needed to keep her happy. If your hormone health seems to be derailing or you've gone off track, use the six-week programme as a reminder to get back to the essentials: a nutrient-dense plate (Chapter 4), balanced blood sugar (Chapter 5), a diverse gut microbiome (Chapter 6), good oestrogen detoxification (Chapter 7), an upgraded HPA axis (Chapter 8), and a healthy thyroid (Chapter 9). The core habits outlined in each week's protocol will have a positive snowball effect.

So, come back to these hormone-friendly habits whenever the need arises to harness your cycle superpowers and thrive. When you know your period, you know your power. Here's to continuing to unleash it!

ACKNOWLEDGEMENTS

I waited to write this until the very end (like an hour before I turned the manuscript in to my editor!), partly because I wanted to make sure I included everyone who was along for the ride, but mostly because finding the words to adequately express my overflowing gratitude for these phenomenal people who helped me throughout this process is, well, basically impossible.

Most important, I want to acknowledge Haden (the Period Guy), for endlessly and many times selflessly supporting me, my business, and all of my dreams. This book would simply not have been possible without you. The fact that you've put up with me over this last year is a testament to the fact that you are the best human I know. Your enduring love, patience, positive attitude, and ability to see the big picture mean more to me than I can convey.

Mom, thank you for your unconditional love and everything you've done for me. The road was long and hard, but we made it! I doubt I would have taken this path were it not for all that we've been through in this lifetime. Dad, I wish more than anything that you were here right now to witness my success. To my sis, Chantal, thank you for your enduring support along the way. What would I do without all your silliness and laughter? To my extended family in Antigua, Guyana, the UK, Trinidad, the United States, and Canada, thank you for cheering me on!

To Arthur, Claudine, Timmy, Nicholas, and Matthew, thank you from the bottom of my heart for letting me hijack your dining table for five weeks straight as I finished this manuscript. Moving out of our apartment at the tail end of this process was not the most brilliant idea, but I am beyond grateful that you opened your home to us! And to the rest of the Ware family, endless thanks for your support and understanding when I was so busy writing and unable to spend as much quality time with you as I would have liked throughout this last year.

For my clients and all the women who are part of the Fix Your Period community all over the world. *You* are the reason I get up every day and do this work. Without you, none of this would be possible. This book is my gift to you and everyone who is still on their healing journey. Special shout-out to my 2019 mastermind and apprenticeship participants. Thanks for your patience with me as I wrote this book and simultaneously led both of these programmes.

I have deep appreciation for the crew of people who helped brainstorm, edit, read, fact check, and cheerlead over the last year. Asking for help is hard, but you all made it easy. Ellie Thomas, you are a queen! Carrie Jones and Angela Heap, y'all are superstars! Heather Pierce, thank you for your yummy recipes! Jessica Drummond, Robin Randisi, Lara Briden, Lisa Hendrickson-Jack, Shawn Tassone, Laura Wershler, Amanda Laird, Holly Grigg-Spall, Adam Kirby, E. M. Grimes-Graeme, Jessica Scheer, Kelsey Knight, Barbara Loomis, Cindy Luquin, and Fiona McCulloch, your contributions were invaluable!

Writing a book is quite a shock to the system. Why didn't anyone tell me? There is no way I could have done this without my "Book Group." Jenny Sansouci and Jenn Racioppi, we are now blood sisters bonded for life after navigating the treacherous seas of being first-time authors together. Here's to birthing our book babies!

This book would not have been possible without my wonderful agent, Wendy Sherman. Thank you for recognising back in 2016 that I needed to write a book (long before I did!) and helping to make it a reality. I have such deep appreciation for your guidance and steadfast support this year. And big thanks to Sheila Oakes for bringing my book proposal to life! A huge thank-you goes out to Hannah

Robinson, my editor at Harper Wave, for seeing the vision and direction from the get-go. You were the best editor a girl could have ever asked for! Massive thanks to Haley Swanson for taking over this project at a critical time, and making the transition seamless. Your support has been invaluable over the last few months. Deep thanks to the rest of the team at Harper Wave, including the publisher, Karen Rinaldi; the marketing and publicity team, Laura Cole, Brian Perrin, and Sophia Lauriello; as well as Nikki Baldauf and Elina Cohen for production and design.

To my talented illustrators, Hannah Coward and Elizabeth Hudy. So grateful for your gifts and your outstanding ability to bring my words to life through imagery.

To the Fix Your Period Team. You kept my business running while I've been writing away for the better part of this year. I truly couldn't have done this without your hard work and dedication. Special thanks to Deirdre, my right-hand lady. And so much appreciation for Emily and everyone else who plays a supporting role in my business.

To all my friends, mentors, and colleagues who are the trailblazers changing the conversation and radically shifting the landscape in women's health and medicine. Dr Christiane Northrup, Dr Sara Gottfried, Dr Aviva Romm, Dr Jessica Drummond, Dr Lara Briden, Dr Carrie Jones, Alexandra Pope, Dr Shawn Tassone, Lisa Hendrickson-Jack, Dr Jolene Brighten, Nat Kringoudis, Dr Kelly Brogan, Kelsey and Emily of the Fifth Vital Sign, Jennifer Weiss Wolf, Sarah Hill, Jennifer Block, Erica Chidi Cohen, Dr Felice Gersh, Marc Sklar, Molly Nichols, Kimberly Johnson, Abby Epstein and Ricki Lake, Caroline Zwickson, Holly Grigg-Spall, Dr Mariza Snyder, Aimee Raupp, Dr Fiona McCulloch, Melissa Ramos, Dr Anna Cabeca, Angelique Panagos, Angela Heap, Charlotte Bulman, and Maisie Hill. I have a huge crush on all of you!

And to my girlfriends. What would this life be without each of you? No doubt, it would suck! Thank you for showing up for me when I needed you the most—for your support, phone calls, texts, pep talks, coaching, tea dates, funny memes, and your ability to talk me off the ledge when I was so sure I couldn't go on. All of it. I am so lucky to have each of you in my life. Shout-out to Jeannine and Molly . . . OMG, I would not have survived this without all your sanity check-ins!

Finally, I want to express my gratitude for the opportunities I've been given in this lifetime. I came to the United States in 2001 from my home country, Antigua, with nothing more than a dream to "make something of myself." With the help of a long list of people over the last eighteen years, I have managed to create a life and business that far exceeds anything I could ever have imagined.

RECIPES

Note: Recipes free of inflammatory foods, and that can be used as part of the gut-healing protocol in week three, are marked with an asterisk (*).

DETOX LEMON ELIXIR

Makes 1 serving

350 to 475 millilitres warm filtered water

Juice of ¼ lemon

Optional add-ins:

1 tablespoon raw apple cider vinegar

Pinch of cinnamon

1 to 2 drops stevia

Add all the ingredients to the water. Stir well and drink immediately.

BREAKFAST

MIX-AND-MATCH FORMULA: BREAKFAST GODDESS BOWL*

Makes 1 serving

75 grams chopped starchy vegetable of your choice: sweet potato, carrots, squash

30 to 60 grams chopped greens of your choice: kale, spring greens, broccoli, chard, spinach

2 organic eggs (replace with turkey or chicken sausages during the Fix Your Period elimination diet)

1/2 small avocado, sliced

1 to 2 tablespoons naturally fermented sauerkraut, or other pickled or "cultured" (fermented) vegetables (optional)

Optional toppings: Extra-virgin olive oil or flaxseed oil, sea salt, freshly ground black pepper, sesame seeds, broccoli sprouts, microgreens, or your favourite spices and condiments

1. Fill a large pan with a few centimetres of water, fit with a steamer basket or steamer pot, and bring to the boil over medium-high heat.

2. Place the starchy vegetables and greens in the steamer basket. Nest eggs (still in shell) on top of the veggies and cover the pan. (If you are using sausages, add to a frying pan and cook until heated through and slightly browned.)

3. Steam vegetables and eggs for 6 to 7 minutes (8 to 9 minutes if you prefer hard yolks), then remove eggs with a slotted spoon, place in a small bowl, and rinse with cool water for 30 seconds. Remove the starchy vegetables and greens from the steamer basket.

4. Assemble your plate with greens, starchy vegetables, avocado slices, and sauerkraut/cultured vegetables if using. Add toppings as desired.

5. Peel the eggs, slice them lengthwise, and place them on the plate.

6. Behold the colourful work of art in front of you before you devour it.

FAVOURITE BREAKFAST GODDESS BOWL COMBOS

- *Broccoli, sweet potato, and pickled beetroot with rocket microgreens*
- *Kale, carrots, and red cabbage sauerkraut with broccoli sprouts*

LOW-SUGAR BERRY SMOOTHIE BOWL*

Makes 1 serving

150 millilitres unsweetened almond milk or any dairy-free milk

50 grams frozen blueberries

35 grams frozen cherries

1 tablespoon flaxseed

1 tablespoon chia seeds

1 tablespoon almond butter

2 scoops collagen protein or 1 serving vanilla protein powder

1 handful spinach

Optional toppings: berries, a small swirl of almond butter, hemp seeds, sunflower seeds, grain-free granola, shredded coconut

1. Place liquid in blender, followed by all the remaining ingredients, and blend until smooth.

2. Serve in a bowl with your favourite toppings.

MIX-AND-MATCH FORMULA: SMOOTHIE*

Makes 1 serving

235 millilitres from "Liquid" list

2 to 3 items from "Bulk and Nutrition" list

1 to 3 items from "Sweetener and Flavour" list

1 to 3 items from "Superfoods" list

LIQUID

Water

Coconut water

Unsweetened almond milk

Coconut milk

BULK AND NUTRITION

125 grams plain non-dairy yoghurt

125 grams pureed pumpkin

1/2 cucumber

3 to 4 stalks kale or spring greens, or 1 handful spinach

1 scoop collagen or 1 scoop protein powder

1/2 avocado

1 to 2 tablespoons natural almond butter

SWEETENER AND FLAVOUR

1/2 banana (frozen is better)

50 grams frozen berries

25 grams frozen mango

1 teaspoon vanilla extract

2-centimetre piece fresh ginger root

1/2 teaspoon ground cinnamon

1/4 teaspoon ground nutmeg

1/2 pear or apple, cored, skin on

Squeeze of fresh lemon juice

SUPERFOODS

2 tablespoons ground flaxseed

2 tablespoons chia seeds

1 small handful microgreens or broccoli sprouts

1 scoop powdered greens

1 tablespoon raw cacao powder

small handful fresh herbs like mint, basil, or coriander

Place liquid in blender, followed by all the remaining ingredients. Blend until smooth and well combined. Add more liquid until the smoothie reaches the desired consistency.

WARM QUINOA BREAKFAST PORRIDGE*

Makes 1 serving

90 grams cooked quinoa or millet

120 millilitres water or almond milk

2 tablespoons raisins

Sprinkle of ground cinnamon

2 tablespoons sunflower seeds

2 tablespoons ground flaxseed

Drizzle of raw honey or maple syrup (optional)

1. Bring the quinoa or millet and water or almond milk to a boil.
2. Lower heat and cook for 5 to 7 minutes, or until creamy.
3. Mix in the raisins, cinnamon, sunflower seeds, and ground flaxseed. Add the raw honey or maple syrup, if desired. Enjoy!

CHICKEN SAUSAGE WITH STIR-FRIED CHARD*

Makes 1 serving

2 to 3 large leaves Swiss chard

1 tablespoon avocado oil

1 shallot, peeled and sliced

Sea salt

1 chicken or turkey sausage, sliced

1. Separate the chard stalks from the leaves. Chop up the stalks. Stack the leaves, roll them up like a cigar, and slice through them to create thin green ribbons.
2. Heat avocado oil in a frying pan over medium heat.
3. Add the shallots and cook for 3 minutes or until soft.
4. Add the chard stalks and a pinch of salt. Cook for 1 minute.
5. Add the chard ribbons, another pinch of salt, and cook for 2 to 3 minutes or until the ribbons become tender to the bite.
6. Move the veggies to the edge of the pan to create a little nest and add the chicken or turkey sausage slices.
7. Cook the sausage slices until they are heated through and slightly browned. Serve with the veggies. For extra protein, use the hot pan to quickly scramble an egg to enjoy on top of your sausage and greens.

COCONUT YOGHURT PARFAIT WITH POMEGRANATE AND PISTACHIOS*

Makes 1 serving

250 grams coconut yoghurt

40 grams pistachios and walnut pieces (or any combination of nuts)

1 tablespoon hemp seeds (or any seeds, e.g. flaxseed or sunflower seeds)

35 grams pomegranate seeds and raspberries (or any berries)

1. Add half of the yoghurt to a bowl or glass.

2. Add a layer of pistachios, walnuts, hemp seeds, pomegranate seeds, and raspberries.

3. Top with the remaining yoghurt.

4. Sprinkle with the remaining nuts, seeds, and berries. Enjoy!

VARIATIONS

- *Sprinkle cinnamon on top.*

- *Substitute the pomegranate and raspberries with blackberries, strawberries, blueberries, or chopped apple.*

- *Add a layer of grain-free granola.*

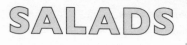

MIX-AND-MATCH FORMULA: SALAD*

Makes 1 serving

30 to 60 grams from "Greens" list

150 grams from "Other Veggies" list

50 grams from "Sweetness" list

2 tablespoons salad dressing (see options under "Dressing")

40 grams from "Richness" list

115 to 170 grams from "Protein" list

GREENS

Rocket

Baby spinach

Mesclun greens

Romaine lettuce

Radicchio

Endive

OTHER VEGGIES

Sweet peppers

Carrots

Cherry tomatoes

Red cabbage

Cucumber

Green beans (cooked)

Roasted red peppers

Marinated artichokes

Roasted beetroot

Roasted root vegetables

SWEETNESS

Raisins

Dried cranberries

Fruit slices

TOASTY/NUTTY FLAVOURS

Toasted nuts

Toasted seeds

DRESSING

Lemon juice and olive oil

Sesame Vinaigrette (see Crunchy Cabbage Salad with Sesame Vinaigrette recipe)

Lemon Dijon (see Kale Salad with Pomegranate or Figs and Lemon Dijon Dressing recipe)

RICHNESS

Avocado slices

Olives

PROTEIN

Chicken

Turkey

Grilled skirt steak

Salmon

Pulses (don't use if you are avoiding them on elimination diet)

Hard-boiled eggs (avoid on elimination diet)

Grilled shrimp (avoid on elimination diet)

Place all ingredients in a bowl and toss with dressing to coat. Enjoy!

KALE SALAD WITH POMEGRANATE OR FIGS AND LEMON DIJON DRESSING*

Makes 2 servings as a main dish, 4 servings as a side dish

1 bunch kale, leaves removed from stems and torn into bite-size pieces

1 tablespoon extra-virgin olive oil

1 tablespoon fresh lemon juice

180 grams cooked and slightly cooled quinoa (optional)

75 grams chopped figs or pomegranate seeds

65 grams pumpkin seeds

110 grams grated carrot

Zest of 1 lemon

FOR THE DRESSING

1 tablespoon Dijon mustard

1 tablespoon fresh lemon juice

2 tablespoons extra-virgin olive oil

1. Add the torn kale to a large bowl and drizzle with olive oil and lemon juice. Massage the kale with your hands until it reduces in size and becomes tender, about 3 to 5 minutes.

2. Add the cooked quinoa (if using), fruit, pumpkin seeds, grated carrot, and lemon zest.

3. Make the dressing: whisk together the mustard, lemon juice, and olive oil.

4. Drizzle the dressing over the salad, toss, and serve. This salad keeps well for up to 2 or 3 days in the fridge.

CRUNCHY CABBAGE SALAD WITH SESAME VINAIGRETTE*

Makes about 4 servings

1 small head savoy cabbage, sliced into thin shreds

1/2 small head red cabbage, sliced into thin shreds

Handful fresh mint, roughly chopped

Handful fresh coriander, roughly chopped

55 grams slivered or sliced almonds, toasted

FOR THE VINAIGRETTE

2 tablespoons extra-virgin olive oil

1 tablespoon toasted sesame oil

1 tablespoon coconut aminos

1 tablespoon brown rice vinegar or fresh lime juice

Toasted sesame seeds (optional)

1. Add the shredded cabbage, mint, coriander, and almonds to a large bowl.

2. Make the vinaigrette: In a small bowl, whisk together the oils, coconut aminos, and vinegar or lime juice until combined.

3. Drizzle dressing over salad and toss to coat.

4. Sprinkle with more almonds and/or sesame seeds and enjoy! Keeps for 3 to 4 days in the fridge.

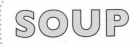

MIX-AND-MATCH FORMULA: SOUP*

Makes about 6 servings

2 tablespoons from the "Fats" list

1 to 3 items from the "Aromatic Veggies" list

150 grams of 1 to 2 items from the "Accent Veggies" list, thinly sliced

600 to 900 grams of any number of items from the "Main Ingredients" list, roughly chopped

Sea salt and freshly ground black pepper, to taste

1 item from the "Liquids" list (amount depends on amount of veggies used)

A sprinkle or dollop of 1 to 3 items from the "Toppings" list

FATS

Butter from grass-fed cows

Avocado oil

Coconut oil

AROMATIC VEGGIES

Minced garlic (3 cloves)

Grated ginger root (2 tbsp)

Sliced leeks (90 g)

Chopped onion (150 g)

Sliced shallots (100 g)

ACCENT VEGGIES

Carrots

Celery

MAIN INGREDIENTS

Asparagus

Broccoli

Cauliflower

Kale

Other root veggies (e.g. parsnips)

Summer squash (courgettes)

Winter squash (butternut)

LIQUIDS

Beef stock

Chicken stock

Vegetable stock

Water

TOPPINGS

Coconut milk

Fresh herbs

Coconut yoghurt

Maple syrup

Spices (curry powder, cinnamon, ginger)

Toasted pumpkin seeds

1. Put the fat in large pan over medium heat.

2. When the fat has melted, add aromatic veggies and cook until they soften, stirring occasionally, about 5 minutes.

3. Add the accent veggies, main ingredients, sea salt, and pepper and stir.

4. Add enough stock or water to cover the vegetables and bring to the boil.

5. Stir, lower the heat to a simmer, and cover until vegetables are tender, 15 to 25 minutes (depending on the water content of the main ingredients and how small you sliced them).

6. Remove pot from heat, puree with a stick blender or add veggies to a blender/food processor using a slotted spoon and blend. Fill blender only three-quarters full and blend in batches if you have to. Warning: DO NOT put the top on a glass blender if the soup is still hot; the glass will explode! Instead, put a dish towel over the top of the blender to let some steam escape and blend veggies on low until smooth. You may need to add liquid from the pot to help it along.

7. Return to pot (if you used the blender/food processor), taste, and adjust the salt and pepper as desired. Add your toppings and any other spices or herbs that tickle your fancy.

CREAMY CARROT SOUP*

Makes 4 to 6 servings

2 tablespoons butter from grass-fed cows or avocado oil

2 shallots or 1 small onion, peeled and sliced

8 to 10 medium-size carrots, peeled and roughly sliced (as they will eventually be pureed)

Sea salt

Freshly ground black pepper

700 millilitres to 1 litre bone broth, low-sodium chicken stock, vegetable stock, or water

Parsley, chopped (optional)

1. Add the butter or avocado oil (if you're completely avoiding dairy) in a large pan over medium heat until the butter melts or the oil is hot. Swirl pan to cover entire bottom with butter or oil.

2. Add the shallots or onions to the pan and cook until soft and slightly brown at some edges, stirring frequently.

3. Add the carrots, a pinch of salt, and a few grinds of fresh pepper. Stir.

4. Add enough stock or water to cover the carrots by 2.5 cm.

5. Turn the heat up to high and bring to the boil.

6. Turn the heat down to a simmer and cover the pan. Cook the carrots for about 15 minutes or until they are tender and easily pierced with a fork. Turn off the heat.

7. Puree the soup: If you have a stick blender, stick it in the pan and blend away until soup is smooth. If you have a traditional blender, use a slotted spoon to transfer the veggies (cooked carrots and shallots or onions) to the blender (fill blender only three-quarters full and blend in batches if you have to). Warning: DO NOT put the top on a glass blender if the soup is still hot; the glass will explode! Instead, put a dish towel over the top of the blender to let some steam escape and blend veggies on low until smooth. You may need to add liquid from the pan to help it along.

8. Return the pureed carrots to the pan, stir, taste, and add more salt if desired.

9. Top with chopped parsley, if desired, and serve. You can also divide the soup into airtight containers (e.g. kilner jars) and store in the fridge for up to a week or in the freezer for up to 3 months. Just make sure you let it completely cool in the fridge before transferring it to the freezer.

CHICKEN SOUP THREE WAYS*

Makes 6 to 8 servings

2 tablespoons butter from grass-fed cows or avocado oil

1 potato (or sweet potato), diced

1 medium onion, diced

2 carrots, diced

2 celery sticks, diced

1 turnip, diced

Sea salt

Freshly ground black pepper

1 400 gram tin chopped tomatoes

2 sprigs thyme

About 1 litre bone broth, chicken stock, or water

1 small head cabbage, shredded

450 grams boneless, skinless chicken breasts or thighs

500 millilitres chicken stock (to cook chicken with)

1. Heat the butter or avocado oil in a large soup pot or enamelled cast-iron pan over medium heat.

2. Add the potato, onion, carrots, celery, turnip, two pinches of sea salt, and pepper, and cook in the butter or oil for about 5 minutes to soften.

3. Add the chopped tomatoes and thyme and cover all the vegetables with the stock or water. Add more liquid if necessary.

4. Bring to the boil, then lower the heat to simmer. Cook until the veggies are tender and easily pierced with a fork.

5. Add the cabbage and another pinch of salt and cook until the cabbage becomes bright green. Remove from heat.

6. In a separate pan, add the chicken and cover with chicken stock. Bring to the boil, then reduce to a simmer and cook for 10 to 15 minutes until the chicken is cooked through.

7. Remove the chicken and shred by hand.

8. Stir the chicken into the cooked soup or keep it in a separate airtight container with a little chicken broth to add to the soup as desired.

VARIATIONS

- *Thai Curry Chicken Soup*

When you add the tinned tomatoes to the soup, add 1 to 2 tablespoons red Thai curry paste and 1 tin of coconut milk.

- *Tortilla Chicken Soup*

When you add the tinned tomatoes to the soup, add 1 tablespoon chopped chipotle peppers in adobo sauce (comes in a jar and can be found in the world foods aisle) and 1 tablespoon chilli powder. When the soup is done, squeeze in the juice of 2 fresh limes.

BONE BROTH*

About 2 to 3 kilograms bones (beef marrow, knuckle bones, meaty rib, neck bones—whatever the butcher will give you)

3 to 4 litres cold water (depends on size of pot)

125 millilitres vinegar (I prefer apple cider vinegar)

2 to 3 onions, coarsely chopped

3 carrots, coarsely chopped

3 celery sticks, coarsely chopped

Several sprigs fresh thyme, tied together

1 teaspoon dried green peppercorns, crushed, or 1 teaspoon black peppercorns

1. Add all the ingredients to a slow cooker or a large stockpot and cook on low for 24 hours.

2. Remove from heat and let the stock cool slightly.

3. Strain all the ingredients with a metal strainer to remove the remaining bones and vegetables.

4. Pour into kilner jars or another airtight container.

5. Chill for 30 to 60 minutes to allow the layer of fat at the top of the broth to solidify. Remove the layer of fat and discard it.

6. Store in fridge for up to 5 days or in the freezer for up to 3 months.

SIDES

PARSNIP FRIES*

Makes 2 to 3 servings

5 medium-sized parsnips

1 to 2 tablespoons grapeseed or coconut oil

Sea salt

1. Preheat the oven to 230°C and line a baking tray with parchment paper.
2. Peel the parsnips, trim off the ends, and discard or compost the peelings. Cut off any skinny parts and set aside. Slice the remaining part of the parsnips in half lengthwise, then again in half lengthwise to create little batons, or "fries."
3. In a large bowl, combine the set-aside pieces of parsnips and the fries and toss with oil and a pinch of sea salt until well coated.
4. Transfer to the baking sheet and roast in the oven for 10 to 15 minutes, tossing once, until slightly browned and tender.
5. Let cool and enjoy!

VARIATION

- *Carrots can be used instead of parsnips*

STIR-FRIED ASPARAGUS WITH CASHEWS*

Makes 4 servings

1 bunch asparagus

1 tablespoon grapeseed or coconut oil

1 tablespoon grated fresh ginger root

75 grams cashews, chopped

2 tablespoons coconut aminos

1 tablespoon toasted sesame oil

1. Remove the ends of the asparagus and cut remaining asparagus into 2.5-cm pieces.

2. Heat the oil in a large frying pan over medium-high heat. Add the ginger and stir-fry for 1 minute.

3. Add the asparagus and stir-fry until crisp and tender, about 4 to 5 minutes.

4. Add chopped cashews, stir in coconut aminos and sesame oil, and serve!

VARIATIONS

- *Replace the cashews with almonds, hazelnuts, walnuts, or pecans.*
- *Replace the asparagus with pak choi or broccoli.*
- *Add diced or shredded chicken to make it a full meal.*
- *Serve over quinoa or rice.*

CRAZY SIMPLE STIR-FRIED GREENS*

Makes 2 servings

5 to 6 large spring green leaves or Swiss chard leaves

1 tablespoon avocado oil

1 shallot, peeled and sliced

Sea salt

1. Separate the spring green or chard leaves from the stalks. Chop up the stalks. Layer the leaves on top of one another, roll them up like a cigar, and slice through them to create thin green ribbons.

2. Heat the avocado oil in a frying pan over medium heat.

3. Add the shallots and cook for 3 minutes until soft.

4. Add the stalks and a pinch of salt and cook for 1 minute.

5. Add the spring greens or chard ribbons and a pinch of salt and cook for 2 to 3 minutes until the greens become tender to the bite, and serve!

MAINS

BUILD-YOUR-OWN GODDESS BOWL*

Makes 1 serving

75 grams roasted root vegetables, quinoa, rice, buckwheat, or millet

30 grams stir-fried, steamed, or raw greens

125 grams protein: leftover chicken, beef burger, steak, fish

Toppings: chopped toasted nuts and seeds, fresh herbs like parsley or coriander, broccoli sprouts, microgreens, avocado slices, lemon juice and olive oil, Sesame Vinaigrette or Lemon Dijon Dressing

Add all the ingredients to a bowl, toss with your favourite dressing, and enjoy! (I love roasted root vegetables, stir-fried spring greens, shredded chicken, avocado, toasted pumpkin seeds, and Lemon Dijon Dressing—but the possibilities are endless.)

CURRIED CHICKEN SALAD WITH CASHEW CREAM MAYO*

Makes 4 servings

FOR THE CASHEW CREAM MAYO

150 grams raw cashews

235 millilitres filtered water

Pinch of salt, plus more to taste

Juice of 1 lemon

1 teaspoon apple cider vinegar

1 teaspoon curry powder

Pinch of sea salt

Freshly ground black pepper, to taste

FOR THE CURRIED CHICKEN SALAD

1 apple, diced

Juice from 1/2 lemon or lime

450 grams leftover cooked chicken breast or thighs

1 celery stick, sliced

25 grams almond slivers, toasted

1 lime, sliced (optional)

Fresh coriander or parsley (optional)

MAKE THE CASHEW CREAM MAYO

1. Soak the cashews in a bowl of water for at least 1 hour. Or soak, covered, in the fridge for up to 24 hours.

2. Drain the soaked cashews and add to a high-speed blender with a fresh cup of filtered water and a pinch of salt. Blend until creamy.

3. Add the lemon juice and vinegar and blend again until combined.

4. Whisk together 125 grams of the mixture with 1 teaspoon curry powder, a pinch of salt, and a few grinds of freshly ground black pepper. Taste and adjust to your liking. (Store extra Cashew Cream Mayo in an airtight container, such as a kilner jar, for up to a week and use as a condiment or dressing.)

MAKE THE CURRIED CHICKEN SALAD

1. In a bowl, combine the apple pieces with the lemon or lime juice to keep them from turning brown.

2. Shred the chicken by hand.

3. Add the shredded chicken, celery, and nuts to the bowl with the apple.

4. Add the Cashew Cream Mayo and mix until well combined.

5. Garnish with an extra squeeze of lime and a sprinkle of coriander or parsley and serve on top of greens or wrapped in a spring greens leaf.

GINGER-LIME COD EN PAPILLOTE*

Makes 1 serving

1 115 grams wild-caught cod fillet

Sea salt

Freshly ground black pepper

1 tablespoon butter from grass-fed cows or ghee

1 teaspoon freshly grated ginger root

1 teaspoon fresh lime zest

Juice from 1/2 fresh lime

1 tablespoon chopped fresh coriander (optional)

1. Preheat oven to 225°C.

2. Cut parchment paper into a 40-cm square. Fold in half to make a crease, then open it again.

3. Place the fish fillet in the middle of one half of the parchment. Season both sides of the fillet with salt and pepper.

4. Place the butter or ghee on top of the fillet and sprinkle it with ginger, lime zest, lime juice, and coriander.

5. Fold over one corner of the crease into a tiny triangle, then continue folding the paper over itself to make little pleats that go all the way around the folded paper, sealing the fish in.

6. Place the packet on a baking tray and bake until the packet puffs up, about 10 to 12 minutes.

7. Open up the packet and serve with your choice of sides!

TURKEY "MOLE" CHILLI WITH BUTTERNUT SQUASH*

Makes 6 to 8 servings

1 tablespoon avocado or grapeseed oil

2 medium-size leeks, rinsed and thinly sliced

2 carrots, grated

900 grams turkey mince

2 teaspoons cumin

2 tablespoons chilli powder

1 tablespoon cacao or cocoa powder (optional, but worth it)

Sea salt, to taste

Freshly ground black pepper, to taste

125 millilitres tomato paste

1 400 gram tin chopped fire-roasted tomatoes

400 millilitres beef stock or water

300 grams chopped butternut squash or 300 grams chopped cauliflower

Garnish options: fresh lime, coriander, avocado, jalapeño

1. Heat oil in a large pan over medium heat.

2. Add the leeks and carrots and cook, stirring frequently, until soft and the leeks are brighter green, about 5 minutes.

3. Add turkey mince and cook, breaking it up with a wooden spoon, until it's just cooked through, about 5 minutes.

4. Add the cumin, chilli powder, cacao or cocoa (if using), a pinch of salt, and a few grinds of pepper. Stir well.

5. Add the tomato paste and stir for 1 minute.

6. Add the chopped tomatoes, beef stock or water, and butternut squash or cauliflower, and bring to the boil.

7. Turn heat down and simmer for 1 to 2 hours to let the flavours develop. The longer it simmers, the deeper the flavours.

8. Remove from the heat and serve over rice or a handful of baby spinach with a squeeze of lime, a sprig of coriander, slices of avocado, and/or jalapeño slices. You can also store the chilli in airtight containers in the fridge for up to 4 days or in the freezer for up to 3 months. Just make sure you let the chilli completely cool before freezing.

VARIATIONS

- *Make it heartier: use beef mince instead of turkey.*
- *Make it spicier: add a teaspoon of cayenne and/or red pepper flakes.*
- *Make it sweeter: add a teaspoon of cinnamon.*

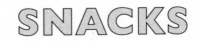

SNACKS

APPLE AND SUNFLOWER BUTTER*

Makes 1 serving

1 apple, cut into slices
2 tablespoons sunflower butter
Pinch of sea salt

Sprinkle each slice with salt and smear with a little sunflower butter!

TAHINI AND VEGGIES*

Makes 1 serving

240 grams shop-bought sesame tahini (look for brands that do not use rapeseed, safflower, or other vegetable oil)

180 millilitres cold water (you may need more for a smoother, more liquid consistency)

Juice of 1/2 a lemon

1 to 3 cloves garlic (if mixing by hand, garlic should be minced)

Pinch of sea salt

Chopped raw veggies of choice (carrots, celery, sweet peppers) or roasted brussels sprouts or carrots

1. Add all ingredients except the veggies to a food processor or high-speed blender. Or you can get an arm workout in and do it by hand with a whisk in a big bowl.

2. Blend or mix ingredients together until creamy. Serve with raw veggies or drizzle over roasted brussels sprouts or carrots. Yum!

3. Keep leftover tahini in an airtight container in the fridge for up to a week.

CHOCOLATE CHIA PUDDING*

Makes 4 servings

600 millilitres unsweetened almond milk or 1 400 millilitre tin coconut milk

2 tablespoons pure maple syrup

1 teaspoon vanilla extract

85 grams chia seeds

2 tablespoons raw cacao powder

Raspberries or sliced strawberries (optional)

1. In a medium bowl or jar, combine the almond or coconut milk, maple syrup, and vanilla extract.

2. Stir or cover and shake the jar to combine.

3. Add the chia seeds and cocoa powder and stir with a whisk to remove all clumps.

4. Cover and place in the refrigerator for 2 to 3 hours (or overnight, which is best), stirring occasionally.

5. Top with raspberries or sliced strawberries if desired.

POWER BALLS*

Makes 4 to 6 servings, 2 balls per serving

250 grams unsalted natural almond or sunflower butter

150 grams ground flaxseed

2 to 3 pitted dates or dried figs

1 tablespoon cacao powder

1/4 teaspoon ground cinnamon

Sea salt

Vanilla extract

2 tablespoons cacao nibs (optional)

20 grams toasted coconut flakes (optional)

1. Add almond or sunflower butter, flaxseed, dates or figs, cacao powder, cinnamon, salt, and vanilla extract to a food processor and pulse until smooth.

2. Mix in cacao nibs (if using) by hand.

3. Scoop out 1 teaspoon and use your hands to roll the mixture into a ball. If it feels too sticky and won't hold together, mix in 1 to 2 teaspoons more ground flaxseed.

4. Roll each ball in coconut flakes (if using) and enjoy!

TESTS FOR HORMONE HEALTH

To say there are a lot of testing methods to measure hormones is an understatement. Some of them are more accurate or appropriate than others, so I've outlined the best options depending on your circumstances and resources. In the UK many of these tests will not be available on the NHS but there are private clinics that will undertake these investigations for a fee.

DUTCH

My preferred testing method today is the Dried Urine Test for Comprehensive Hormones, or DUTCH, which collects a large amount of data, including oestrogen, progesterone, testosterone, DHEA, and cortisol, and a variety of other helpful indicators such as melatonin and neurotransmitters. DUTCH also tells you what's going on with your hormone metabolites for oestrogen, progesterone, androgens, and cortisol, showing how your liver is processing or breaking down these hormones. In other words, it provides you with more insights into why you might be experiencing your symptoms, especially if previous tests came back as normal. (Oestrogen metabolites are covered in detail in Chapter 7.) DUTCH offers a few different test options, you can order the test on your own, and it can be performed at home. That being said, I strongly recommend working with a doctor who understands this test, as the results are complicated. DUTCH does not test your thyroid; thyroid testing is done only via blood. (See "Thyroid Tests" in this appendix.)

BLOOD TESTS

Basic Hormone Tests

If DUTCH is not an option for you, ask your doctor for the following blood hormone tests. If you are cycling, these tests should be done between days 19 and 21 of a 28-day cycle, or approximately 5 to 7 days after you've ovulated. This will help determine accurate levels of progesterone following ovulation. (After all, there's no point in testing progesterone if you haven't ovulated yet.) In the UK, these tests may not be available on demand from the NHS, and you may have to pursue this testing through private clinics.

- Oestradiol
- Progesterone
- Testosterone
- DHEA-S

Additional Hormones and Other Tests

Test between days 2 and 4 of your cycle to get a clearer picture of your fertility. Note: oestradiol can be tested at this time of the cycle as well.

- FSH levels should be tested between days 2 and 4 of your cycle (during your period).
- LH levels should be tested between days 2 and 4 with FSH, or near ovulation, to see if your LH level is rising correctly.

- Oestradiol should be tested between days 2 and 4. If your oestradiol is high then, it could be artificially suppressing FSH, giving you a less-than-accurate picture of FSH levels.

TEST ANYTIME IN YOUR CYCLE

- Vitamin D should be tested because many people are deficient and this vitamin has a broad impact on multiple body systems. I don't recommend supplementing without knowing if you are deficient.

- Prolactin should be tested to ensure it is not too high; high levels can disrupt or stop ovulation.

- Sex hormone-binding globulin, or SHBG, binds up oestrogen and testosterone. High SHBG binds too much of these hormones, making them unavailable for use by the body, and low SHBG causes them to be higher.

- A test for blood sugar markers should test glucose tolerance, fasting insulin, fasting glucose, and hemoglobin A1c.

THYROID TESTS

- TSH (thyroid-stimulating hormone)
- Free T_4
- Free T_3
- Reverse T_3
- Thyroid peroxidase antibody (TPO) and thyroglobulin antibody (TGAB)

Keep in mind, hormone blood testing can be helpful but doesn't always give the full picture or allow you to see levels for more than a brief moment in time. For example, testing cortisol by blood doesn't make much sense because it doesn't allow you to see your cortisol curve happening throughout the day. Testing cortisol is best done via DUTCH or through a saliva cortisol panel. You can order the latter from an at-home testing site such as ZRT Laboratory.

ADVANCED TESTING

Sometimes your symptoms require a little more detective work, and you'll need to do some advanced testing to get a more specific diagnosis. Here are some recommendations to guide you. Work with a functional medicine or naturopathic doctor to help identify the root cause(s) of your issues.

For PCOS or Irregular Periods

In addition to the "Basic Hormone Tests," ask for the following markers to be checked:

- Have your blood sugar markers tested; this should include the glucose tolerance test, fasting insulin, fasting glucose, and hemoglobin A1c.

- Get your androgens tested; this would include testing for total testosterone, free testosterone, androstenedione, dihydrotestosterone (DHT), and DHEA-S.

- Test your FSH, LH, SHBG, and prolactin, which, if dysregulated, can cause anovulation or irregular cycles.

- Get a full thyroid panel.

- Get the cortisol awakening response (CAR) test from DUTCH, which includes cortisol right upon awakening and a diurnal cortisol test. You'll collect samples throughout the day to see what your cortisol does from morning to evening.

- Get your vitamin D levels tested to determine if there is a deficiency. As discussed in Chapter 10, vitamin D is important for proper menstrual cycle function.

- Get an adrenal stress index (ASI) done. This tests levels of 17-hydroxyprogesterone, which, if high, could indicate congenital adrenal hyperplasia (CAH), a condition that presents similarly to PCOS. This will help you get a proper diagnosis.

For Amenorrhoea or Potential Infertility

In addition to the "Basic Hormone Tests":

- Get a pregnancy test.

- Test for FSH, LH, SHBG, and prolactin, which can all cause anovulation if dysregulated.

- Test for anti-Müllerian hormone (AMH). Along with FSH, this test will give you more information on your ovarian reserve. Please keep in mind that AMH is just one test and not a reflection of your overall fertility. As you now know, there is a lot that can be done to improve your menstrual cycle and fertility.

- Get a coeliac panel. As discussed in Chapter 6, coeliac disease can cause periods to disappear and fertility trouble.

- Get an MRI to test for a possible pituitary tumour. A pituitary tumour can be the cause of high prolactin levels and subsequently missing or very irregular periods.

- Have a full thyroid panel done.

- Get the cortisol awakening response (CAR) test from DUTCH, which includes cortisol right upon awakening and a diurnal cortisol test. You'll collect samples throughout the day to see what your cortisol does from morning to evening.

- Test your vitamin D levels.

NICOLE'S HEALTHY RESOURCES

Connect with me online. Here are all the ways to find me and get even more hormone- and period-lovin' content:

- Visit my website (nicolejardim.com).
- Take the Period Quiz (nicolejardim.com/quiz).
- Listen to my podcast, *The Period Party*, which you can find on all major podcast platforms.
- Find me on Instagram (instagram.com/nicolemjardim/ or @nicolemjardim).
- Find me on Facebook (facebook.com/nicolemjardim).

NICOLE'S FIX YOUR PERIOD DOWNLOADABLE RESOURCES

Visit fixyourperiod.com for all the downloadable resources I've mentioned throughout the book and other exclusive material.

FOR FURTHER READING

Fertility Awareness and Cycle Tracking

The Fifth Vital Sign, by Lisa Hendrickson-Jack

The Garden of Fertility and *Honoring Our Cycles*, by Katie Singer

Taking Charge of Your Fertility, by Toni Weschler

Periods and the Menstrual Cycle

Beautiful You, by Dr Nat Kringoudis

Beyond the Pill, by Dr Jolene Brighten

Code Red, by Lisa Lister

Heavy Flow, by Amanda Laird

Her Blood Is Gold, by Lara Owen

No Period. Now What?, by Dr Nicola J. Rinaldi

Period Power, by Maisie Hill

Period Repair Manual, by Dr Lara Briden

Periods Gone Public, by Jennifer Weiss-Wolf

The Pill: Are You Sure It's for You?, by Jane Bennett and Alexandra Pope

Seeing Red, by Kirsten Karchmer

Sweetening the Pill, by Holly Grigg-Spall

Wild Power, by Alexandra Pope and Sjanie Hugo Wurlitzer

Women's Health

The Adrenal Thyroid Revolution, by Dr Aviva Romm

The Balance Plan, by Angelique Panagos

8 Steps to Reverse Your PCOS, by Dr Fiona McCulloch

The Essential Oils Hormone Solution, by Dr Mariza Snyder

Hashimoto's Thyroiditis: Lifestyle Interventions for Finding and Treating the Root Cause, by Izabella Wentz

Healing PCOS, by Amy Medling

The Hormone Cure, by Dr Sara Gottfried

Keto for Women, by Leanne Vogel

A Mind of Your Own, by Kelly Brogan, MD

Moody Bitches, by Julie Holland

PCOS SOS Fertility Fast Track, by Dr. Felice Gersh

The Stress Remedy, by Dr. Doni Wilson

The Upside of Stress, by Kelly McGonigal

Women's Bodies, Women's Wisdom, by Christiane Northrup, MD

Pelvic Pain and Endometriosis

Beating Endo, by Iris Kerin Orbuch, MD, and Amy Stein, DPT

Ending Female Pain, by Isa Herrera

Outsmart Endo, by Dr. Jessica Drummond

Connecting to Your Feminine Energy

The Book of SHE, by Sara Avant Stover

Goddesses in Everywoman, by Jean Shinoda Bolen

Ignite Your Inner Goddess, by Marina Schroeder

Wild Feminine, by Tami Lynn Kent

Women Who Run with the Wolves, by Clarissa Pinkola Estés

WEBSITES

Functional Medicine or Naturopathic Doctor

The American Association of Naturopathic Physicians (naturopathic.org)

The Institute for Functional Medicine (ifm.org)

Certified Women's Health Coach

The Integrative Women's Health Institute (integrativewomens healthinstitute.com): choose "Women's Health Coach Certified" from their provider directory

UK Health Coaches Association (ukhealthcoaches.com)

Nutritional Therapist or Nutrition Consultant

Bauman College (baumancollege.org): search their alumni directory

Nutritional Therapy Association (nutritionaltherapy.com)

British Association for Nutrition and Lifestyle Medicine (bant.org.uk): search their practitioner directory

Naturopathic Nutrition Association (nna-uk.com.)

Hormone and Other Tests

DiagnosTechs Adrenal Stress Index (diagnostechs.com)

DUTCH (dutchtest.com)

Let'sGetChecked at-home testing kits (letsgetchecked.com)

MediChecks (medichecks.com)

Thriva (thriva.co)

Fertility Awareness Method (FAM)
Further Education and Resources

Websites

Association of Fertility Awareness Professionals (fertilityawareness professionals.com)

Taking Charge of Your Fertility (tcoyf.com)

The Natural Family Planning Teachers Association (nfpta.org.uk)

WORKBOOKS

Fertility Awareness Mastery Charting Workbook, by Lisa Hendrickson-Jack

Honoring Our Cycles: A Natural Family Planning Workbook, by Katie Singer

PRODUCTS

Blood Glucose Test Kits

There are a variety of blood glucose monitors on the market and many are available online. Make sure to purchase a monitor, needles, and test strips in order to test your blood sugar. Check the price of the test strips before purchasing the monitor, as those tend to be expensive. The supplements listed are widely available online.

Supplements

ASHWAGANDHA

Gaia Herbs Ashwagandha

NOW Foods Ashwagandha

Seeking Health Ashwagandha

B-COMPLEX

Designs for Health B-Supreme

Seeking Health B Complex Plus

Seeking Health B-Minus (free of B_{12} and folate for people who don't tolerate methylated B vitamins)

Thorne Research Basic B Complex

BETAINE HCL

Bluebonnet HCl Plus Pepsin

Now Foods Betaine HCl

COD LIVER OIL

Rosita Real Foods Extra Virgin Cod Liver Oil

Green Pasture Fermented Cod Liver Oil

COLLAGEN

Bulletproof Upgraded Collagen

Great Lakes Collagen Hydrolysate

Vital Proteins Collagen Peptides

DIGESTIVE ENZYMES

Integrative Therapeutics Bio-Zyme

Pure Encapsulations Digestive Enzymes Ultra

DIINDOLYLMETHANE (DIM)

Designs for Health DIM-Evail

FISH OIL

Carlson Elite Super Omega-3

Designs for Health OmegAvail Ultra

Nordic Naturals ProOmega

Nordic Naturals Ultimate Omega

GELATIN

Great Lakes Gelatin

Vital Proteins Beef Gelatin

GLUTATHIONE

Designs for Health S-Acetyl Glutathione Synergy with NAC

LivOn Labs Liposomal Glutathione

GUT HEALING

Apex Energetics RepairVite

Designs for Health GI Revive

Microbiome Labs MegaMucosa

IRON

Designs for Health Ferrochel

Seeking Health Optimal Iron

MAGNESIUM

Natural Vitality Calm Magnesium Citrate (for constipation)

Seeking Health Magnesium Glycinate Powder

Seeking Health Optimal Magnesium Capsules

Sunfood Magnesium Oil Spray

MILK THISTLE

Designs for Health Milk Thistle

Gaia Herbs Milk Thistle Seed

N-ACETYL CYSTEINE (NAC)

Integrative Therapeutics NAC

Pure Encapsulations NAC

Thorne Research NAC

PHOSPHATIDYLSERINE

Klaire Labs Phosphatidyl Serine

Now Foods Phosphatidyl Serine

PROBIOTICS

Just Thrive Probiotic & Antioxidant

Klaire Labs Ther-Biotic Complete

Microbiome Labs MegaSporeBiotic

Seeking Health HistaminX (can be helpful if you have a histamine intolerance)

Seeking Health ProBiota 12

PROBIOTICS TO SUPPORT VAGINAL HEALTH

Garden of Life RAW Probiotics Vaginal Care

Integrative Therapeutics Pro-Flora Women's Probiotic

Jarrow Formulas Fem-Dophilus

Nature's Way Primadophilus Optima Women's 90 Billion Active Probiotics

Seeking Health ProBiota Woman

RHODIOLA

Gaia Herbs Rhodiola Rosea

Thorne Research Rhodiola

SELENIUM

Klaire Labs Seleno Met

Pure Encapsulations Selenium (Selenomethionine)

Thorne Research Selenomethionine

SULFORAPHANE GLUCOSINOLATE (SGS)

Thorne Research Crucera-SGS

TURMERIC

Designs for Health Curcum-Evail

VITAMIN C

LivOn Labs Liposomal Vitamin C

Seeking Health Vitamin C Powder

VITAMIN D

Seeking Health Vitamin D_3 + K_2 Capsules

Seeking Health Vitamin D_3 + K_2 Drops

VITAMIN E

Designs for Health Ultra Gamma E Complex

Now Foods Advanced Gamma E Complex

ZINC

Seeking Health Zinc Lozenge

Thorne Research Zinc Picolinate

NOTES

Introduction: What's Up with Your Period?

1. Stella Iacovides et al., "What We Know About Primary Dysmenorrhea Today: A Critical Review," *Human Reproduction Update* 21, no. 6 (Nov./Dec. 2015): 762–78, doi:10.1093/humupd/dmv039; Giovanni Grandi et al., "Prevalence of Menstrual Pain in Young Women: What Is Dysmenorrhea?," *Journal of Pain Research* 5 (June 2012): 169–74, doi:10.2147/JPR .S30602.

2. Rachel K. Jones, "Beyond Birth Control: The Overlooked Benefits of Oral Contraceptive Pills," Guttmacher Institute, 2011, https://www.gutt macher.org/sites/default/files/report_pdf/beyond-birth-control.pdf.

3. Elizabeth Siegel Watkins, "How the Pill Became a Lifestyle Drug: The Pharmaceutical Industry and Birth Control in the United States Since 1960," *American Journal of Public Health* 102, no. 8 (Aug. 2012): 1462–72, doi:10.2105/AJPH.2012.300706.

4. Danielle B. Cooper and Heba Mahdy, "Oral Contraceptive Pills," StatPearls (Aug. 14, 2019), https://www.ncbi.nlm.nih.gov/books/NBK430882/; R. Rivera et al., "The Mechanism of Action of Hormonal Contraceptives and Intrauterine Contraceptive Devices," *American Journal of Obstetrics and Gynecology* 181, no. 5 (Nov. 1999): 1263–9, https://www.ncbi.nlm.nih.gov /pubmed/10561657; Sarah Horvath et al., "Contraception," Endotext (Jan. 17, 2018), https://www.ncbi.nlm.nih.gov/books/NBK279148/.

5. Horvath et al., "Contraception"; Filipa de Castro Coelho and Cremilda Barros, "The Potential of Hormonal Contraception to Influence Female Sexuality," *International Journal of Reproductive Medicine* (March 3, 2019), https://www.ncbi.nlm.nih.gov/pmc/articles/PMC6421036/.

1. Committee Opinion No. 651: "Menstruation in Girls and Adolescents: Using the Menstrual Cycle as a Vital Sign," *Obstetrics and Gynecology* 126, no. 6 (Dec. 2015): e143–46, doi:10.1097/AOG.0000000000001215.

2. Pilar Vigil, Carolina Lyon, Betsi Flores, Hernán Rioseco, and Felipe Serrano. "Ovulation, A Sign of Health," *The Linacre Quarterly* 84, no. 4 (Nov. 2017), 343–355, doi:10.1080/00243639.2017.1394053

3. S. Novella et al., "Mechanisms Underlying the Influence of Oestrogen on Cardiovascular Physiology in Women," *The Journal of Physiology* (Aug. 2019): 4873–86, doi:10.1113/JP278063.

4. R. Kaaks et al., "Serum Sex Steroids in Premenopausal Women and Breast Cancer Risk Within the European Prospective Investigation into Cancer and Nutrition (EPIC)," *Journal of the National Cancer Institute* 97, no. 10 (May 2005): 755–65, doi:10.1093/jnci/dji132.

5. A. Shieh et al., "Estradiol and Follicle-Stimulating Hormone as Predictors of Onset of Menopause Transition-Related Bone Loss in Pre- and Perimenopausal Women," *Journal of Bone and Mineral Research* (Aug. 2019): 2246–53, doi:10.1002/jbmr.3856.

6. S. V. Khadilkar et al., "Sex Hormones and Cognition: Where Do We Stand?," *The Journal of Obstetrics and Gynecology of India* 69, no. 4 (Aug. 2019): 303–12, doi:10.1007/s13224-019-01223-5; A. N. Siddiqui et al., "Neuroprotective Role of Steroidal Sex Hormones: An Overview," *CNS Neuroscience and Therapeutics* 22, no. 5 (May 2016): 342–50, doi:10.1111/cns.12538; R. C. Melcangi et al., "Levels and Actions of Progesterone and Its Metabolites in the Nervous System During Physiological and Pathological Conditions," *Progress in Neurobiology* 113 (Feb. 2014): 56–69, doi:10.1016/j.pneurobio.2013.07.006.

7. Sonya S. Dasharathy et al., "Menstrual Bleeding Patterns Among Regularly Menstruating Women," *American Journal of Epidemiology* 175, no. 6 (Feb. 2012): 536–45, doi:10.1093/aje/kwr356; Yixin Wang, et al. "Menstrual cycle regularity and length and risk of mortality: a prospective cohort study." *Fertility and Sterility* 112, no. 3 (September 2019), e437-e438, doi:10.1016/j.fertnstert.2019.08.019; Pilar Vigil, Carolina Lyon, Betsi Flores, Hernán Rioseco, and Felipe Serrano, "Ovulation, A Sign of Health," *The Linacre Quarterly* 84, no. 4 (Nov. 2017): 343–355, doi:10.1080/002436 39.2017.1394053.

8. Salvatore Giovanni Vitale et al., "The Impact of Lifestyle, Diet, and Psychological Stress on Female Fertility," *Oman Medical Journal* 32, no. 5

(Sept. 2017): 443–44, doi:10.5001/omj.2017.85; Sunni L. Mumford et al., "Serum Antioxidants Are Associated with Serum Reproductive Hormones and Ovulation Among Healthy Women," *The Journal of Nutrition* 146, no. 1 (Nov. 2015), 98–106, doi:10.3945/jn.115.217620.

9. K. D. Ballard et al., "Can Symptomatology Help in the Diagnosis of Endometriosis? Findings from a National Case-Control Study—Part 1," *BJOG* 115, no. 11 (Oct. 2008): 1382–91, doi:10.1111/j.1471-0528.2008.01878.x; Jason Abbott, "Optimal Management of Chronic Cyclical Pelvic Pain: An Evidence-Based and Pragmatic Approach," *International Journal of Women's Health*, August 2010, 263–277, doi:10.2147/ijwh.s7991.

10. Anna B. Livdans-Forret et al., "Menorrhagia: A Synopsis of Management Focusing on Herbal and Nutritional Supplements, and Chiropractic," *The Journal of the Canadian Chiropractic Association* 51, no. 4 (Dec. 2007): 235–46.

11. Chrisandra L. Shufelt et al., "Hypothalamic Amenorrhea and the Long-Term Health Consequences," *Seminars in Reproductive Medicine* 35, no. 3 (May 2017): 256–62, doi:10.1055/s-0037-1603581.

12. R. Hampl et al., "Antimüllerian Hormone (AMH) Not Only a Marker for Prediction of Ovarian Reserve," *Physiological Research* 60 (2011): 217–23, http://www.biomed.cas.cz/physiolres/pdf/60/60_217.pdf.

13. Beverly G. Reed and Bruce Carr, "The Normal Menstrual Cycle and the Control of Ovulation," Endotext (Aug. 5, 2018), https://www.ncbi.nlm.nih.gov/books/NBK279054/.

14. L. L. Espey and H. Lipner, "Ovulation," in E. Knobil and J. D. Neill, eds., *The Physiology of Reproduction* (New York: Raven, 1994), 725.

15. J. Depares et al., "Ovarian Ultrasonography Highlights Precision of Symptoms of Ovulation as Markers of Ovulation," *British Medical Journal* (Clinical Research Ed.) 292, no. 6535 (June 1986): 1562, doi:10.1136/bmj.292.6535.1562.

16. M. Fukuda et al., "Right-Sided Ovulation Favours Pregnancy More than Left-Sided Ovulation," *Human Reproduction* 15, no. 9 (Sept. 2000): 1921–26, doi:10.1093/humrep/15.9.1921.

17. Catherine E. Keefe et al., "The Evaluation and Treatment of Cervical Factor Infertility: A Medical-Moral Analysis," *Linacre Quarterly* 79, no. 4 (Nov. 2012): 409–25, https://doi.org/10.1179/002436312804827127.

18. Tolga B. Mesen et al., "Progesterone and the Luteal Phase: A Requisite to Reproduction," *Obstetrics and Gynecology Clinics of North America* 42, no. 1 (March 2015): 135–51, doi:10.1016/j.ogc.2014.10.003.

19. C. K. Welt et al., "Control of Follicle-Stimulating Hormone by Estradiol and the Inhibins: Critical Role of Estradiol at the Hypothalamus During the Luteal-Follicular Transition," *The Journal of Clinical Endocrinology and Metabolism* 88, no. 4 (April 2003): 1766–71, doi:10.1210/jc.2002 -021516.

20. G. D. Niswender and T. M. Nett, "The Corpus Luteum and Its Control in Infraprimate Species," in E. Knobil and J. D. Neill, eds., *The Physiology of Reproduction* (New York: Raven, 1994), 781.

21. Hsiu-Wei Su et al., "Detection of Ovulation: A Review of Currently Available Methods," *Bioengineering and Translational Medicine* 2, no. 3 (May 2017): 238–46, doi:10.1002/btm2.10058.

22. Reed and Carr, "The Normal Menstrual Cycle and the Control of Ovulation."

23. Nicola Davis, "'We Don't Need to Bleed': Why Many Women Are Giving Up on Periods," *The Guardian*, July 18, 2019, https://www.theguardian .com/lifeandstyle/2019/jul/18/women-dont-need-to-bleed-why-many -more-of-us-are-giving-up-periods; Ashley Oerman, "Here's How to Stop Your Period from Coming If You're Sick of This Sh*t Every Month," *Cosmopolitan*, Feb. 26, 2019, https://www.cosmopolitan.com/health-fitness /a26516622/how-to-stop-your-period-from-coming/.

24. Richard Fehring et al., "Variability in the Phases of the Menstrual Cycle," *Journal of Obstetric, Gynecologic, and Neonatal Nursing* 35 (May/June 2006): 376–84, doi:10.1111/j.1552-6909.2006.00051.x.

25. Mesen et al., "Progesterone and the Luteal Phase: A Requisite to Reproduction," 135–51.

26. Fehring et al., "Variability in the Phases of the Menstrual Cycle," 376–84.

27. G. Boutzios et al., "Common Pathophysiological Mechanisms Involved in Luteal Phase Deficiency and Polycystic Ovary Syndrome: Impact on Fertility," *Endocrine* 43, no. 2 (April 2013): 314–17, doi:10.1007/s12020-012 -9778-9.

28. Fehring et al., "Variability in the Phases of the Menstrual Cycle," 376– 84; K. Münster et al., "Length and Variation in the Menstrual Cycle— A Cross-Sectional Study from a Danish County," *BJOG* 99, no. 5 (May 1992): 422–29, doi:10.1111/j.1471-0528.1992.tb13762.x; Mitchell D. Creinin, Sharon Keverline, and Leslie A. Meyn, "How Regular Is Regular? An Analysis of Menstrual Cycle Regularity," *Contraception* 70, no. 4 (2004), 289–92, doi:10.1016/j.contraception.2004.04.012.

29. Dasharathy et al., "Menstrual Bleeding Patterns Among Regularly Menstruating Women," 536–45

30. Nanette Santoro et al., "Menopausal Symptoms and Their Management," *Endocrinology and Metabolism Clinics of North America* 44, no. 3 (Sept. 2015): 497–515, doi:10.1016/j.ecl.2015.05.001.

31. D. A. Koutras, "Disturbances of Menstruation in Thyroid Disease," *Annals of the New York Academy of Sciences* 816 (June 1997): 280–84, doi:10.1111/j.1749-6632.1997.tb52152.x.

32. Dasharathy et al., "Menstrual Bleeding Patterns Among Regularly Menstruating Women," 536–45; Julia L. Magnay et al., "A Systematic Review of Methods to Measure Menstrual Blood Loss," *BMC Women's Health* 18, no. 142 (Aug. 2018), doi:10.1186/s12905-018-0627-8; I. S. Fraser et al., "Estimating Menstrual Blood Loss in Women with Normal and Excessive Menstrual Fluid Volume," *Obstetrics and Gynecology* 98, no. 5, part 1 (Nov. 2001): 806–14, https://doi.org/10.1097/00006250-200111000-00017.

33. Dasharathy et al., "Menstrual Bleeding Patterns Among Regularly Menstruating Women," 536–45.

34. Magnay et al, "A Systematic Review of Methods to Measure Menstrual Blood Loss"; Katrina M. Wyatt et al., "Determination of Total Menstrual Blood Loss," *Fertility and Sterility* 76, no. 1 (July 2001): 125–31, https://doi.org/10.1016/s0015-0282(01)01847-7.

35. Wyatt et al., "Determination of Total Menstrual Blood Loss," 125–31.

36. Dan Apter et al., "Follicular Growth in Relation to Serum Hormonal Patterns in Adolescent Compared with Adult Menstrual Cycles," *Fertility and Sterility* 47, no. 1 (Jan. 1987): 82–88, doi:10.1016/S0015-0282(16)49940-1.

37. Fehring et al., "Variability in the Phases of the Menstrual Cycle," 376–84.

38. G. E. Hale et al., "Endocrine Features of Menstrual Cycles in Middle and Late Reproductive Age and the Menopausal Transition Classified According to the Staging of Reproductive Aging Workshop (STRAW) Staging System," *The Journal of Clinical Endocrinology and Metabolism* 92, no. 8 (Aug. 2007): 3060–67, doi:10.1210/jc.2007-0066; N. Santoro et al., "Factors Related to Declining Luteal Function in Women During the Menopausal Transition," *The Journal of Clinical Endocrinology and Metabolism* 93, no. 5 (May 2008): 1711–21, doi:10.1210/jc.2007-2165.

39. Pilar Vigil et al., "The Importance of Fertility Awareness in the Assessment of a Woman's Health: A Review," *Linacre Quarterly* 79, no. 4 (Nov. 2012): 426–50, doi:10.1179/002436312804827109.

2 The Hormonal Hierarchy

1. David H. Wasserman, "Four Grams of Glucose," *American Journal of Physiology: Endocrinology and Metabolism* 296, no. 1 (Jan. 2009): E11–21, doi:10.1152/ajpendo.90563.2008.

2. S. M. Haffner, "Sex Hormone-Binding Protein, Hyperinsulinemia, Insulin Resistance and Noninsulin-Dependent Diabetes," *Hormone Research in Paediatrics* 45, no 3–5 (1996): 233–37.

3. M. Vallée et al., "Role of Pregnenolone, Dehydroepiandrosterone and Their Sulfate Esters on Learning and Memory in Cognitive Aging," *Brain Research Reviews* 37, no. 1–3 (Nov. 2001): 301–12.

4. I. J. Osuji et al., "Pregnenolone for Cognition and Mood in Dual Diagnosis Patients," *Psychiatric Research* 178, no. 2 (July 2010): 309–12, doi:10.1016/j.psychres.2009.09.006.

5. A. M. Traish et al., "Dehydroepiandrosterone (DHEA): A Precursor Steroid or an Active Hormone in Human Physiology," *The Journal of Sexual Medicine* 8, no. 11 (Nov. 2011): 2960–82, doi:10.1111/j.1743-6109.2011.02523.x; O. M. Wolkowitz et al., "Dehydroepiandrosterone (DHEA) Treatment of Depression," *Biological Psychiatry* 41, no. 3 (Feb. 1997): 311–18, doi:10.1016/s0006-3223(96)00043-1.

6. N. Orentreich et al., "Age Changes and Sex Differences in Serum Dehydroepiandrosterone Sulfate Concentrations Throughout Adulthood," *The Journal of Clinical Endocrinology and Metabolism* 59, no. 3 (Sept. 1984): 551–55, doi:10.1210/jcem-59-3-551.

7. N. Heldring et al., "Estrogen Receptors: How Do They Signal and What Are Their Targets," *Physiological Reviews* 87, no. 3 (July 2007): 905–31, doi:10.1152/physrev.00026.2006.

8. Reed and Carr, "The Normal Menstrual Cycle and the Control of Ovulation."

9. Michael Schumacher et al., "Progesterone Synthesis in the Nervous System: Implications for Myelination and Myelin Repair," *Frontiers in Neuroscience* 6 (Feb. 2012): 10, doi:10.3389/fnins.2012.00010.

10. M. Datta et al., "Thyroid Hormone Stimulates Progesterone Release from Human Luteal Cells by Generating a Proteinaceous Factor," *Journal of Endocrinology* 158, no. 3 (Sept. 1998): 319–25.

11. Ari Shechter and Diane B. Boivin, "Sleep, Hormones, and Circadian Rhythms Throughout the Menstrual Cycle in Healthy Women and Women

with Premenstrual Dysphoric Disorder," *International Journal of Endocrinology* (2010): 259345, doi:10.1155/2010/259345.

12. Mary Barron, "Light Exposure, Melatonin Secretion, and Menstrual Cycle Parameters: An Integrative Review," *Biological Research for Nursing* 9, no. 1 (July 2007): 49–69, doi:10.1177/1099800407303337.

3 Decoding Your Period:
What Your Period Problems Are Trying to Tell You

1. L. M. Dickerson et al., "Premenstrual Syndrome," *American Family Physician* 67, no. 8 (April 2003): 1743–52.

2. Ashraf Direkvand-Moghadam et al., "The Worldwide Prevalence of Premenstrual Syndrome: A Systematic Review and Meta-analysis Study," *Iranian Journal of Obstetrics, Gynecology and Infertility* 16, no. 65 (Sept. 2013): 8–17.

3. S. Tschudin et al., "Prevalence and Predictors of Premenstrual Syndrome and Premenstrual Dysphoric Disorder in a Population-Based Sample," *Archives of Women's Mental Health* 13, no. 6 (Dec. 2010): 485–94, doi:10.1007/s00737-010-0165-3; José Luis Dueñas et al., "Prevalence of Premenstrual Syndrome and Premenstrual Dysphoric Disorder in a Representative Cohort of Spanish Women of Fertile Age," *European Journal of Obstetrics and Gynecology and Reproductive Biology* 156, no. 1 (May 2011): 72–77, doi:10.1016/j.ejogrb.2010.12.013.

4. Liisa Hantsoo and C. N. Epperson. "Premenstrual Dysphoric Disorder: Epidemiology and Treatment," *Current Psychiatry Reports* 17, no. 11 (Nov. 2015), doi:10.1007/s11920-015-0628-3.

5. Kimberly A. Yonkers et al., "Epidemiology and Pathogenesis of Premenstrual Syndrome and Premenstrual Dysphoric Disorder," UpToDate, https://www.uptodate.com/contents/epidemiology-and-pathogenesis-of-premenstrual-syndrome-and-premenstrual-dysphoric-disorder.

6. U. Halbreich et al., "The Prevalence, Impairment, Impact, and Burden of Premenstrual Dysphoric Disorder (PMS/PMDD)," *Psychoneuroendocrinology* 28, no. 3 (Aug. 2003): 1–23, doi:10.1016/s0306-4530(03)00098-2.

7. Tschudin et al., "Prevalence and Predictors of Premenstrual Syndrome and Premenstrual Dysphoric Disorder in a Population-Based Sample," 485–94.

8. John Fauber, "Lowering the Bar: How PMDD Went from an Idea to a Diagnosis," MedPageToday, Nov. 16, 2016, https://www.medpagetoday.com/special-reports/loweringthebar/61457.

9.   Iacovides et al., "What We Know About Primary Dysmenorrhea Today," 762–78; Grandi et al., "Prevalence of Menstrual Pain in Young Women," 169–74.

10. Hong Ju et al., "The Prevalence and Risk Factors of Dysmenorrhea," *Epidemiologic Reviews* 36, no. 1 (2014): 104–13, doi:10.1093/epirev/mxt009.

11. Iacovides et al., "What We Know About Primary Dysmenorrhea Today," 762–78.

12. M. Pall et al., "Induction of Delayed Follicular Rupture in the Human by the Selective COX-2 Inhibitor Rofecoxib: A Randomized Double-Blind Study," *Human Reproduction* 16, no. 7 (July 2001): 1323–28, doi:10.1093/humrep/16.7.1323.

13. Kathryn A. McInerney et al., "Preconception Use of Pain Relievers and Time to Pregnancy: A Prospective Cohort Study," *Human Reproduction* 32, no. 1 (Jan. 2017): 103–11, doi:10.1093/humrep/dew272; M. Gaytan et al., "Non-steroidal Anti-inflammatory Drugs (NSAIDs) and Ovulation: Lessons from Morphology," *Histology and Histopathology* 21, no. 5 (May 2006): 541–56, doi:10.14670/HH-21.541.

14. Tasuku Harada, "Dysmenorrhea and Endometriosis in Young Women," *Yonago Acta Medica* 56, no. 4 (Nov. 2013): 81–84.

15. Amimi S. Osayande and Suarna Mehulic, "Diagnosis and Initial Management of Dysmenorrhea," *American Family Physician* 89, no. 5 (March 2014): 341–46, https://www.aafp.org/afp/2014/0301/p341.html.

16. V. H. Eisenberg et al., "Epidemiology of Endometriosis: A Large Population-Based Database Study from a Healthcare Provider with 2 Million Members," *BJOG* 125, no. 1 (Jan. 2018): 55–62, doi:10.1111/1471-0528.14711.

17. E. A. Stewart et al., "Epidemiology of Uterine Fibroids: A Systematic Review," *BJOG* 124, no. 10 (Sept. 2017): 1501–12, doi:10.1111/1471-0528.14640.

18. Jin-Jiao Li, Jacqueline P. Chung, Sha Wang, Tin-Chiu Li, and Hua Duan, "The Investigation and Management of Adenomyosis in Women Who Wish to Improve or Preserve Fertility," *BioMed Research International* 2018 (March 2018), 1–12, doi:10.1155/2018/6832685.

19. Ibid.

20. Kristen Kreisel et al., "Prevalence of Pelvic Inflammatory Disease in Sexually Experienced Women of Reproductive Age—United States, 2013–2014," *Morbidity and Mortality Weekly Report* 66, no. 3 (Jan. 2017): 80–83, doi:10.15585/mmwr.mm6603a3.

21. J. H. Hobby et al., "Effect of Baseline Menstrual Bleeding Pattern on Copper Intrauterine Device Continuation," *American Journal of Obstetrics and Gynecology* 219, no. 5 (Nov. 2018): 465, doi:10.1016/j.ajog.2018.08.028.

22. Selin Elmaoğulları and Zehra Aycan, "Abnormal Uterine Bleeding in Adolescents," *Journal of Clinical Research in Pediatric Endocrinology* 10, no. 3 (Sept. 2018): 191–97, doi:10.4274/jcrpe.0014; Nanette Santoro, "Perimenopause: From Research to Practice," *Journal of Women's Health* 25, no. 4 (April 2016): 332–39, doi:10.1089/jwh.2015.5556.

23. P. A. Regidor, "Progesterone in Peri- and Postmenopause: A Review," *Geburtshilfe und Frauenheilkunde* 74, no. 11 (Oct. 2014): 995–1002, doi:10 .1055/s-0034-1383297.

24. Dharani K. Hapangama and Judith N Bulmer, "Pathophysiology of Heavy Menstrual Bleeding," *Women's Health* 12, no. 1 (Jan. 2016): 3-13, doi: 10.2217/whe.15.81.

25. Dilip Gude, "Thyroid and Its Indispensability in Fertility," *Journal of Human Reproductive Sciences* 4, no. 1 (Jan.–April 2011): 59–60, doi:10.4103 /0974-1208.82368.

26. Jacques Donnez and Marie-Madeleine Dolmans, "Uterine Fibroid Management: From the Present to the Future," *Human Reproduction Update* 22, no. 6 (Nov. 2016): 665–86, doi:10.1093/humupd/dmw023.

27. Charles J. Lockwood, "Mechanisms of Normal and Abnormal Endometrial Bleeding," *Menopause* 18, no. 4 (April 2011): 408–11, doi:10.1097 /GME.0b013e31820bf288.

28. Jennifer Villavicencio and Rebecca H. Allen, "Unscheduled Bleeding and Contraceptive Choice: Increasing Satisfaction and Continuation Rates," *Open Access Journal of Contraception* 7 (March 2016): 43–52, doi:10.2147 /OAJC.S85565.

29. Hapangama and Bulmer, "Pathophysiology of Heavy Menstrual Bleeding," 3–13; Giancarlo Castaman and Silvia Linari, "Diagnosis and Treatment of von Willebrand Disease and Rare Bleeding Disorders," *Journal of Clinical Medicine* 6, no. 4 (April 2017): 45, doi:10.3390/jcm6040045.

30. Elmaoğulları and Aycan, "Abnormal Uterine Bleeding in Adolescents," 191–97.

31. G. L. Hammond, "Plasma Steroid-Binding Proteins: Primary Gatekeepers of Steroid Hormone Action," *Journal of Endocrinology* 230, no. 1 (July 2016): R13–25, doi:10.1530/JOE-16-0070.

32. Lindsay T. Fourman and Pouneh K. Fazeli, "Neuroendocrine Causes of Amenorrhea: An Update," *The Journal of Clinical Endocrinology and Metabolism* 100, no. 3 (Jan. 2015): 812–24, doi:10.1210/jc.2014-3344.

33. A. Cassidy et al., "Biological Effects of a Diet of Soy Protein Rich in Isoflavones on the Menstrual Cycle of Premenopausal Women," *The American Journal of Clinical Nutrition* 60, no. 3 (Sept. 1994): 333–40, doi:10.1093/ajcn/60.3.333.

34. Cassidy et al., "Biological Effects of a Diet of Soy Protein Rich in Isoflavones on the Menstrual Cycle of Premenopausal Women," 333–40.

35. C. M. Gordon et al., "Functional Hypothalamic Amenorrhea: An Endocrine Society Clinical Practice Guideline," *The Journal of Clinical Endocrinology and Metabolism* 102, no. 5 (May 2017): 1413–39, doi:10.1210/jc.2017-00131.

36. F. Parazzini et al., "Lifelong Menstrual Pattern and Risk of Breast Cancer," *Oncology* 50, no. 4 (July 1993): 222–25, doi:10.1159/000227183.

37. Sunni L. Mumford et al., "The Utility of Menstrual Cycle Length as an Indicator of Cumulative Hormonal Exposure," *The Journal of Clinical Endocrinology and Metabolism* 97, no. 10 (Oct. 2012): E1871–79, doi:10.1210/jc.2012-1350.

38. Ibid.

39. Ibid.

40. Anne Marie Zaura Jukic et al., "Lifestyle and Reproductive Factors Associated with Follicular Phase Length," *Journal of Women's Health* 16, no. 9 (Nov. 2007): 1340–47, doi:10.1089/jwh.2007.0354.

41. D. A. Klein, "Amenorrhea: An Approach to Diagnosis and Management," *American Family Physician* 87, no. 11 (June 2013): 781–88.

42. "What Causes Amenorrhea?," National Institute of Child Health and Human Development, https://www.nichd.nih.gov/health/topics/amenorrhea/conditioninfo/causes.

43. R. Rojas-Walsson and R. Cardoso, "Diagnosis and Management of Post-pill Amenorrhea," *The Journal of Family Practice* 13, no. 2 (Aug. 1981): 165–69.

44. Daria La Torre and Alberto Falorni, "Pharmacological Causes of Hyperprolactinemia," *Therapeutics and Clinical Risk Management* 3, no. 5 (Oct. 2007): 929–51.

45. Chiara Tersigni et al., "Celiac Disease and Reproductive Disorders: Meta-analysis of Epidemiologic Associations and Potential Pathogenic

Mechanisms," *Human Reproduction Update* 20, no. 4 (July/Aug. 2014): 582–93, doi:10.1093/humupd/dmu007.

46. Shufelt et al., "Hypothalamic Amenorrhea and the Long-Term Health Consequences," 256–62.

47. S. Schrager, "Abnormal Uterine Bleeding Associated with Hormonal Contraception," *American Family Physician* 65, no. 10 (May 2002): 2073–80.

48. F. Uguz et al., "Antidepressants and Menstruation Disorders in Women: A Cross-Sectional Study in Three Centers," *General Hospital Psychiatry* 34, no. 5 (Sept.–Oct. 2012): 529–33, doi:10.1016/j.genhosppsych.2012.03 .014; Marianne M. Casilla-Lennon et al., "The Effect of Antidepressants on Fertility," *American Journal of Obstetrics and Gynecology* 215, no. 3 (2016): 314.e1–314.e5, doi:10.1016/j.ajog.2016.01.170.

49. Giuliano Bedoschi et al., "Chemotherapy-Induced Damage to Ovary: Mechanisms and Clinical Impact," *Future Oncology* 12, no. 20 (Oct. 2016): 2333–44, doi:10.2217/fon-2016-0176.

50. M. P. Murke et al., "Study of Menstrual Irregularities in Patients Receiving Antipsychotic Medications," *Indian Journal of Psychiatry* 53, no. 1 (Jan.– March 2011): 79–80, doi:10.4103/0019-5545.75550.

51. A. E. W. McLachlan and Donald D. Brown, "The Effects of Penicillin Administration on Menstrual and Other Sexual Cycle Functions," *British Journal of Venereal Diseases* (March 1947): 1–10, doi:10.1136/sti.23.1.1, https://sti.bmj.com/content/sextrans/23/1/1.full.pdf.

52. Shufelt et al., "Hypothalamic Amenorrhea and the Long-Term Health Consequences," 256–62.

53. Lockwood, "Mechanisms of Normal and Abnormal Endometrial Bleeding," 408–11.

54. M. E. Pennant et al., "Premenopausal Abnormal Uterine Bleeding and Risk of Endometrial Cancer," *BJOG* 124, no. 3 (Feb. 2017): 404–11, doi:10.1111/1471-0528.14385.

55. Susan Sirmans and Kristen Pate, "Epidemiology, Diagnosis, and Management of Polycystic Ovary Syndrome," *Clinical Epidemiology* 6, no. 1 (Dec. 2013): 1–13, doi:10.2147/clep.s37559; B. Trivax and R. Azziz, "Diagnosis of Polycystic Ovary Syndrome," *Clinical Obstetrics and Gynecology* 50, no. 1 (March 2007): 166–77, doi:10.1097/GRF.0b013e31802f351b.

56. Andrew A. Bremer, "Polycystic Ovary Syndrome in the Pediatric Population," *Metabolic Syndrome and Related Disorders* 8, no. 5 (Oct. 2010): 375–94, doi:10.1089/met.2010.0039.

57. Angela Boss and Evelina Weidman, *Living with PCOS* (Omaha, NE: Addicus Books, 2001), 3.

58. Suvarna Satish Khadilkar, "Polycystic Ovarian Syndrome: Is It Time to Rename PCOS to HA-PODS?," *Journal of Obstetrics and Gynaecology of India* 66, no. 2 (April 2016): 81–87, https://www.ncbi.nlm.nih.gov/pmc /articles/PMC4818834/.

59. Walter Futterweit and George Ryan, *A Patient's Guide to PCOS: Understanding and Reversing Polycystic Ovary Syndrome* (New York: Henry Holt and Company, 2006), 11.

60. Joselyn Rojas et al., "Polycystic Ovary Syndrome, Insulin Resistance, and Obesity: Navigating the Pathophysiologic Labyrinth," *International Journal of Reproductive Medicine* 2014 (2014): 719050, doi:10.1155/2014/719050; N. K. Stepto et al., "Women with Polycystic Ovary Syndrome Have Intrinsic Insulin Resistance on Euglycaemic-Hyperinsulaemic Clamp," *Human Reproduction* 28, no. 3 (March 2013): 777–84, doi:10.1093/humrep/des463.

61. Michelle R. Jones, Ning Xu, and Mark O. Goodarzi, "Recent Advances in the Genetics of Polycystic Ovary Syndrome," *Polycystic Ovary Syndrome*, April 2013, 29–52, doi:10.1007/978-1-4614-8394-6_3.

62. Richard O Burney and Linda C Giudice, "Pathogenesis and Pathophysiology of Endometriosis," *Fertility and Sterility* 98, no. 3 (Sep. 2012): 511–9, doi:10.1016/j.fertnstert.2012.06.029.

63. M. Cervigni and F. Natale, "Gynecological Disorders in Bladder Pain Syndrome/Interstitial Cystitis Patients," *International Journal of Urology* 21, no. 1 (April 2014): 85–88, doi:10.1111/iju.12379.

64. G D Adamson, et al., "Creating Solutions in Endometriosis: Global Collaboration Through the World Endometriosis Research Foundation," *Journal of Endometriosis and Pelvic Pain Disorders* 2, no. 1 (Jan. 2010): 3-6. doi: 10.1177/228402651000200102; P. A. Rogers et al., "Priorities for Endometriosis Research: Recommendations from an International Consensus Workshop," *Reproductive Science* 16, no. 4 (April 2009): 335–46, doi:10.1177/1933719108330568.

65. Carlo Bulletti et al., "Endometriosis and Infertility," *Journal of Assisted Reproduction and Genetics* 27, no. 8 (Aug. 2010): 441–47, doi:10.1007/s10815 -010-9436-1.

66. G. K. Husby et al., "Diagnostic Delay in Women with Pain and Endometriosis," *Acta Obstetricia et Gynecologica Scandinavica* 82, no. 7 (July 2003): 649–53, doi:10.1034/j.1600-0412.2003.00168.x.

67. Richard O. Burney and Linda C. Giudice, "Pathogenesis and Pathophysiology of Endometriosis," *Fertility and Sterility* 98, no. 3 (Sept. 2012): 511–19, doi:10.1016/j.fertnstert.2012.06.029.

4 Week One: Enlist the Power of Food to Feed Your Hormones

1. David Zeevi et al., "Personalized Nutrition by Prediction of Glycemic Responses," *Cell* 163, no. 5 (Nov. 2015): 1079–93, doi:10.1016/j.cell.2015.11.001.

2. Maris Coelho et al., "Biochemistry of Adipose Tissue: An Endocrine Organ," *Archives of Medical Science* 9, no. 2 (April 2013): 191–200, doi:10.5114/aoms.2013.33181.

3. A. Booth et al., "Adipose Tissue: An Endocrine Organ Playing a Role in Metabolic Regulation," *Hormone Molecular Biology and Clinical Investigation* 26, no. 1 (April 2016): 25–42, doi:10.1515/hmbci-2015-0073.

4. Fatemeh Shobeiri et al., "Effect of Calcium on Premenstrual Syndrome: A Double-Blind Randomized Clinical Trial," *Obstetrics and Gynecology Science* 60, no. 1 (Jan. 2017): 100–105, doi:10.5468/ogs.2017.60.1.100.

5. F. Abdi et al., "A Systematic Review of the Role of Vitamin D and Calcium in Premenstrual Syndrome," *Obstetrics and Gynecology Science* 62, no. 2 (March 2019): 73–86, doi:10.5468/ogs.2019.62.2.73.

6. Marieke ten Bolscher et al., "Estrogen Regulation of Intestinal Calcium Absorption in the Intact and Ovariectomized Adult Rat," *Journal of Bone and Mineral Research* 14, no. 7 (Dec. 2009): 1197–202, doi:10.1359/jbmr.1999.14.7.1197.

7. M. Moslehi et al., "The Association Between Serum Magnesium and Premenstrual Syndrome: A Systematic Review and Meta-analysis of Observational Studies," *Biological Trace Element Research* 192, no. 2 (Dec. 2019): 145–52, doi:10.1007/s12011-019-01672-z.

8. Kia A. Saeedian et al., "The Association Between the Risk of Premenstrual Syndrome and Vitamin D, Calcium, and Magnesium Status Among University Students: A Case Control Study," *Health Promotion Perspectives* 5, no. 3 (Oct. 2015): 225–30, doi:10.15171/hpp.2015.027.

9. Elizabeth M. Miller, "The Reproductive Ecology of Iron in Women," *American Journal of Physical Anthropology* 159 (2016), 172–95, doi:10.1002/ajpa.22907.

10. Livdans-Forret et al., "Menorrhagia: A Synopsis of Management Focusing on Herbal and Nutritional Supplements, and Chiropractic," 235–46.

11. Delia McCabe and Marc Colbeck, "The Effectiveness of Essential Fatty Acid, B Vitamin, Vitamin C, Magnesium and Zinc Supplementation for Managing Stress in Women: A Systematic Review Protocol," *JBI Database of Systematic Reviews and Implementation Reports* 13, no. 7 (July 2015): 104–18, http://journals.lww.com/jbisrir/Fulltext/2015/13070/The_effectiveness_of_essential_fatty_acid,_B.10.aspx.

12. A. J. Gaskins et al., "The Impact of Dietary Folate Intake on Reproductive Function in Premenopausal Women: A Prospective Cohort Study," *PLOS One* 7, no. 9 (2012): e46276, doi:10.1371/journal.pone.0046276.

13. Z. Asemi et al., "Effects of Long-Term Folate Supplementation on Metabolic Status and Regression of Cervical Intraepithelial Neoplasia: A Randomized, Double-Blind, Placebo-Controlled Trial," *Nutrition* 32, no. 6 (June 2016): 681–86, doi:10.1016/j.nut.2015.12.028.

14. B. Teucher et al., "Enhancers of Iron Absorption: Ascorbic Acid and Other Organic Acids," *International Journal for Vitamin and Nutrition Research* 74, no. 6 (Nov. 2004): 403–19, doi:10.1024/0300-9831.74.6.403.

15. Sunni L. Mumford et al., "Serum Antioxidants Are Associated with Serum Reproductive Hormones and Ovulation Among Healthy Women," *The Journal of Nutrition* 146, no. 1 (Jan. 2016): 98–106, doi:10.3945/jn.115.217620.

16. D. Cao et al., "Association Between Vitamin C Intake and the Risk of Cervical Neoplasia: A Meta-analysis," *Nutrition and Cancer* 68, no. 1 (2016): 48–57, doi:10.1080/01635581.2016.1115101; F. H. Thomas, K. A. Walters, and E. E. Telfer, "How to Make a Good Oocyte: An Update on in-Vitro Models to Study Follicle Regulation," *Human Reproduction Update* 9, no. 6 (2003): 541–55, https://doi.org/10.1093/humupd/dmg042.

17. N. Santanam et al., "Antioxidant Supplementation Reduces Endometriosis-Related Pelvic Pain in Humans," *Translational Research* 161, no. 3 (March 2013): 189–95, doi:10.1016/j.trsl.2012.05.001.

18. M. Kashanian et al., "Evaluation of the Effect of Vitamin E on Pelvic Pain Reduction in Women Suffering from Primary Dysmenorrhea," *The Journal of Reproductive Medicine* 58, no. 1–2 (Jan.–Feb. 2013): 34–38.

19. Livdans-Forret et al., "Menorrhagia: A Synopsis of Management Focusing on Herbal and Nutritional Supplements, and Chiropractic," 235–46.

20. S. Q. Wang et al., "Indole-3-Carbinol (I3C) and Its Major Derivatives: Their Pharmacokinetics and Important Roles in Hepatic Protection," *Current Drug Metabolism* 17, no. 4 (2016): 401–9.

21. P. Felker et al., "Concentrations of Thiocyanate and Goitrin in Human Plasma, Their Precursor Concentrations in Brassica Vegetables, and Associated Potential Risk for Hypothyroidism," *Nutrition Reviews* 74, no. 4 (April 2016): 248–58, doi:10.1093/nutrit/nuv110.

22. M. McMillan et al., "Preliminary Observations on the Effect of Dietary Brussels Sprouts on Thyroid Function," *Human Toxicology* 5, no. 1 (Jan. 1986): 15–19, doi:10.1177/096032718600500104.

23. M. S. Baggish et al., "Urinary Oxalate Excretion and Its Role in Vulvar Pain Syndrome," *American Journal of Obstetrics and Gynecology* 177, no. 3 (Sept. 1997): 507–11, doi:10.1016/s0002-9378(97)70137-6.

24. J. W. Fahey, Y. Zhang, and P. Talalay, "Broccoli Sprouts: An Exceptionally Rich Source of Inducers of Enzymes That Protect Against Chemical Carcinogens," *Proceedings of the National Academy of Sciences* 94, no. 19 (Sep. 1997), 10367–10372, doi:10.1073/pnas.94.19.10367.

25. Don James, Sridevi Devaraj, Prasad Bellur, Shantala Lakkanna, John Vicini, and Sekhar Boddupalli, "Novel Concepts of Broccoli Sulforaphanes and Disease: Induction of Phase Ii Antioxidant and Detoxification Enzymes by Enhanced-Glucoraphanin Broccoli," *Nutrition Reviews* 70, no. 11 (Nov. 2012), 654–65, doi:10.1111/j.1753-4887.2012.00532.x.

26. J. V. Higdon et al., "Cruciferous Vegetables and Human Cancer Risk: Epidemiologic Evidence and Mechanistic Basis," *Pharmacological Research* 55, no. 3 (March 2007): 224–36, doi:10.1016/j.phrs.2007.01.009.

27. Z. Xiao et al., "Assessment of Vitamin and Carotenoid Concentrations of Emerging Food Products: Edible Microgreens," *Journal of Agricultural and Food Chemistry* 60, no. 31 (Aug. 2012): 7644–51, doi:10.1021/jf300459b; Edgar Pinto et al., "Comparison Between the Mineral Profile and Nitrate Content of Microgreens and Mature Lettuces," *Journal of Food Composition and Analysis* 37 (Feb. 2015): 38–43, doi:10.1016/j.jfca.2014.06.018.

28. P. O. Chocano-Bedoya et al., "Dietary B Vitamin Intake and Incident Premenstrual Syndrome," *The American Journal of Clinical Nutrition* 93, no. 5 (May 2011): 1080–86, doi:10.3945/ajcn.110.009530; N. Wolak et al., "Vitamins B1, B2, B3 and B9: Occurrence, Biosynthesis Pathways and Functions in Human Nutrition," *Mini-Reviews in Medicinal Chemistry* 17, no. 12 (2017): 1075–111, doi:10.2174/13895575166661607 25095729.

29. Sukanya Jaroenporn et al., "Effects of Pantothenic Acid Supplementation on Adrenal Steroid Secretion from Male Rats," *Biological and Pharmaceutical Bulletin* 31, no. 6 (2008): 1205–8, https://doi.org/10.1248/bpb.31.1205.

30. D. P. Rose, "The Interactions Between Vitamin B6 and Hormones," *Vitamins and Hormones* 36 (1978): 53–99.

31. Nahid Fathizadeh et al., "Evaluating the Effect of Magnesium and Magnesium Plus Vitamin B6 Supplement on the Severity of Premenstrual Syndrome," *Iranian Journal of Nursing and Midwifery Research* 15, suppl. 1 (Dec. 2010): 401–5.

32. J. Holley et al., "Effects of Vitamin B_6 Nutritional Status on the Uptake of [³H]-oestradiol into the Uterus, Liver and Hypothalamus of the Rat," *Journal of Steroid Biochemistry* 18, no. 2 (Feb. 1983): 161–65, doi:10.1016/0022-4731(83)90082-1; Livdans-Forret et al., "Menorrhagia: A Synopsis of Management Focusing on Herbal and Nutritional Supplements, and Chiropractic," 235–46; Fatemeh Shobeiri et al., "Clinical Effectiveness of Vitamin E and Vitamin B6 for Improving Pain Severity in Cyclic Mastalgia," *Iranian Journal of Nursing and Midwifery Research* 20, no. 6 (Nov.–Dec. 2015): 723–27, doi:10.4103/1735-9066.170003; M. C. De Souza et al., "A Synergistic Effect of a Daily Supplement for 1 Month of 200 mg Magnesium Plus 50 mg Vitamin B6 for the Relief of Anxiety-Related Premenstrual Symptoms: A Randomized, Double-Blind, Crossover Study," *Journal of Women's Health and Gender-Based Medicine* 9, no. 2 (March 2000): 131–39, doi:10.1089/152460900318623.

33. L. Shi et al., "Changes in Levels of Phytic Acid, Lectins and Oxalates During Soaking and Cooking of Canadian Pulses," *Food Research International* 107 (May 2018): 660–68, doi:10.1016/j.foodres.2018.02.056.

34. Keng-Wen Lien et al., "Assessing Aflatoxin Exposure Risk from Peanuts and Peanut Products Imported to Taiwan," *Toxins* 11, no. 2 (Feb. 2019): 80, doi:10.3390/toxins11020080.

35. "Soy," Non-GMO Project, https://www.nongmoproject.org/high-risk/soy/#easy-footnote-2-1012.

36. "Recent Trends in GE Adoption," graph, United States Department of Agriculture Economic Research Service, https://www.ers.usda.gov/data-products/adoption-of-genetically-engineered-crops-in-the-us/recent-trends-in-ge-adoption.aspx.

37. Heather B. Patisaul and Wendy Jefferson, "The Pros and Cons of Phytoestrogens," *Frontiers in Neuroendocrinology* 31, no. 4 (March 2010): 400–419, doi:10.1016/j.yfrne.2010.03.003.

38. C. Barmeyer et al., "Long-Term Response to Gluten-Free Diet as Evidence for Non-celiac Wheat Sensitivity in One Third of Patients with Diarrhea-Dominant and Mixed-Type Irritable Bowel Syndrome," *Interna-*

tional Journal of Colorectal Disease 32, no. 1 (Jan. 2017): 29–39, doi:10.1007/s00384-016-2663-x.

39. Stephan C. Bischoff et al., "Intestinal Permeability: A New Target for Disease Prevention and Therapy," *BMC Gastroenterology* 14 (Nov. 2014): 189, doi:10.1186/s12876-014-0189-7.

40. Pekka Collin et al., "Autoimmune Thyroid Disorders and Coeliac Disease," *European Journal of Endocrinology* 130, no. 2 (Feb. 1994): 137–40, doi:10.1530/eje.0.1300137; M. N. Akcay and G. Akcay, "The Presence of the Antigliadin Antibodies in Autoimmune Thyroid Diseases," *Hepato-Gastroenterology* 50, suppl. 2 (Dec. 2003): cclxxix–cclxxx.

41. "Corn," Non-GMO Project, https://www.nongmoproject.org/high-risk/corn/.

42. A. S. Jackson et al., "The Effect of Sex, Age and Race on Estimating Percentage Body Fat from Body Mass Index: The Heritage Family Study," *International Journal of Obesity* 26, no. 6 (June 2002): 789–96, doi:10.1038/sj.ijo.0802006.

43. C. Y. Chang et al., "Essential Fatty Acids and Human Brain," *Acta Neurologica Taiwanica* 18, no. 4 (Dec. 2009): 231–41.

44. Mandana Zafari et al., "Comparison of the Effect of Fish Oil and Ibuprofen on Treatment of Severe Pain in Primary Dysmenorrhea," *Caspian Journal of Internal Medicine* 2, no. 3 (Summer 2011): 279–82; F. Sampalis et al., "Evaluation of the Effects of Neptune Krill Oil on the Management of Premenstrual Syndrome and Dysmenorrhea," *Alternative Medicine Review* 8, no. 2 (May 2003): 171–79; M. G. Brush et al., "Abnormal Essential Fatty Acid Levels in Plasma of Women with Premenstrual Syndrome," *American Journal of Obstetrics and Gynecology* 150, no. 4 (Oct. 1984): 363–66, doi:10.1016/s0002-9378(84)80139-8.

45. Elisa Gonzales et al., "Omega-3 Fatty Acids Improve Behavioral Coping to Stress in Multiparous Rats," *Behavioural Brain Research* 279 (Feb. 2015): 129–38, doi:10.1016/j.bbr.2014.11.010.

46. A. P. Simopoulos, "The Importance of the Ratio of Omega-6/Omega-3 Essential Fatty Acids," *Biomedicine and Pharmacotherapy* 56, no. 8 (Oct. 2002): 365–79, doi:10.1016/S0753-3322(02)00253-6.

47. Iacovides et al., "What We Know About Primary Dysmenorrhea Today," 762–78.

48. Azadeh Nadjarzadeh et al., "The Effect of Omega-3 Supplementation on Androgen Profile and Menstrual Status in Women with Polycystic Ovary Syndrome: A Randomized Clinical Trial," *Iranian Journal of Reproductive Medicine* 11, no. 8 (Aug. 2013): 665–72.

49. Thomas Larrieu and Sophie Layé, "Food for Mood: Relevance of Nutritional Omega-3 Fatty Acids for Depression and Anxiety," *Frontiers in Physiology* 9 (Aug. 2018): 1047, doi:10.3389/fphys.2018.01047.

50. N. Rahbar et al., "Effect of Omega-3 Fatty Acids on Intensity of Primary Dysmenorrhea," *The International Journal of Gynecology and Obstetrics* 117, no. 1 (April 2012): 45–47, doi:10.1016/j.ijgo.2011.11.019.

51. B. C. Davis et al., "Achieving Optimal Essential Fatty Acid Status in Vegetarians: Current Knowledge and Practical Implications," *The American Journal of Clinical Nutrition* 78, no. 3 (Sept. 2003): 640S–46S, doi:10.1093/ajcn/78.3.640S.

52. M. Piourde and S. C. Cunnane, "Extremely Limited Synthesis of Long Chain Polyunsaturates in Adults: Implications for Their Dietary Essentiality and Use as Supplements," *Applied Physiology, Nutrition, and Metabolism* 32, no. 4 (Aug. 2007): 619–34, doi:10.1139/H07-034.

53. R. A. Gibson et al., "Docosahexaenoic Acid Synthesis from Alpha-Linolenic Acid Is Inhibited by Diets High in Polyunsaturated Fatty Acids," *Prostaglandins, Leukotrienes and Essential Fatty Acids* 88, no. 1 (Jan. 2013): 139–46, doi:10.1016/j.plefa.2012.04.003; H. Gerster, "Can Adults Adequately Convert Alpha-Linolenic Acid (18:3n-3) to Eicosapentaenoic Acid (20:5n-3) and Docosahexaenoic Acid (22:6n-3)?," *International Journal for Vitamin and Nutrition Research* 68, no. 3 (1998): 159–73.

54. Lynette P. Shek et al., "Role of Dietary Long-Chain Polyunsaturated Fatty Acids in Infant Allergies and Respiratory Diseases," *Clinical and Developmental Immunology* 5, suppl. 2 (Aug. 2012): 730568, doi:10.1155/2012/730568.

55. Jorge E. Chavarro et al., "Dietary Fatty Acid Intakes and the Risk of Ovulatory Infertility," *The American Journal of Clinical Nutrition* 85, no. 1 (Jan. 2007): 231–37, doi:10.1093/ajcn/85.1.231; Jorge E. Chavarro et al., "Diet and Lifestyle in the Prevention of Ovulatory Disorder Infertility," *Obstetrics and Gynecology* 110, no. 5 (Nov. 2007): 1050–58, doi:10.1097/01.AOG.0000287293.25465.e1.

56. University of Adelaide, "Women's Fertility Linked to Detox Element in Diet," ScienceDaily, Nov. 17, 2014, https://www.sciencedaily.com/releases/2014/11/141117111008.htm.

57. X. Tian and F. J. Diaz, "Zinc Depletion Causes Multiple Defects in Ovarian Function During the Periovulatory Period in Mice," *Endocrinology* 153, no. 2 (Feb. 2012): 873–86, doi:10.1210/en.2011-1599; X. Tian and F. J.

Diaz, "Acute Dietary Zinc Deficiency Before Conception Compromises Oocyte Epigenetic Programming and Disrupts Embryonic Development," *Developmental Biology* 376, no. 1 (April 2013): 51–61, doi:10.1016/j.ydbio .2013.01.015.

58. Trine Maxel et al., "Expression Patterns and Correlations with Metabolic Markers of Zinc Transporters ZIP14 and ZNT1 in Obesity and Polycystic Ovary Syndrome," *Frontiers in Endocrinology* 8 (March 2017): 38, doi:10.3389/fendo.2017.00038.

59. Ambooken Betsy et al., "Zinc Deficiency Associated with Hypothyroidism: An Overlooked Cause of Severe Alopecia," *International Journal of Trichology* 5, no. 1 (Jan.–March 2013): 40–42, doi:10.4103/0974-7753.114714; Ananda S. Prasad, "Zinc Is an Antioxidant and Anti-inflammatory Agent: Its Role in Human Health," *Frontiers in Nutrition* 1 (Sept. 2014): 14, doi:10.3389/fnut.2014.00014.

60. Ewelina Pałkowska-Goździk, "Effects of Dietary Protein on Thyroid Axis Activity." *Nutrients* 10, no. 1 (Dec. 2017), 5. doi:10.3390/nu10010005; Adel Pezeshki, Rizaldy C. Zapata, Arashdeep Singh, Nicholas J. Yee, and Prasanth K. Chelikani, "Low Protein Diets Produce Divergent Effects on Energy Balance," *Scientific Reports* 6, no. 1 (April 2016), doi:10.1038 /srep25145.

61. A. Jabbar et al., "Vitamin B12 Deficiency Common in Primary Hypothyroidism," *The Journal of the Pakistan Medical Association* 58, no. 5 (May 2008): 258–61.

62. Heidi Lynch et al., "Plant-Based Diets: Considerations for Environmental Impact, Protein Quality, and Exercise Performance," *Nutrients* 10, no. 12 (Dec. 2018): 1841, doi:10.3390/nu10121841.

63. Kazumi Maruyama, Tomoe Oshima, and Kenji Ohyama, "Exposure to Exogenous Oestrogen Through Intake of Commercial Milk Produced from Pregnant Cows," *Pediatrics International* 52, no. 1 (Feb. 2010), 33–38, doi:10.1111/j.1442-200x.2009.02890.x; Maya M. Jeyaraman, Ahmed M. Abou-Setta, Laurel Grant, Farnaz Farshidfar, Leslie Copstein, Justin Lys, Tania Gottschalk et al., "Dairy Product Consumption and Development of Cancer: An Overview of Reviews." *BMJ Open* 9, no. 1 (Jan. 2019), e023625, doi:10.1136/bmjopen-2018-023625.

64. Alexandre Lamas et al., "Tracing Recombinant Bovine Somatotropin Ab(Use) Through Gene Expression in Blood, Hair Follicles, and Milk Somatic Cells: A Matrix Comparison," *Molecules* 23, no. 7 (July 2018): 1708, doi:10.3390/molecules23071708.

65. Keewan Kim et al., "Dairy Food Intake Is Associated with Reproductive Hormones and Sporadic Anovulation Among Healthy Premenopausal Women," *The Journal of Nutrition* 147, no. 2 (Feb. 2017): 218–26, doi:10.3945/jn.116.241521.

66. M. Aghasi et al., "Dairy Intake and Acne Development: A Meta-analysis of Observational Studies," *Clinical Nutrition* 38, no. 3 (June 2019): 1067–75, doi:10.1016/j.clnu.2018.04.015; B. C. Melnik, "Evidence for Acne-Promoting Effects of Milk and Other Insulinotropic Dairy Products," *Nestlé Nutrition Institute Workshop Series Pediatric Program* 67 (2011): 131–45, doi:10.1159/000325580.

67. Simon Brooke-Taylor et al., "Systematic Review of the Gastrointestinal Effects of A1 Compared with A2 β-Casein," *Advances in Nutrition* 8, no. 5 (Sept. 2017): 739–48, doi:10.3945/an.116.013953.

5 Week Two: Step Off the Blood Sugar Roller Coaster

1. Bryan J. Neth and Suzanne Craft, "Insulin Resistance and Alzheimer's Disease: Bioenergetic Linkages," *Frontiers in Aging Neuroscience* 9 (Oct. 2017): 345, doi:10.3389/fnagi.2017.00345; Etan Orgel and Steven D. Mittelman, "The Links Between Insulin Resistance, Diabetes, and Cancer," *Current Diabetes Reports* 13, no. 2 (April 2013): 213–22, doi:10.1007/s11892-012-0356-6.

2. Richard J. Johnson et al., "Theodore E. Woodward Award—The Evolution of Obesity: Insights from the Mid-Miocene," *Transactions of the American Clinical and Climatological Association* 121 (2010): 295–308.

3. "New CDC Report: More than 100 Million Americans Have Diabetes or Prediabetes," CDC, July 18, 2017, https://www.cdc.gov/media/releases/2017/p0718-diabetes-report.html.

4. "WHO Calls on Countries to Reduce Sugars Intake Among Adults and Children," World Health Organization, March 4, 2015, https://www.who.int/mediacentre/news/releases/2015/sugar-guideline/en/.

5. M. I. Miranda et al., "The Role of Dopamine D2 Receptors in the Nucleus Accumbens During Taste-Aversive Learning and Memory Extinction After Long-Term Sugar Consumption," *Neuroscience* 359 (Sept. 2017): 142–50, doi:10.1016/j.neuroscience.2017.07.009; David A. Wiss et al., "Sugar Addiction: From Evolution to Revolution," *Frontiers in Psychiatry* 9 (Nov. 2018): 545, doi:10.3389/fpsyt.2018.00545.

6. Magalie Lenoir et al., "Intense Sweetness Surpasses Cocaine Reward," *PloS One* 2, no. 8 (Aug. 2007): e698, doi:10.1371/journal.pone.0000698.

7. J. J. DiNicolantonio et al. (2018). "Not Salt But Sugar as Aetiological in Osteoporosis: A Review," *Missouri Medicine* 115, no. 3, 247–52.

8. Gilbert G. G. Donders et al., "Impaired Tolerance for Glucose in Women with Recurrent Vaginal Candidiasis," *American Journal of Obstetrics and Gynecology* 187, no. 4 (Oct. 2002): 989–93, doi:10.1067/mob.2002.126285.

9. Marie E. Thoma et al., "Bacterial Vaginosis Is Associated with Variation in Dietary Indices," *The Journal of Nutrition*, 141, no. 9 (Sept. 2011): 1698–704, doi:10.3945/jn.111.140541.

10. Gloria González-Saldivar et al., "Skin Manifestations of Insulin Resistance: From a Biochemical Stance to a Clinical Diagnosis and Management," *Dermatology and Therapy* 7, no. 1 (March 2017): 37–51, doi:10.1007/s13555-016-0160-3.

11. Etan Orgel and Steven D. Mittelman, "The Links Between Insulin Resistance, Diabetes, and Cancer," *Current Diabetes Reports* 13, no. 2 (April 2013), 213–222, doi:10.1007/s11892-012-0356-6.

12. Mohammad G. Saklayen, "The Global Epidemic of the Metabolic Syndrome," *Current Hypertension Reports* 20, no. 2 (Feb. 2018): 12, doi:10.1007/s11906-018-0812-z; James M. Rippe and Theodore J. Angelopoulos, "Relationship Between Added Sugars Consumption and Chronic Disease Risk Factors: Current Understanding," *Nutrients* 8, no. 11 (Nov. 2016): 697, doi:10.3390/nu8110697.

13. Wasserman, "Four Grams of Glucose," E11–21.

14. A. Vambergue et al., "Pathophysiology of Gestational Diabetes," *Journal de Gynécologie Obstétrique et Biologie de la Reproduction* 31, suppl. 6 (Oct. 2002): 4S3–4S10; O. Pedersen, "Insulin Resistance: A Physiopathological Condition with Numerous Sequelae: Non-insulin-dependent Diabetes Mellitus (NIDDM), Android Obesity, Essential Hypertension, Dyslipidemia and Atherosclerosis," *Ugeskrift for Læger* 154, no. 20 (May 1992): 1411–16.

15. Rojas et al., "Polycystic Ovary Syndrome, Insulin Resistance, and Obesity," 719050; E. J. Graham et al., "A Model of Ovulatory Regulation Examining the Effects of Insulin-Mediated Testosterone Production on Ovulatory Function," *Journal of Theoretical Biology* 416 (March 2017): 149–60, doi:10.1016/j.jtbi.2017.01.007.

16. J. Dupont et al., "Insulin Signalling and Glucose Transport in the Ovary and Ovarian Function During the Ovarian Cycle," *Biochemical Journal* 473, no. 11 (June 2016): 1483–501, doi:10.1042/BCJ20160124.

17. P. Moghetti, "Insulin Resistance and Polycystic Ovary Syndrome," *Current Pharmaceutical Design* 22, no. 36 (2016): 5526–34.

18. Dupont et al., "Insulin Signalling and Glucose Transport in the Ovary and Ovarian Function During the Ovarian Cycle," 1483–501; S. Franks and H. D. Mason, "Polycystic Ovary Syndrome: Interaction of Follicle Stimulating Hormone and Polypeptide Growth Factors in Oestradiol Production by Human Granulosa Cells," *The Journal of Steroid Biochemistry and Molecular Biology* 40, no. 1–3 (1991): 405–9, doi:10.1016/0960-0760(91)90208-m.

19. G. Strain et al., "The Relationship Between Serum Levels of Insulin and Sex Hormone-Binding Globulin in Men: The Effect of Weight Loss," *The Journal of Clinical Endocrinology and Metabolism* 79, no. 4 (Oct. 1994): 1173–76, doi:10.1210/jcem.79.4.7962291.

20. M. G. Sweet et al., "Evaluation and Management of Abnormal Uterine Bleeding in Premenopausal Women," *American Family Physician* 85, no. 1 (Jan. 2012): 35–43.

21. S. R. Ferreira and A. B. Motta, "Uterine Function: From Normal to Polycystic Ovarian Syndrome Alterations," *Current Medicinal Chemistry* 25, no. 15 (2018): 1792–804, doi:10.2174/0929867325666171205144119.

22. Y. Liang and S. Yao, "Potential Role of Oestrogen in Maintaining the Imbalanced Sympathetic and Sensory Innervation in Endometriosis," *Molecular and Cellular Endocrinology* 424 (March 2016): 42–49, doi:10.1016/j.mce.2016.01.012.

23. N. Luo et al., "Estrogen-Mediated Activation of Fibroblasts and Its Effects on the Fibroid Cell Proliferation," *Translational Research* 163, no. 3 (March 2014): 232–41, doi:10.1016/j.trsl.2013.11.008.

24. P. G. Cohen, "Aromatase, Adiposity, Aging and Disease: The Hypogonadal-Metabolic-Atherogenic-Disease and Aging Connection," *Medical Hypotheses* 56, no. 6 (June 2001): 702–8, doi:10.1054/mehy.2000.1169.

25. Sudha Ambiger et al., "Role of Leutenising Hormone LH and Insulin Resistance in Polycystic Ovarian Syndrome," *International Journal of Reproduction, Contraception, Obstetrics and Gynecology* 6, no. 9 (Aug. 2017): 3892–96, doi:10.18203/2320-1770.ijrcog20174029.

26. Pratap Kumar and Sameer Farouk Sait, "Luteinizing Hormone and Its Dilemma in Ovulation Induction," *Journal of Human Reproductive Sciences* 4, no. 1 (Jan.–April 2011): 2–7, doi:10.4103/0974-1208.82351.

27. Espey and Lipner, "Ovulation," 725.

28. E. A. MacGregor and A. Hackshaw, "Prevalence of Migraine on Each Day of the Natural Menstrual Cycle," *Neurology* 63, no. 2 (July 2004), 351–53, doi:10.1212/01.wnl.0000133134.68143.2e.

29. J. Parantainen et al., "Relevance of Prostaglandins in Migraine," *Cephalalgia* 5, suppl. 2 (May 1985): 93–97, doi:10.1177/03331024850050S217; P. L. Durham et al., "Changes in Salivary Prostaglandin Levels During Menstrual Migraine with Associated Dysmenorrhea," *Headache: The Journal of Headache and Face Pain* 50, no. 5 (May 2010): 844–51, doi:10.1111/j.1526 -4610.2010.01657.x.

30. G. Nattero et al., "Relevance of Prostaglandins in True Menstrual Migraine," *Headache: The Journal of Headache and Face Pain* 29, no. 4 (April 1989): 233–38, doi:10.1111/j.1526-4610.1989.hed22904233.x.

31. T. J. Hartman et al., "Alcohol Consumption and Urinary Oestrogens and Oestrogen Metabolites in Premenopausal Women," *Hormones and Cancer* 7, no. 1 (Feb. 2016): 65–74, doi:10.1007/s12672-015-0249-7.

32. Hanne Frydenberg et al., "Alcohol Consumption, Endogenous Oestrogen and Mammographic Density Among Premenopausal Women," *Breast Cancer Research* 17 (Aug. 2015): 103, doi:10.1186/s13058-015-0620-1.

33. "Alcohol and Sleep: How Drinking Disrupts the Body's Circadian Rhythm," Chronobiology, https://www.chronobiology.com/alcohol-and -sleep-how-drinking-disrupts-the-bodys-circadian-rhythm/.

34. C. P. Rowan et al., "Aerobic Exercise Training Modalities and Prediabetes Risk Reduction," *Medicine and Science in Sports and Exercise* 49, no. 3 (March 2017): 403–12, doi:10.1249/MSS.0000000000001135.

35. C. L. Hwang et al., "Novel All-Extremity High-Intensity Interval Training Improves Aerobic Fitness, Cardiac Function and Insulin Resistance in Healthy Older Adults," *Experimental Gerontology* 82 (Sept. 2016): 112–19, doi:10.1016/j.exger.2016.06.009; K. Marcinko et al., "High Intensity Interval Training Improves Liver and Adipose Tissue Insulin Sensitivity," *Molecular Metabolism* 4, no. 12 (Oct. 2015): 903–15, doi:10.1016/j.molmet .2015.09.006.

36. W. L. Westcott, "Resistance Training Is Medicine: Effects of Strength Training on Health," *Current Sports Medicine Reports* 11, no. 4 (July–Aug. 2012): 209–16, doi:10.1249/JSR.0b013e31825dabb8.

37. S. Di Meo et al., "Improvement of Obesity-Linked Skeletal Muscle Insulin Resistance by Strength and Endurance Training," *Journal of Endocrinology* 234, no. 3 (Sept. 2017): R159–81, doi:10.1530/JOE-17-0186.

38. H. T. Vinutha et al., "Effect of Integrated Approach of Yoga Therapy on Autonomic Functions in Patients with Type 2 Diabetes," *Indian Journal of Endocrinology and Metabolism* 19, no. 5 (Sept.–Oct. 2015): 653–57, doi:10.4103/2230-8210.163194; Ashwini Sham Tikhe et al., "Yoga: Managing Overweight in Mid-life T2DM," *Journal of Mid-Life Health* 6, no. 2 (April–June 2015): 81–84, doi:10.4103/0976-7800.158959.

39. I. Stelzer et al., "Ultra-endurance Exercise Induces Stress and Inflammation and Affects Circulating Hematopoietic Progenitor Cell Function," *Scandinavian Journal of Medicine and Science in Sports* 25, no. 5 (Oct. 2015): e442–50, doi:10.1111/sms.12347.

40. J. S. Fuqua and A. D. Rogol, "Neuroendocrine Alterations in the Exercising Human: Implications for Energy Homeostasis," *Metabolism* 62, no. 7 (July 2013): 911–21, doi:10.1016/j.metabol.2013.01.016.

41. J. M. Escalante Pulido and M. Alpizar Salazar, "Changes in Insulin Sensitivity, Secretion and Glucose Effectiveness During Menstrual Cycle," *Archives of Medical Research* 30, no. 1 (Jan.–Feb. 1999): 19–22; Sue A. Brown, Boyi Jiang, Molly McElwee-Malloy, Christian Wakeman, and Marc D. Breton. "Fluctuations of Hyperglycemia and Insulin Sensitivity Are Linked to Menstrual Cycle Phases in Women with T1D." *Journal of Diabetes Science and Technology* 9, no. 6 (Oct. 2015), 1192–1199, doi:10.1177/1932296815608400.

42. Edwina H. Yeung et al., "Longitudinal Study of Insulin Resistance and Sex Hormones over the Menstrual Cycle: The BioCycle Study," *The Journal of Clinical Endocrinology and Metabolism* 95, no. 12 (Dec. 2010): 5435–42, doi:10.1210/jc.2010-0702.

43. G. Allais et al., "Estrogen, Migraine, and Vascular Risk," *Neurological Sciences* 39, suppl. 1 (June 2018): 11–20, doi:10.1007/s10072-018-3333-2.

44. G. Fink et al., "Estrogen Control of Central Neurotransmission: Effect on Mood, Mental State, and Memory," *Cellular and Molecular Neurobiology* 16, no. 3 (June 1996): 325–44.

45. Srinaree Kaewrudee et al., "Vitamin or Mineral Supplements for Premenstrual Syndrome," *Cochrane Database of Systematic Reviews* 2018, no. 1 (Jan. 2018): CD012933, doi:10.1002/14651858.CD012933; Saeedian et al., "The Association Between the Risk of Premenstrual Syndrome and Vitamin D, Calcium, and Magnesium Status Among University Students," 225–30; A. Girman et al., "An Integrative Medicine Approach to Premenstrual Syndrome," *American Journal of Obstetrics and Gynecology* 188, suppl. 5 (May 2003): S56–65; Hannah Retallick-Brown, Julia Rucklidge, and Neville

Blampied, "Study Protocol for a Randomized Double Blind, Treatment Control Trial Comparing the Efficacy of a Micronutrient Formula to a Single Vitamin Supplement in the Treatment of Premenstrual Syndrome."

46. G. E. Abraham, "Nutritional Factors in the Etiology of the Premenstrual Tension Syndromes," *The Journal of Reproductive Medicine* 28, no. 7 (July 1983), 446–64.

47. W. Li et al., "Sex Steroid Hormones Exert Biphasic Effects on Cytosolic Magnesium Ions in Cerebral Vascular Smooth Muscle Cells: Possible Relationships to Migraine Frequency in Premenstrual Syndromes and Stroke Incidence," *Brain Research Bulletin* 54, no. 1 (Jan. 2001): 83–89, doi:10.1016/s0361-9230(00)00428-7.

6 Week Three: Fix Your Gut, Fix Your Hormones

1. J. M. Baker et al., "Estrogen–Gut Microbiome Axis: Physiological and Clinical Implications," *Maturitas* 103 (Sept. 2017): 45–53, doi:10.1016/j.maturitas.2017.06.025.

2. Claudia S. Plottel and Martin J. Blaser, "Microbiome and Malignancy," *Cell Host and Microbe* 10, no. 4 (Oct. 2011): 324–35, doi:10.1016/j.chom.2011.10.003.

3. P. C. Konturek et al., "Stress and the Gut: Pathophysiology, Clinical Consequences, Diagnostic Approach, and Treatment Options," *Journal of Physiology and Pharmacology* 62, no. 6 (2011): 591–99, http://www.jpp.krakow.pl/journal/archive/12_11/pdf/591_12_11_article.pdf.

4. M. J. Tetel et al., "Steroids, Stress and the Gut Microbiome–Brain Axis," *Journal of Neuroendocrinology* 30, no. 2 (2018), doi:10.1111/jne.12548.

5. C. Hubinont and F. Debieve, "Prevention of Preterm Labour: 2011 Update on Tocolysis," *Journal of Pregnancy* 2011 (Nov. 2011): 941057, doi: 10.1155/2011/941057.

6. J. Evans and L. A. Salamonsen, "Inflammation, Leukocytes and Menstruation," *Reviews in Endocrine and Metabolic Disorders* 13, no. 4 (Dec. 2012): 277–88, doi:10.1007/s11154-012-9223-7.

7. A. Fasano, "Intestinal Permeability and Its Regulation by Zonulin: Diagnostic and Therapeutic Implications," *Clinical Gastroenterology and Hepatology* 10, no. 10 (Oct. 2012): 1096–100, doi:10.1016/j.cgh.2012.08.012.

8. Claire L. Boulangé et al., "Impact of the Gut Microbiota on Inflammation, Obesity, and Metabolic Disease," *Genome Medicine* 8, no. 1 (April 2016): 42, doi:10.1186/s13073-016-0303-2.

9. Alberto Caminero et al., "Mechanisms by Which Gut Microorganisms Influence Food Sensitivities," *Nature Reviews: Gastroenterology and Hepatology* 16 (2019): 7–18.

10. A. Nishida et al., "Gut Microbiota in the Pathogenesis of Inflammatory Bowel Disease," *Clinical Journal of Gastroenterology* 11, no. 1 (Feb. 2018): 1–10, doi:10.1007/s12328-017-0813-5.

11. Stacy Menees and William Chey, "The Gut Microbiome and Irritable Bowel Syndrome," *F1000Research* 7 (July 2018): 1029, doi:10.12688/f1000 research.14592.1.

12. C. Virili et al., "Gut Microbiota and Hashimoto's Thyroiditis," *Reviews in Endocrine and Metabolic Disorders* 19, no. 4 (Dec. 2018): 292–300, doi: 10.1007/s11154-018-9467-y.

13. L. Sacchetti and C. Nardelli, "Gut Microbiome Investigation in Celiac Disease: From Methods to Its Pathogenetic Role," *Clinical Chemistry and Laboratory Medicine* (2019), doi:10.1515/cclm-2019-0657.

14. O. Vaarala, "Gut Microbiota and Type 1 Diabetes," *The Review of Diabetic Studies* 9, no. 4 (Winter 2012): 251–59, doi:10.1900/RDS.2012.9.251.

15. A. Budhram et al., "Breaking Down the Gut Microbiome Composition in Multiple Sclerosis," *Multiple Sclerosis Journal* 23, no. 5 (April 2017): 628–36, doi:10.1177/1352458516682105.

16. Ravinder Nagpal et al., "Obesity-Linked Gut Microbiome Dysbiosis Associated with Derangements in Gut Permeability and Intestinal Cellular Homeostasis Independent of Diet," *Journal of Diabetes Research* 2018 (Sept. 2018), doi:10.1155/2018/3462092.

17. Katherine Harmon Courage, "Fiber-Famished Gut Microbes Linked to Poor Health," *Scientific American*, March 23, 2015, https://www.scientific american.com/article/fiber-famished-gut-microbes-linked-to-poor -health1/.

18. J. C. Bode et al., "Jejunal Microflora in Patients with Chronic Alcohol Abuse," *Hepato-Gastroenterology* 31, no. 1 (Feb. 1984): 30–34.

19. M. Lyte et al., "Stress at the Intestinal Surface: Catecholamines and Mucosa-Bacteria Interactions," *Cell and Tissue Research* 343, no. 1 (Jan. 2011): 23–32, doi:10.1007/s00441-010-1050-0.

20. Robin C. Spiller, "Hidden Dangers of Antibiotic Use: Increased Gut Permeability Mediated by Increased Pancreatic Proteases Reaching the Colon," *Cellular and Molecular Gastroenterology and Hepatology* 6, no. 3 (July 2018): 347–48.e1, doi:10.1016/j.jcmgh.2018.06.005.

21. Hamed Khalili, "Risk of Inflammatory Bowel Disease with Oral Contraceptives and Menopausal Hormone Therapy: Current Evidence and Future Directions," *Drug Safety* 39, no. 3 (March 2016): 193–97, doi:10.1007/s40264-015-0372-y.

22. Sharon L. Achilles and Sharon L. Hillier, "The Complexity of Contraceptives: Understanding Their Impact on Genital Immune Cells and Vaginal Microbiota," *AIDS* 27, suppl. 1 (Oct. 2013): S5–15, doi:10.1097/QAD.0000000000000058.

23. Deepshika Ramanan and Ken Cadwell, "Intrinsic Defense Mechanisms of the Intestinal Epithelium," *Cell Host & Microbe* 19, no. 4 (March 2016), 434–441, doi:10.1016/j.chom.2016.03.003.

24. Nazanin Samadi et al., "The Role of Gastrointestinal Permeability in Food Allergy," *Annals of Allergy, Asthma and Immunology* 121, no. 2 (Aug. 2018): 168–73, doi:10.1016/j.anai.2018.05.010.

25. Qinghui Mu et al., "Leaky Gut as a Danger Signal for Autoimmune Diseases," *Frontiers in Immunology* 8 (May 2017): 598, doi:10.3389/fimmu.2017.00598.

26. Bischoff et al., "Intestinal Permeability: A New Target for Disease Prevention and Therapy," 189.

27. John R. Kelly et al., "Breaking Down the Barriers: The Gut Microbiome, Intestinal Permeability and Stress-Related Psychiatric Disorders," *Frontiers in Cellular Neuroscience* 9 (Oct. 2015): 392, doi:10.3389/fncel.2015.00392.

28. M. G. Clemente et al., "Early Effects of Gliadin on Enterocyte Intracellular Signalling Involved in Intestinal Barrier Function," *Gut* 52, no. 2 (Feb. 2003): 218–23, doi:10.1136/gut.52.2.218.

29. Faraz Bishehsari et al., "Alcohol and Gut-Derived Inflammation," *Alcohol Research: Current Reviews* 38, no. 2 (2017): 163–71.

30. Hamed Khalili et al., "Association Between Long-Term Oral Contraceptive Use and Risk of Crohn's Disease Complications in a Nationwide Study," *Gastroenterology* 150, no. 7 (June 2016): 1561–67.e1, doi:10.1053/j.gastro.2016.02.041.

31. Spiller, "Hidden Dangers of Antibiotic Use," 347–48.e1.

32. Erika Utzeri and Paolo Usai, "Role of Non-steroidal Anti-inflammatory Drugs on Intestinal Permeability and Nonalcoholic Fatty Liver Disease," *World Journal of Gastroenterology* 23, no. 22 (June 2017): 3954–63, doi:10.3748/wjg.v23.i22.3954.

33. Qixing Mao et al., "The Ramazzini Institute 13-Week Pilot Study on Glyphosate and Roundup Administered at Human-Equivalent Dose to Sprague Dawley Rats: Effects on the Microbiome," *Environmental Health: A Global Access Science Source* 17 (May 2018): 50, doi:10.1186/s12940-018-0394-x; Veronica L. Lozano et al., "Sex-Dependent Impact of Roundup on the Rat Gut Microbiome," *Toxicology Reports* 5 (2018): 96–107, doi:10.1016/j.toxrep.2017.12.005; Yassine Aitbali et al., "Glyphosate-Based Herbicide Exposure Affects Gut Microbiota, Anxiety and Depression-Like Behaviors in Mice," *Neurotoxicology and Teratology* 67 (May–June 2018): 44–49, doi:10.1016/j.ntt.2018.04.002.

34. Plottel and Blaser, "Microbiome and Malignancy," 324–35.

35. R. Flores et al., "Fecal Microbial Determinants of Fecal and Systemic Oestrogens and Oestrogen Metabolites: A Cross-Sectional Study," *Journal of Translational Medicine* 10 (Dec. 2012): 253, doi:10.1186/1479-5876-10-253.

36. Baker et al., "Estrogen–Gut Microbiome Axis: Physiological and Clinical Implications," 45–53.

37. Boulangé et al., "Impact of the Gut Microbiota on Inflammation, Obesity, and Metabolic Disease," 42.

38. F. Magata et al., "Lipopolysaccharide in Ovarian Follicular Fluid Influences the Steroid Production in Large Follicles of Dairy Cows," *Animal Reproduction Science* 144, no. 1–2 (Jan. 2014): 6–13, doi:10.1016/j.anireprosci.2013.11.005; E. J. Williams et al., "The Effect of Escherichia Coli Lipopolysaccharide and Tumour Necrosis Factor Alpha on Ovarian Function," *American Journal of Reproductive Immunology* 60, no. 5 (Nov. 2008): 462–73; K. Tremellen et al., "Metabolic Endotoxemia—A Potential Novel Link Between Ovarian Inflammation and Impaired Progesterone Production," *Gynecological Endocrinology* 31, no. 4 (2015): 309–12.

39. K. M. Lammers et al., "Gliadin Induces an Increase in Intestinal Permeability and Zonulin Release by Binding to the Chemokine Receptor CXCR3," *Gastroenterology* 135, no. 1 (July 2008): 194–204.e3, doi:10.1053/j.gastro.2008.03.023.

40. Prashant Singh et al., "Global Prevalence of Celiac Disease: Systematic Review and Meta-analysis," *Clinical Gastroenterology and Hepatology* 16, no. 6 (June 2018): 823–36, doi:10.1016/j.cgh.2017.06.037.

41. Catalina Ortiz et al., "Celiac Disease, Non-celiac Gluten Sensitivity and Wheat Allergy: Comparison of 3 Different Diseases Triggered by the Same Food," *Revista Chilena de Pediatría* 88, no. 3 (June 2017): 417–23, doi:10 .4067/S0370-41062017000300017.

42. Ilaria Parzanese et al., "Celiac Disease: From Pathophysiology to Treatment," *World Journal of Gastrointestinal Pathophysiology* 8, no. 2 (May 2017): 27–38, doi:10.4291/wjgp.v8.i2.27.

43. Janet M. Choi et al., "Increased Prevalence of Celiac Disease in Patients with Unexplained Infertility in the United States," *The Journal of Reproductive Medicine* 56, no. 5–6 (May–June 2011): 199–203.

44. Hugh-James Freeman, "Reproductive Changes Associated with Celiac Disease," *World Journal of Gastroenterology* 16, no. 46 (Dec. 2010): 5810– 14, doi:10.3748/wjg.v16.i46.5810; A. S. Khashan et al., "The Impact of Maternal Celiac Disease on Birthweight and Preterm Birth: A Danish Population-Based Cohort Study," *Human Reproduction* 25, no. 2 (Feb. 2010): 528–34, doi:10.1093/humrep/dep409.

45. Hilary Jericho and Stefano Guandalini, "Extra-intestinal Manifestation of Celiac Disease in Children," *Nutrients* 10, no. 6 (June 2018): 755, doi:10.3390/nu10060755.

46. Choi et al., "Increased Prevalence of Celiac Disease in Patients with Unexplained Infertility in the United States," 199–203.

47. Javier Barbuzano, "Understanding How the Intestine Replaces and Repairs Itself," *Harvard Gazette.* Last modified June 13, 2019. https://news .harvard.edu/gazette/story/2017/07/understanding-how-the-intestine -replaces-and-repairs-itself/.

48. Rahul Mittal et al., "Neurotransmitters: The Critical Modulators Regulating Gut-Brain Axis," *Journal of Cellular Physiology* 232, no. 9 (Sept. 2017): 2359–72, doi:10.1002/jcp.25518.

49. Marilia Carabotti et al., "The Gut-Brain Axis: Interactions Between Enteric Microbiota, Central and Enteric Nervous Systems," *Annals of Gastroenterology* 28, no. 2 (April–June 2015): 203–9.

50. Mittal et al., "Neurotransmitters: The Critical Modulators Regulating Gut-Brain Axis," 2359–72.

51. Tamaki Matsumoto, Takahisa Ushiroyama, Tetsuya Kimura, Tatsuya-Hayashi, and Toshio Moritani, "Altered Autonomic Nervous System Activity as a Potential Etiological Factor of Premenstrual Syndrome and Premenstrual Dysphoric Disorder," *BioPsychoSocial Medicine* 1, no. 1 (Dec. 2007), 24, doi:10.1186/1751-0759-1-24.

52. C. Park et al., "Probiotics for the Treatment of Depressive Symptoms: An Anti-inflammatory Mechanism?," *Brain, Behavior, and Immunity* 73 (Oct. 2018): 115–24, doi:10.1016/j.bbi.2018.07.006.

53. V. H. Eisenberg et al., "Is There an Association Between Autoimmunity and Endometriosis?," *Autoimmunity Reviews* 11, no. 11 (Sept. 2012): 806–14, doi:10.1016/j.autrev.2012.01.005.

54. K. N. Khan et al., "17β-Estradiol and Lipopolysaccharide Additively Promote Pelvic Inflammation and Growth of Endometriosis," *Reproductive Sciences* 22, no. 5 (May 2015): 585–94, doi:10.1177/1933719114556487.

55. J. R. Mathias et al., "Relation of Endometriosis and Neuromuscular Disease of the Gastrointestinal Tract: New Insights," *Fertility and Sterility* 70, no. 1 (July 1998): 81–88, doi:10.1016/s0015-0282(98)00096-x; M. W. Laschke et al., "The Gut Microbiota: A Puppet Master in the Pathogenesis of Endometriosis?," *American Journal of Obstetrics and Gynecology* 215, no. 1 (July 2016): 68e1–4, doi:10.1016/j.ajog.2016.02.036.

56. Laschke et al., "The Gut Microbiota," 68e1–4.

57. N. C. Polpeta et al., "Clinical and Therapeutic Aspects of Vulvodynia: The Importance of Physical Therapy," *Minerva Ginecologica* 64, no. 5 (Oct. 2012): 437–45.

58. L. A. Sadownik, "Etiology, Diagnosis, and Clinical Management of Vulvodynia," *International Journal of Women's Health* 6 (May 2014): 437–39, doi:10.2147/IJWH.S37660.

59. Laura Maintz and Natalija Novak, "Histamine and Histamine Intolerance," *The American Journal of Clinical Nutrition* 85, no. 5 (May 2007): 1185–96, doi:10.1093/ajcn/85.5.1185.

60. T. H. Zhu et al., "Estrogen Is an Important Mediator of Mast Cell Activation in Ovarian Endometriomas," *Reproduction* 155, no. 1 (Jan. 2016): 73–83, doi:10.1530/REP-17-0457; D. Kempuraj et al., "Increased Numbers of Activated Mast Cells in Endometriosis Lesions Positive for Corticotropin-Releasing Hormone and Urocortin," *American Journal of Reproductive Immunology* 52, no. 4 (2004): 267–75, doi:10.1111/j.1600-0897.2004.00224.x.

61. V. Anaf et al., "Pain, Mast Cells, and Nerves in Peritoneal, Ovarian, and Deep Infiltrating Endometriosis," *Fertility and Sterility* 86, no. 5 (Nov. 2006): 1336–43, doi:10.1016/j.fertnstert.2006.03.057.

62. Lawrence B. Afrin et al., "Successful Mast-Cell-Targeted Treatment of Chronic Dyspareunia, Vaginitis, and Dysfunctional Uterine Bleeding," *Journal of Obstetrics and Gynaecology* 39, no. 5 (July 2019): 664–69.

63. M. M. Binda et al., "Targeting Mast Cells: A New Way to Treat Endometriosis," *Expert Opinion on Therapeutic Targets* 21, no. 1 (Jan. 2017): 67–75, doi:10.1080/14728222.2017.1260548.

64. M. Gajdacs et al., "Resistance Levels and Epidemiology of Non-fermenting Gram-Negative Bacteria in Urinary Tract Infections of Inpatients and Outpatients (RENFUTI): A 10-Year Epidemiological Snapshot," *Antibiotics* (Basel) 8, no. 3 (Sept. 2019): ii, E143, doi:10.3390/antibiotics8030143.

65. N. Paalanne et al., "Intestinal Microbiome as a Risk Factor for Urinary Tract Infections in Children," *European Journal of Clinical Microbiology and Infectious Diseases* 37, no. 10 (Oct. 2018): 1881–91, doi:10.1007/s10096-018-3322-7.

66. Yulan Liu et al., "Therapeutic Potential of Amino Acids in Inflammatory Bowel Disease," *Nutrients* 9, no. 9 (Aug. 2017): 920, doi:10.3390/nu9090920; L. R. Lopetuso et al., "The Therapeutic Management of Gut Barrier Leaking: The Emerging Role for Mucosal Barrier Protectors," *European Review for Medical and Pharmacological Sciences* 19, no. 6 (2015): 1066–76.

7 Week Four: Love Up Your Liver

1. Institute of Medicine, "The Challenge: Chemicals in Today's Society," chap. 2 in *Identifying and Reducing Environmental Health Risks of Chemicals in Our Society: Workshop Summary* (Washington, DC: National Academies Press, 2014).

2. A. Correa et al., "Ethylene Glycol Ethers and Risks of Spontaneous Abortion and Subfertility," *American Journal of Epidemiology* 143, no. 7 (April 1996): 707–17, doi:10.1093/oxfordjournals.aje.a008804; Pau-Chung Chen et al., "Prolonged Time to Pregnancy in Female Workers Exposed to Ethylene Glycol Ethers in Semiconductor Manufacturing," *Epidemiology* 13, no. 2 (2002): 191–96, http://www.jstor.org/stable/3703912.

3. Lisa M. Weatherly and Julie A. Gosse, "Triclosan Exposure, Transformation, and Human Health Effects," *Journal of Toxicology and Environmental*

Health, Part B: Critical Reviews 20, no. 8 (2017): 447–69, doi:10.1080/1093 7404.2017.1399306.

4.   Xin-Yuan Cao et al., "Impact of Triclosan on Female Reproduction Through Reducing Thyroid Hormones to Suppress Hypothalamic Kisspeptin Neurons in Mice," *Frontiers in Molecular Neuroscience* 19 (Jan. 2018), doi:10.3389/fnmol.2018.00006.

5.   Roger T. Engeli et al., "Interference of Paraben Compounds with Oestrogen Metabolism by Inhibition of 17β-Hydroxysteroid Dehydrogenases," *International Journal of Molecular Sciences* 18, no. 9 (Sept. 2017): 2007, doi: 10.3390/ijms18092007.

6.   John D. Meeker et al., "Phthalates and Other Additives in Plastics: Human Exposure and Associated Health Outcomes," *Philosophical Transactions of the Royal Society of London: Series B, Biological Sciences* 364, no. 1526 (July 2009): 2097–113, doi:10.1098/rstb.2008.0268; Sailas Benjamin et al., "Phthalates Impact Human Health: Epidemiological Evidences and Plausible Mechanism of Action," *Journal of Hazardous Materials* 340 (Oct. 2017): 360–83, doi:10.1016/j.jhazmat.2017.06.036; Lauren E. Parlett et al., "Women's Exposure to Phthalates in Relation to Use of Personal Care Products," *Journal of Exposure Science and Environmental Epidemiology* 23, no. 2 (March 2013): 197–206, doi:10.1038/jes.2012.105.

7.   Tatsuya Kunisue et al., "Urinary Concentrations of Benzophenone-Type UV Filters in U.S. Women and Their Association with Endometriosis," *Environmental Science and Technology* 46, no. 8 (March 2012): 4624–32, doi: 10.1021/es204415a.

8.   Mehmet Demır et al., "Effects of Acute Toluene Toxicity on Different Regions of Rabbit Brain," *Analytical Cellular Pathology* 2017 (March 2017): 2805370, doi:10.1155/2017/2805370.

9.   "Dioxins and Their Effects on Human Health," World Health Organization, Oct. 4, 2016, https://www.who.int/en/news-room/fact-sheets/detail /dioxins-and-their-effects-on-human-health.

10. "Dioxins and Their Effects on Human Health," World Health Organization.

11. A. Venerosi et al., "Sex Dimorphic Behaviors as Markers of Neuroendocrine Disruption by Environmental Chemicals: The Case of Chlorpyrifos," *NeuroToxicology* 33, no. 6 (Dec. 2012): 1420–26, doi:10.1016/j. neuro.2012.08.009; T. A. Slotkin, "Does Early-Life Exposure to Organophosphate Insecticides Lead to Prediabetes and Obesity?," *Reproductive Toxicology* 31, no. 3 (April 2011): 297–301, doi:10.1016/j.reprotox.2010.07.012.

12. Tyrone B. Hayes et al., "Atrazine Induces Complete Feminization and Chemical Castration in Male African Clawed Frogs (Xenopus Laevis)," *Proceedings of the National Academy of Sciences* 107, no. 10 (March 2010): 4612–17.

13. R. L. Cooper et al., "Atrazine and Reproductive Function: Mode and Mechanism of Action Studies," *Birth Defects Research, Part B: Developmental and Reproductive Toxicology* 80, no. 2 (April 2007): 96–112, doi:10.1002 /bdrb.20110; N. Benachour et al., "Cytotoxic Effects and Aromatase Inhibition by Xenobiotic Endocrine Disrupters Alone and in Combination," *Toxicology and Applied Pharmacology* 222, no. 2 (July 2007): 129–40, doi:10.1016/j .taap.2007.03.033; Tyrone B. Hayes, "There Is No Denying This: Defusing the Confusion About Atrazine," *BioScience* 54, no. 12 (Dec. 2004): 1138–49, doi:10.1641/0006-3568(2004)054[1138:TINDTD]2.0.CO;2.

14. Laura N. Vandenberg et al., "Hormones and Endocrine-Disrupting Chemicals: Low-Dose Effects and Nonmonotonic Dose Responses," *Endocrine Reviews* 33, no. 3 (June 2012): 378–455, doi:10.1210/er.2011-1050.

15. P. Connett, "50 Reasons to Oppose Fluoridation," *Medical Veritas* 1 (2004): 70–80, doi:10.1588/medver.2004.01.00014.

16. Tolga Unüvar and Atilla Büyükgebiz, "Fetal and Neonatal Endocrine Disruptors," *Journal of Clinical Research in Pediatric Endocrinology* 4, no. 2 (June 2012): 51–60, doi:10.4274/jcrpe.569.

17. Paloma Alonso-Magdalena et al., "The Oestrogenic Effect of Bisphenol A Disrupts Pancreatic β-Cell Function *In Vivo* and Induces Insulin Resistance," *Environmental Health Perspectives* 114, no. 1 (Jan. 2006): 106–12, doi:10.1289/ehp.8451; Mauri José Piazza and Almir Antônio Urbanetz, "Environmental Toxins and the Impact of Other Endocrine Disrupting Chemicals in Women's Reproductive Health," *JBRA Assisted Reproduction* 23, no. 2 (April 2019): 154–64, doi:10.5935/1518-0557.20190016; Vandenberg et al., "Hormones and Endocrine-Disrupting Chemicals," 378–455.

18. Monika Rönn et al., "Bisphenol A Is Related to Circulating Levels of Adiponectin, Leptin and Ghrelin, but Not to Fat Mass or Fat Distribution in Humans," *Chemosphere* 112 (Oct. 2014): 42–48, doi:10.1016/j.chemo sphere.2014.03.042.

19. B. S. Rubin et al., "The Case for BPA as an Obesogen: Contributors to the Controversy," *Frontiers in Endocrinology* 10 (Feb. 2019): 30, doi:10.3389 /fendo.2019.00030.

20. Patricia A. Hunt et al., "Bisphenol A Alters Early Oogenesis and Follicle Formation in the Fetal Ovary of the Rhesus Monkey," *Proceedings of the*

National Academy of Sciences 109, no. 43 (Oct. 2012): 17525–30, doi:10.1073/pnas.1207854109.

21. Jackye Peretz et al., "Bisphenol A Impairs Follicle Growth, Inhibits Steroidogenesis, and Downregulates Rate-Limiting Enzymes in the Estradiol Biosynthesis Pathway," *Toxicological Sciences* 119, no. 1 (Jan. 2011): 209–17, doi:10.1093/toxsci/kfq319.

22. Wei Wang et al., "In Utero Bisphenol A Exposure Disrupts Germ Cell Nest Breakdown and Reduces Fertility with Age in the Mouse," *Toxicology and Applied Pharmacology* 276, no. 2 (April 2014): 157–64, doi:10.1016/j.taap.2014.02.009.

23. M. S. Kurzer and X. Xu, "Dietary Phytoestrogens," *Annual Review of Nutrition* 17 (July 1997): 353–81, doi:10.1146/annurev.nutr.17.1.353.

24. F. Branca and S. Lorenzetti, "Health Effects of Phytoestrogens," *Forum of Nutrition* 57 (2005): 100–11; M. Bryant et al., "Effect of Consumption of Soy Isoflavones on Behavioural, Somatic and Affective Symptoms in Women with Premenstrual Syndrome," *British Journal of Nutrition* 93, no. 5 (May 2005): 731–39, doi:10.1079/bjn20041396.

25. W. R. Phipps et al., "Effect of Flax Seed Ingestion on the Menstrual Cycle," *The Journal of Clinical Endocrinology and Metabolism* 77, no. 5 (Nov. 1993): 1215–19, doi:10.1210/jcem.77.5.8077314.

26. Ivonee M. C. M. Rietjens et al., "The Potential Health Effects of Dietary Phytoestrogens," *British Journal of Pharmacology* 174, no. 11 (June 2017): 1263–80, doi:10.1111/bph.13622.

27. Bryant et al., "Effect of Consumption of Soy Isoflavones on Behavioural, Somatic and Affective Symptoms in Women with Premenstrual Syndrome," 731–39.

28. Margaret E. Sears et al., "Arsenic, Cadmium, Lead, and Mercury in Sweat: A Systematic Review," *Journal of Environmental and Public Health* 2012 (2012): 184745, doi:10.1155/2012/184745.

29. Xinsheng Gu and Jose E. Manautou, "Molecular Mechanisms Underlying Chemical Liver Injury," *Expert Reviews in Molecular Medicine* 14 (Feb. 2012): e4, doi:10.1017/S1462399411002110.

30. Erin Jackson et al., "Adipose Tissue as a Site of Toxin Accumulation," *Comprehensive Physiology* 7, no. 4 (Sept. 2017): 1085–135, doi:10.1002/cphy.c160038.

31. Samavat H. Kurzer MS, "Estrogen Metabolism and Breast Cancer," *Cancer Lett.* 2015;356:231–43, doi:10.1016/j.canlet.2014.04.018.

32. Ercole L. Cavalieri and Eleanor G. Rogan, "Depurinating Oestrogen-DNA Adducts, Generators of Cancer Initiation: Their Minimization Leads to Cancer Prevention," *Clinical and Translational Medicine* 5, no. 1 (March 2016): 12, doi:10.1186/s40169-016-0088-3.

33. Hamed Samavat and Mindy S. Kurzer, "Estrogen Metabolism and Breast Cancer," *Cancer Letters* 356, no. 2, part A (Jan. 2015): 231–43, doi:10.1016/j.canlet.2014.04.018.

34. N. J. Lakhani, M/ A. Sarkar, J. Venitz, W. D. Figg, "2-Methoxyestradiol, A Promising Anticancer Agent," *Pharmacotherapy* 23 (2003), 165–72. 10.1592/phco.23.2.165.32088.

35. James D. Yager, "Catechol-O-Methyltransferase: Characteristics, Polymorphisms and Role in Breast Cancer," *Drug Discovery Today: Disease Mechanisms* 9, no. 1–2 (June 2012), e41-e46. doi:10.1016/j.ddmec.2012.10.002; C. Worda, "Influence of the Catechol-O-Methyltransferase (COMT) Codon 158 Polymorphism on Oestrogen Levels in Women," *Human Reproduction* 18, no. 2 (Feb. 2003), 262–66, doi:10.1093/humrep/deg059.

36. B. Regland et al., "Increased Concentrations of Homocysteine in the Cerebrospinal Fluid in Patients with Fibromyalgia and Chronic Fatigue Syndrome," *Scandinavian Journal of Rheumatology* 26, no. 4 (1997): 301–7, doi:10.3109/03009749709105320; Nebojsa Knezevic, Tatiana Tverdohleb, Ivana Knezevic, and Kenneth Candido, "The Role of Genetic Polymorphisms in Chronic Pain Patients," *International Journal of Molecular Sciences* 19, no. 6 (June 2018), 1707, doi:10.3390/ijms19061707.

37. R. Mukhopadhyay et al., "*MTHFR C677T* and *Factor V Leiden* in Recurrent Pregnancy Loss: A Study Among an Endogamous Group in North India," *Genetic Testing and Molecular Biomarkers* 13, no. 6 (Dec. 2009): 861–65, doi:10.1089/gtmb.2009.0063; María del Rosario Rodríguez-Guillén et al., "Maternal MTHFR Polymorphisms and Risk of Spontaneous Abortion," *Salud Pública de México* 51, no. 1 (Jan.–Feb. 2009): 19–25.

38. "Non-alcoholic Fatty Liver Disease," Genetics Home Reference, https://ghr.nlm.nih.gov/condition/non-alcoholic-fatty-liver-disease#statistics.

39. Nancy Vargas-Mendoza et al., "Hepatoprotective Effect of Silymarin," *World Journal of Hepatology* 6, no. 3 (March 2014): 144–49, doi:10.4254/wjh.v6.i3.144.

8 Week Five: Stress Hacks in the Age of Chronic Overstimulation

1. Chaojuan Zhu et al., "Exogenous Melatonin in the Treatment of Pain: A Systematic Review and Meta-analysis," *Oncotarget* 8, no. 59 (Oct. 2017): 100582–92, doi:10.18632/oncotarget.21504.

2. Shechter and Boivin, "Sleep, Hormones, and Circadian Rhythms Through-out the Menstrual Cycle in Healthy Women and Women with Premen-strual Dysphoric Disorder," 259345; Jacqueline D. Kloss et al., "Sleep, Sleep Disturbance, and Fertility in Women," *Sleep Medicine Reviews* 22 (Aug. 2015): 78–87, doi:10.1016/j.smrv.2014.10.005.

3. M. Attarchi et al., "Characteristics of Menstrual Cycle in Shift Workers," *Global Journal of Health Science* 5, no. 3 (Feb. 2013): 163–72, doi:10.5539 /gjhs.v5n3p163; C. C. Lawson et al., "Rotating Shift Work and Men-strual Cycle Characteristics," *Epidemiology* 22, no. 3 (May 2011): 305–12, doi:10.1097/EDE.0b013e3182130016.

4. Hiroshi Tamura et al., "The Role of Melatonin as an Antioxidant in the Fol-licle," *Journal of Ovarian Research* 5 (Jan. 2012): 5, doi:10.1186/1757-2215-5-5.

5. Kloss et al., "Sleep, Sleep Disturbance, and Fertility in Women," 78–87.

6. S. Whirledge and J. A. Cidlowski, "Glucocorticoids, Stress, and Fertility," *Minerva Endocrinologica* 35, no. 2 (2010): 109–25.

7. C. Tsigos and G. P. Chrousos, "Hypothalamic–Pituitary–Adrenal Axis, Neuroendocrine Factors and Stress," *Journal of Psychosomatic Research* 53, no. 4 (Oct. 2002): 865–71, doi:10.1016/s0022-3999(02)00429-4; D. Toufexis et al., "Stress and the Reproductive Axis," *Journal of Neuroendocrinology* 26, no. 9 (Sept. 2014): 573–86, doi:10.1111/jne.12179.

8. J. R. Roney and Z. L. Simmons, "Elevated Psychological Stress Predicts Reduced Estradiol Concentrations in Young Women," *Adaptive Human Be-havior and Physiology* 1, no. 30 (March 2015): 30–40, doi:10.1007/s40750 -014-0004-2.

9. Whirledge and Cidlowski, "Glucocorticoids, Stress, and Fertility," 109–25.

10. A. E. Michael et al., "Direct Inhibition of Ovarian Steroidogenesis by Cor-tisol and the Modulatory Role of 11 β-Hydroxysteroid Dehydrogenase," *Clinical Endocrinology* 38, no. 6 (June 1993): 641–44, doi:10.1111/j.1365 -2265.1993.tb02147.x.

11. Michael et al., "Direct Inhibition of Ovarian Steroidogenesis by Cortisol and the Modulatory Role of 11 β-Hydroxysteroid Dehydrogenase," 641–44; Tsigos and Chrousos, "Hypothalamic–Pituitary–Adrenal Axis, Neuro-endocrine Factors and Stress," 865–71.

12. Joyce C. L. Leo et al., "Glucocorticoid and Mineralocorticoid Cross-Talk with Progesterone Receptor to Induce Focal Adhesion and Growth In-hibition in Breast Cancer Cells," *Endocrinology* 145, no. 3 (March 2004): 1314–21, https://doi.org/10.1210/en.2003-0732.

13. P. Jimena et al., "Adrenal Hormones in Human Follicular Fluid," *Acta Endocrinologica* (Copenhagen) 127, no. 5 (Nov. 1992): 403–6, doi:10.1530 /acta.0.1270403.

14. Tsigos and Chrousos, "Hypothalamic–Pituitary–Adrenal Axis, Neuroendocrine Factors and Stress," 865–71.

15. Ibid.

16. R. Kadiyala et al., "Thyroid Dysfunction in Patients with Diabetes: Clinical Implications and Screening Strategies," *The International Journal of Clinical Practice* 64, no. 8 (July 2010): 1130–39, doi:10.1111/j.1742 -1241.2010.02376.x.

17. Alexandru Tatomir et al., "The Impact of Stress and Glucocorticoids on Memory," *Clujul Medical* 87, no. 1 (Jan. 2014): 3–6, doi:10.15386/cjm .2014.8872.871.at1cm2; Panagiotis Anagnostis et al., "The Pathogenetic Role of Cortisol in the Metabolic Syndrome: A Hypothesis," *The Journal of Clinical Endocrinology and Metabolism* 94, no. 8 (Aug. 2009): 2692–701, doi:10.1210/jc.2009-0370.

18. Kelly et al., "Breaking Down the Barriers," 392.

19. S. E. Taylor et al., "Biobehavioral Responses to Stress in Females: Tend-and-Befriend, Not Fight-or-Flight," *Psychological Review* 107, no. 3 (July 2000): 411–29, http://dx.doi.org/10.1037/0033-295X.107.3.411.

20. Daniel J. Powell and Wolff Schlotz, "Daily Life Stress and the Cortisol Awakening Response: Testing the Anticipation Hypothesis," *PlOS One* 7, no. 12 (Dec. 2012): e52067, doi:10.1371/journal.pone.0052067.

21. Powell and Schlotz, "Daily Life Stress and the Cortisol Awakening Response," e52067.

22. James L. Oschman et al., "The Effects of Grounding (Earthing) on Inflammation, the Immune Response, Wound Healing, and Prevention and Treatment of Chronic Inflammatory and Autoimmune Diseases," *Journal of Inflammation Research* 8 (March 2015): 83–96, doi:10.2147/ JIR.S69656; Gaétan Chevalier et al., "Earthing: Health Implications of Reconnecting the Human Body to the Earth's Surface Electrons," *Journal of Environmental and Public Health* 2012 (Jan. 2012): 291541, doi:10.1155/2012/291541.

23. Chevalier et al., "Earthing: Health Implications of Reconnecting the Human Body to the Earth's Surface Electrons," 291541.

24. M. H. Smolensky et al., "Circadian Disruption: New Clinical Perspective of Disease Pathology and Basis for Chronotherapeutic Intervention,"

Chronobiology International 33, no. 8 (2016): 1101–19, doi:10.1080/0742052
8.2016.1184678.

25. M. Kayaba et al., "The Effect of Nocturnal Blue Light Exposure from Light-Emitting Diodes on Wakefulness and Energy Metabolism the Following Morning," *Environmental Health and Preventive Medicine* 19, no. 5 (Sept. 2014): 354–61, doi:10.1007/s12199-014-0402-x.

26. Paul D. Loprinzi and Bradley J. Cardinal, "Association Between Objectively Measured Physical Activity and Sleep, NHANES 2005–2006," *Mental Health and Physical Activity* 4, no. 2 (Dec. 2011): 65–69, doi:10.1016/j.mhpa.2011.08.001; L. Larun et al., "Exercise Therapy for Chronic Fatigue Syndrome," *Cochrane Database of Systematic Reviews* 12 (Dec. 2016): CD003200, doi:10.1002/14651858.CD003200.pub6.

27. I. O. Ebrahim et al., "Alcohol and Sleep I: Effects on Normal Sleep," *Alcoholism: Clinical and Experimental Research* 37, no. 4 (April 2013): 539–49, doi:10.1111/acer.12006.

9   Week Six: Support Your Thyroid for Healthier Periods

1. M. P. J. Vanderpump et al., "'The Incidence of Thyroid Disorders in the Community: A Twenty-Year Follow-Up of the Whickham Survey," *Clinical Endocrinology* 43, no. 1 (July 1995): 55–68, doi:10.1111/j.1365-2265.1995.tb01894.x.

2. Koutras, "Disturbances of Menstruation in Thyroid Disease," 280–84.

3. Ibid.

4. Ibid.

5. J. B. Rugge et al., "Screening and Treatment of Thyroid Dysfunction: An Evidence Review for the U.S. Preventive Services Task Force," *Annals of Internal Medicine* 162, no. 1 (Jan. 2015): 35–45, doi:10.7326/M14-1456.

6. Vahab Fatourechi, "Subclinical Hypothyroidism: An Update for Primary Care Physicians," *Mayo Clinic Proceedings* 84, no. 1 (Jan. 2009): 65–71, doi:10.1016/S0025-6196(11)60809-4.

7. J. S. Fedail et al., "Roles of Thyroid Hormones in Follicular Development in the Ovary of Neonatal and Immature Rats," *Endocrine* 46, no. 3 (Aug. 2014): 594–604, doi:10.1007/s12020-013-0092-y.

8. K. Poppe et al., "Thyroid Disease and Female Reproduction," *Clinical Endocrinology* 66, no. 3 (March 2007): 309–21, doi:10.1111/j.1365-2265.2007.02752.x.

9. J. Rodríguez-Castelán et al., "Hypothyroidism Reduces the Size of Ovarian Follicles and Promotes Hypertrophy of Periovarian Fat with Infiltration of Macrophages in Adult Rabbits," *BioMed Research International* 2017 (2017): 3795950, doi:10.1155/2017/3795950.

10. M. Gierach et al., "Insulin Resistance and Thyroid Disorders," *Endokrynologia Polska* 65, no. 1 (2014): 70–76, doi:10.5603/EP.2014.0010.

11. Qun Yu and Jin-Bei Wang, "Subclinical Hypothyroidism in PCOS: Impact on Presentation, Insulin Resistance, and Cardiovascular Risk," *BioMed Research International* 2016 (2016): 2067087, doi:10.1155/2016/2067087.

12. David M. Selva et al., "Thyroid Hormones Act Indirectly to Increase Sex Hormone-Binding Globulin Production by Liver via Hepatocyte Nuclear Factor-4α," *Journal of Molecular Endocrinology* 43, no. 1 (July 2009): 19–27, doi:10.1677/JME-09-0025.

13. S. C. Dumoulin et al., "Opposite Effects of Thyroid Hormones on Binding Proteins for Steroid Hormones (Sex Hormone-Binding Globulin and Corticosteroid-Binding Globulin) in Humans," *European Journal of Endocrinology* 132, no. 5 (May 1995): 594–98, doi:10.1530/eje.0.1320594.

14. Amanda Jefferys et al., "Thyroid Dysfunction and Reproductive Health," *The Obstetrician and Gynaecologist* 17, no. 1 (2015): 39–45, https://doi.org/10.1111/tog.12161.

15. A. Squizzato et al., "Thyroid Dysfunction and Effects on Coagulation and Fibrinolysis: A Systematic Review," *The Journal of Clinical Endocrinology and Metabolism* 92, no. 7 (July 2007): 2415–20, doi:10.1210/jc.2007-0199; P. P. Vescovi et al., "The Spectrum of Coagulation Abnormalities in Thyroid Disorders," *Seminars in Thrombosis and Hemostasis* 37, no. 1 (Feb. 2011): 7–10, doi:10.1055/s-0030-1270065.

16. Miller, Elizabeth M. "The Reproductive Ecology of Iron in Women," *American Journal of Physical Anthropology* 159 (2016), 172–95, doi:10.1002/ajpa.22907.

17. W. C. Allan et al., "Maternal Thyroid Deficiency and Pregnancy Complications: Implications for Population Screening," *Journal of Medical Screening* 7, no. 3 (2000): 127–30, doi:10.1136/jms.7.3.127.

18. A. Stagnaro-Green, "Overt Hyperthyroidism and Hypothyroidism During Pregnancy," *Clinical Obstetrics and Gynecology* 54, no. 3 (Sept. 2011): 478–87, doi:10.1097/GRF.0b013e3182272f32.

19. Yaron Tomer and Amanda Huber, "The Etiology of Autoimmune Thyroid Disease: A Story of Genes and Environment," *Journal of Autoimmunity* 32, no. 3–4 (May 2009): 231–39, doi:10.1016/j.jaut.2009.02.007.

20. María L. Vélez et al., "Bacterial Lipopolysaccharide Stimulates the Thyrotropin-Dependent Thyroglobulin Gene Expression at the Transcriptional Level by Involving the Transcription Factors Thyroid Transcription Factor-1 and Paired Box Domain Transcription Factor 8," *Endocrinology* 147, no. 7 (July 2006): 3260–75, http://doi.org/10.1210/en.2005-0789; K. Mori et al., "Does the Gut Microbiota Trigger Hashimoto's Thyroiditis?," *Discovery Medicine* 14, no. 78 (Nov. 2012): 321–26.

21. N. V. Yaglova, "Regulation of Thyroid and Pituitary Function by Bacterial Lipopolysaccharide," *Biomeditsinskaya Khimiya* 56 (Jan. 2010): 179–86, doi:10.18097/pbmc20105602179.

22. Ana Paula Santin and Tania Weber Furlanetto, "Role of Oestrogen in Thyroid Function and Growth Regulation," *Journal of Thyroid Research* 2011 (May 2011): 875125, doi:10.4061/2011/875125.

23. J. E. Gunton et al., "Iodine Deficiency in Ambulatory Participants at a Sydney Teaching Hospital: Is Australia Truly Iodine Replete?," *The Medical Journal of Australia* 171, no. 9 (Nov. 1999): 467–70.

24. Ryoko Katagiri et al., "Effect of Excess Iodine Intake on Thyroid Diseases in Different Populations: A Systematic Review and Meta-analyses Including Observational Studies," *PlOS One* 12, no. 3 (May 2017): e0173722, doi:10.1371/journal.pone.0173722.

25. Kimberly N. Walter et al., "Elevated Thyroid Stimulating Hormone Is Associated with Elevated Cortisol in Healthy Young Men and Women," *Thyroid Research* 5, no. 1 (2012): 13, https://doi.org/10.1186/1756-6614-5-13; Dana L. Helmreich et al., "Relation Between the Hypothalamic-Pituitary-Thyroid (HPT) Axis and the Hypothalamic-Pituitary-Adrenal (HPA) Axis During Repeated Stress," *Neuroendocrinology* 81, no. 3 (2005): 183–92, https://doi.org/10.1159/000087001.

26. Mary E. Turyk et al., "Relationships of Thyroid Hormones with Polychlorinated Biphenyls, Dioxins, Furans, and DDE in Adults," *Environmental Health Perspectives* 115, no. 8 (Aug. 2007): 1197–203, doi:10.1289/ehp.10179.

27. J. Wolff, "Perchlorate and the Thyroid Gland," *Pharmacological Reviews* 50, no. 1 (March 1998): 89–105.

28. Lisa Nainggolan, "Are Flame Retardants Driving Some of Thyroid Cancer Increase?," Medscape, April 1, 2017, https://www.medscape.com/viewarticle/878087.

29. Kenji Moriyama et al., "Thyroid Hormone Action Is Disrupted by Bisphenol A as an Antagonist," *The Journal of Clinical Endocrinology and Metabolism* 87, no. 11 (Nov. 2002): 5185–90, doi:10.1210/jc.2002-020209.

30. R. Thomas Zoeller, "Environmental Chemicals as Thyroid Hormone Analogues: New Studies Indicate that Thyroid Hormone Receptors Are Targets of Industrial Chemicals?," *Molecular and Cellular Endocrinology* 242 (2005): 10–15, http://citeseerx.ist.psu.edu/viewdoc/download?doi =10.1.1.326.6016&rep=rep1&type=pdf.

31. B. A. Jereczek-Fossa et al., "Radiotherapy-Induced Thyroid Disorders," *Cancer Treatment Reviews* 30, no. 4 (June 2004): 369–84, doi:10.1016/j .ctrv.2003.12.003.

32. M. A. Han et al., "Diagnostic X-Ray Exposure and Thyroid Cancer Risk: Systematic Review and Meta-analysis," *Thyroid* 28, no. 2 (Feb. 2018): 220– 28, doi:10.1089/thy.2017.0159.

33. Seyed Mortavazi et al., "Alterations in TSH and Thyroid Hormones Following Mobile Phone Use," *Oman Medical Journal* 24, no. 4 (Oct. 2009): 274–78, doi:10.5001/omj.2009.56.

34. Leanne M. Redman and Eric Ravussin, "Caloric Restriction in Humans: Impact on Physiological, Psychological, and Behavioral Outcomes," *Antioxidants & Redox Signaling* 14, no. 2 (January 2011), 75–87. doi:10.1089 /ars.2010.3253.

35. S. Fallah et al., "Effect of Contraceptive Pill on the Selenium and Zinc Status of Healthy Subjects," *Contraception* 80, no. 1 (July 2009): 40–43, doi:10.1016/j.contraception.2009.01.010.

36. Khalili, "Risk of Inflammatory Bowel Disease with Oral Contraceptives and Menopausal Hormone Therapy," 193–97.

37. Carolyn L. Westhoff et al., "Using Changes in Binding Globulins to Assess Oral Contraceptive Compliance," *Contraception* 87, no. 2 (Feb. 2013): 176–81, doi:10.1016/j.contraception.2012.06.003.

38. C. Sategna-Guidetti et al., "Prevalence of Thyroid Disorders in Untreated Adult Celiac Disease Patients and Effect of Gluten Withdrawal: An Italian Multicenter Study," *The American Journal of Gastroenterology* 96, no. 3 (March 2001): 751–57, doi:10.1111/j.1572-0241.2001.03617.x.

39. S. Nishiyama et al., "Zinc Supplementation Alters Thyroid Hormone Metabolism in Disabled Patients with Zinc Deficiency," *Journal of the American College of Nutrition* 13, no. 1 (1994): 62–67, https://doi.org/10.1080/073 15724.1994.10718373.

40. Mara Ventura et al., "Selenium and Thyroid Disease: From Pathophysiology to Treatment," *International Journal of Endocrinology* 2017 (2017): 1–9, https://doi.org/10.1155/2017/1297658.

41. Ronak Ghiya and Shema Ahmad, "SUN-591 Severe Iron-Deficiency Anemia Leading to Hypothyroidism," *Journal of the Endocrine Society* 3, suppl. 1 (April–May 2019), https://doi.org/10.1210/js.2019-sun-591.

42. Janet R. Hunt, "Bioavailability of Iron, Zinc, and Other Trace Minerals from Vegetarian Diets," *The American Journal of Clinical Nutrition* 78, no. 3 (Sep. 2003), 633S-39S, doi:10.1093/ajcn/78.3.633s.

43. Kunling Wang et al., "Severely Low Serum Magnesium Is Associated with Increased Risks of Positive Anti-thyroglobulin Antibody and Hypothyroidism: A Cross-Sectional Study," *Scientific Reports* 8, no. 1 (July 2, 2018), doi:10.1038/s41598-018-28362-5.

44. Mahdieh Abbasalizad Farhangi et al., "The Effect of Vitamin A Supplementation on Thyroid Function in Premenopausal Women," *Journal of the American College of Nutrition* 31, no. 4 (2012): 268–74. https://doi.org/10.10 80/07315724.2012.10720431; Julie Brossaud et al., "Vitamin A, Endocrine Tissues and Hormones: Interplay and Interactions," *Endocrine Connections* 6, no. 7 (Aug. 9, 2017): R121–30, doi:10.1530/EC-17-0101.

45. V. Rodrigo Mora et al., "Vitamin Effects on the Immune System: Vitamins A and D Take Centre Stage," *Nature Reviews: Immunology* 8, no. 9 (Sept. 2008): 685–98.

10 After the Six Weeks

1. Ethan Russo, "Cannabis Treatments in Obstetrics and Gynecology: A Historical Review," *Journal of Cannabis Therapeutics* 2, no. 3–4 (2002): 5–35, doi: 10.1300/J175v02n03_02.

2. O. S. Walker et al., "The Role of the Endocannabinoid System in Female Reproductive Tissues," *Journal of Ovarian Research* 12, no. 3 (2019), doi:10.1186 /s13048-018-0478-9; Jerome Bouaziz et al., "The Clinical Significance of Endocannabinoids in Endometriosis Pain Management," *Cannabis and Cannabinoid Research* 2, no. 1 (Dec. 2017), http://doi.org/10.1089/can.2016.0035.

3. Juliane Hellhammer et al., "A Soy-Based Phosphatidylserine/Phosphatidic Acid Complex (PAS) Normalizes the Stress Reactivity of Hypothalamus-Pituitary-Adrenal-Axis in Chronically Stressed Male Subjects: A Randomized, Placebo-Controlled Study," *Lipids in Health and Disease* 13 (July 31, 2014): 121, doi:10.1186/1476-511X-13-121.

4. David A. Camfield et al., "The Effects of Multivitamin Supplementation on Diurnal Cortisol Secretion and Perceived Stress," *Nutrients* 5, no. 11 (Nov. 2013): 4429–50, doi:10.3390/nu5114429.

5. Jaroenporn et al., "Effects of Pantothenic Acid Supplementation on Adrenal Steroid Secretion from Male Rats," 1205–8.

6. P. Patak et al., "Vitamin C Is an Important Cofactor for Both Adrenal Cortex and Adrenal Medulla," *Endocrine Research* 30, no. 4 (Nov. 2004): 871–75.

7. Hirofumi Henmi et al., "Effects of Ascorbic Acid Supplementation on Serum Progesterone Levels in Patients with a Luteal Phase Defect," *Fertility and Sterility* 80, no. 2 (Aug. 2003): 459–61, doi:10.1016/S0015-0282(03)00657-5.

8. Narendra Singh et al., "An Overview on Ashwagandha: A Rasayana (Rejuvenator) of Ayurveda," *African Journal of Traditional, Complementary, and Alternative Medicines* 8, suppl. 5 (2011): 208–13, doi:10.4314/ajtcam.v8i5S.9.

9. Case Adams, "Ashwagandha Can Treat More than 50 Medical Conditions," Heal Naturally, Feb. 5, 2013, http://www.realnatural.org/over-fifty-recent-studies-prove-ashwagandhas-potential-for-treating-a-myriad-of-conditions/.

10. Eric W. Manheimer et al., "Paleolithic Nutrition for Metabolic Syndrome: Systematic Review and Meta-analysis," *The American Journal of Clinical Nutrition* 102, no. 4 (Oct. 2015): 922–32, doi:10.3945/ajcn.115.113613; Ian Spreadbury, "Comparison with Ancestral Diets Suggests Dense Acellular Carbohydrates Promote an Inflammatory Microbiota, and May Be the Primary Dietary Cause of Leptin Resistance and Obesity," *Diabetes, Metabolic Syndrome and Obesity: Targets and Therapy* 5 (2012): 175–89, doi:10.2147/DMSO.S33473.

11. Vittorio Unfer et al., "Effects of Inositol(s) in Women with PCOS: A Systematic Review of Randomized Controlled Trials," *International Journal of Endocrinology* 2016 (2016): 1849162, doi:10.1155/2016/1849162.

12. M. Nordio and E. Proietti, "The Combined Therapy with Myo-inositol and D-chiro-inositol Reduces the Risk of Metabolic Disease in PCOS Overweight Patients Compared to Myo-inositol Supplementation Alone," *European Review for Medical and Pharmacological Sciences* 16, no. 5 (May 2012): 578–81.

13. C. Leigh Broadhurst and Philip Domenico, "Clinical Studies on Chromium Picolinate Supplementation in Diabetes Mellitus—A Review," *Diabetes Technology and Therapeutics* 8, no. 6 (Dec. 2006): 677–87.

14. M. Jamilian et al., "Effects of Zinc Supplementation on Endocrine Outcomes in Women with Polycystic Ovary Syndrome: A Randomized, Double-Blind, Placebo-Controlled Trial," *Biological Trace Element Research* 170, no. 2 (April 2016): 271–78, doi:10.1007/s12011-015-0480-7.

15. F. Foroozanfard et al., "Effects of Zinc Supplementation on Markers of Insulin Resistance and Lipid Profiles in Women with Polycystic Ovary Syndrome: A Randomized, Double-Blind, Placebo-Controlled Trial," *Experimental and Clinical Endocrinology and Diabetes* 123, no. 4 (April 2015): 215–20, doi:10.1055/s-0035-1548790.

16. Y. H. M. Krul-Poel et al., "Vitamin D and Metabolic Disturbances in Polycystic Ovary Syndrome (PCOS): A Cross-Sectional Study, " *PlOS One* 13, no. 12 (Dec. 4, 2018): e0204748, doi:10.1371/journal.pone.02 04748.

17. Ming-Wei Lin and Meng-Hsing Wu, "The Role of Vitamin D in Polycystic Ovary Syndrome," *The Indian Journal of Medical Research* 142, no. 3 (Sept. 2015): 238–40, doi:10.4103/0971-5916.166527.

18. Y. Zhang et al., "Curcumin Inhibits Endometriosis Endometrial Cells by Reducing Estradiol Production," *Iranian Journal of Reproductive Medicine* 11, no. 5 (May 2013): 415–22.

19. Maria Grazia Porpora et al., "A Promise in the Treatment of Endometriosis: An Observational Cohort Study on Ovarian Endometrioma Reduction by N-acetylcysteine," *Evidence-Based Complementary and Alternative Medicine* 2013 (2013): 240702, doi:10.1155/2013/240702.

20. Korosh Khanaki et al., "Evaluation of the Relationship Between Endometriosis and Omega-3 and Omega-6 Polyunsaturated Fatty Acids," *Iranian Biomedical Journal* 16, no. 1 (Jan. 2012): 38–43, doi:10.6091/IBJ.1025.2012; Jennifer L. Herington et al., "Dietary Fish Oil Supplementation Inhibits Formation of Endometriosis-Associated Adhesions in a Chimeric Mouse Model," *Fertility and Sterility* 99, no. 2 (Feb. 2013): 543–50, doi:10.1016/j.fertnstert.2012.10.007.

21. IuB Lishmanov et al., "Plasma Beta-Endorphin and Stress Hormones in Stress and Adaptation," *Bulletin of Experimental Biology and Medicine* 103, no. 4 (April 1987): 422–24.

22. R. Brown et al., "Rhodiola Rosea: A Phytomedicinal Overview," *HerbalGram* 56 (2002): 40–52, http://cms.herbalgram.org/herbalgram/issue56/article2333.html.

23. Kerrie L. Moreau, Brian L. Stauffer, Wendy M. Kohrt, and Douglas R. Seals, "Essential Role of Oestrogen for Improvements in Vascular Endothelial Function with Endurance Exercise in Postmenopausal Women," *The Journal of Clinical Endocrinology & Metabolism* 98, no. 11 (Nov. 2013), 4507–15, doi:10.1210/jc.2013-2183.

11 Harness the Power of Your Cycle

1. Kieran Pender, "Ending Period 'Taboo' Gave USA Marginal Gain at World Cup," *The Telegraph*, July 13, 2019, https://www.telegraph.co.uk /world-cup/2019/07/13/revealed-next-frontier-sports-science-usas -secret-weapon-womens/.

2. D. Eschenbach et al., "Influence of the Normal Menstrual Cycle on Vaginal Tissue, Discharge, and Microflora," *Clinical Infectious Diseases* 30, no. 6 (June 2000): 901–7.

3. E. Sung et al., "Effects of Follicular Versus Luteal Phase–Based Strength Training in Young Women," *SpringerPlus* 3 (Nov. 2014): 668, doi:10.1186 /2193-1801-3-668; N. R. Geiker et al., "A Weight-Loss Program Adapted to the Menstrual Cycle Increases Weight Loss in Healthy, Overweight, Premenopausal Women: A 6-Mo Randomized Controlled Trial," *The American Journal of Clinical Nutrition* 104, no. 1 (July 2016): 15–20, doi: 10.3945/ajcn.115.126565.

4. J. R. Roney and Z. L. Simmons, "Hormonal Predictors of Sexual Motivation in Natural Menstrual Cycles," *Hormones and Behavior* 63, no. 4 (April 2013): 636–45, doi:10.1016/j.yhbeh.2013.02.013.

5. Robert Lustig, *The Hacking of the American Mind: The Science Behind the Corporate Takeover of Our Bodies and Brains* (New York: Avery, 2017), 50–51.

6. Linda A. Bean et al., "Estrogen Receptors, the Hippocampus, and Memory," *The Neuroscientist* 20, no. 5 (Oct. 2014): 534–45.

7. P. M. Maki et al., "Implicit Memory Varies Across the Menstrual Cycle: Oestrogen Effects in Young Women," *Neuropsychologia* 40, no. 5 (2002): 518–29, doi:10.1016/s0028-3932(01)00126-9.

8. Katy Vincent and Irene Tracey, "Hormones and Their Interaction with the Pain Experience," *Reviews in Pain* 2, no. 2 (Dec. 2008): 20–24.

9. Simone D. Herzberg et al., "The Effect of Menstrual Cycle and Contraceptives on ACL Injuries and Laxity: A Systematic Review and Meta-analysis," *Orthopaedic Journal of Sports Medicine* 5, no. 7 (July 2017), 232596711771878, doi:10.1177/2325967117718781.

10. Cheryl A. Frye et al., "Progesterone Can Enhance Consolidation and/ or Performance in Spatial, Object and Working Memory Tasks in Long-Evans Rats," *Animal Behaviour* 78, no. 92 (Aug. 2009): 279–86.

11. A. Salonia et al., "Menstrual Cycle-Related Changes in Plasma Oxytocin Are Relevant to Normal Sexual Function in Healthy Women," *Hormones and Behavior* 47, no. 2 (Feb. 2005): 164–69, doi:10.1016/j.yhbeh.2004.10.002.

12   Better Birth Control

1. Holly Grigg-Spall, *Sweetening the Pill: Or How We Got Hooked on Hormonal Birth Control* (Alresford, Hants, UK: Zer0 Books, 2013), 41.

2. Kimberly Daniels et al., "Current Contraceptive Use and Variation by Selected Characteristics Among Women Aged 15–44: United States, 2011–2013," National Health Statistics Reports no. 86, Nov. 2015, https://www.cdc.gov/nchs/data/nhsr/nhsr086.pdf.

3. Carolin A. Lewis, Ann-Christin S. Kimmig, Rachel G. Zsido, Alexander Jank, Birgit Derntl, and Julia Sacher, "Effects of Hormonal Contraceptives on Mood: A Focus on Emotion Recognition and Reactivity, Reward Processing, and Stress Response," *Current Psychiatry Reports* 21, no. 11 (Nov. 2019), doi:10.1007/s11920-019-1095-z; Anouk E. De Wit, Sanne H. Booij, Erik J. Giltay, Hadine Joffe, Robert A. Schoevers, and Albertine J. Oldehinkel, "Association of Use of Oral Contraceptives with Depressive Symptoms Among Adolescents and Young Women," *JAMA Psychiatry*, (Oct. 2019), doi:10.1001/jamapsychiatry.2019.2838; Petra M. Casey, Kathy L. MacLaughlin, and Stephanie S. Faubion, "Impact of Contraception on Female Sexual Function," *Journal of Women's Health* 26, no. 3 (March 2017), 207–13, doi:10.1089/jwh.2015.5703; Filipa De Castro Coelho and Cremilda Barros, "The Potential of Hormonal Contraception to Influence Female Sexuality," *International Journal of Reproductive Medicine* 2019 (March 2019), 1–9, doi:10.1155/2019/9701384; M. Palmery, A. Saraceno, A. Vaiarelli, G. Carlomagno, "Oral Contraceptives and Changes in Nutritional Requirements," *European Review for Medical and Pharmacological Sciences* 2013;17:1804–1813.

4. Vigil et al., "The Importance of Fertility Awareness in the Assessment of a Woman's Health," 426–50.

5. Allen J. Wilcox, Clarice R. Weinberg, and Donna D. Baird, "Timing of Sexual Intercourse in Relation to Ovulation," *Obstetrical & Gynecological Survey* 51, no. 6 (Dec. 1995), 357–58, doi:10.1097/00006254-1996 06000-00016.

6. P. Frank-Herrmann et al., "The Effectiveness of a Fertility Awareness-Based Method to Avoid Pregnancy in Relation to a Couple's Sexual Behaviour

During the Fertile Time: A Prospective Longitudinal Study," *Human Reproduction* 22, no. 5 (May 2007): 1310–19, doi:10.1093/humrep/dem003.

7. Frank-Herrmann et al., "The Effectiveness of a Fertility Awareness Based Method to Avoid Pregnancy in Relation to a Couple's Sexual Behaviour During the Fertile Time," 1310–19.

8. "How Effective Is Pulling Out?," Planned Parenthood, https://www.planned parenthood.org/learn/birth-control/withdrawal-pull-out-method/how -effective-is-withdrawal-method-pulling-out.

9. Z. Zukerman et al., "Does Preejaculatory Penile Secretion Originating from Cowper's Gland Contain Sperm?," *Journal of Assisted Reproduction and Genetics* 20, no. 4 (April 2003): 157–59, doi:10.1023/a:1022933320700; G. Ilaria, "Detection of HIV-1 DNA Sequences in Pre-Ejaculatory Fluid." *The Lancet* 340, no. 8833 (Dec. 1992), 1469, doi:10.1016/0140-6736(92)92658-3.

10. Stephen R. Killick et al., "Sperm Content of Pre-ejaculatory Fluid," *Human Fertility* 14, no. 1 (March 2011): 48–52, doi:10.3109/14647273.2010.520798; E. Kovavisarach et al., "Presence of Sperm in Pre-Ejaculatory Fluid of Healthy Males," *Journal of the Medical Association of Thailand.* Feb. 2016, 99: S38–41.

11. Bliss Kaneshiro et al., "Long-Term Safety, Efficacy, and Patient Acceptability of the Intrauterine Copper T-380A Contraceptive Device," *International Journal of Women's Health* 2 (Aug. 2010), 211–20, doi:10.2147/ijwh .s6914.

12. Paragard prescribing information pamphlet.

13. Sharon L. Achilles et al., "Impact of Contraceptive Initiation on Vaginal Microbiota," *American Journal of Obstetrics and Gynecology* 218, no. 6 (June 2018): 622.e1–622.e10, doi:10.1016/j.ajog.2018.02.017; Paragard prescribing information pamphlet.

14. "Contraception," CDC, https://www.cdc.gov/reproductivehealth/contra ception/index.htm?.

15. Shahideh Jahanian Sadatmahalleh et al., "Menstrual Pattern Following Tubal Ligation: A Historical Cohort Study," *International Journal of Fertility and Sterility* 9, no. 4 (Jan.–March 2016): 477–82, doi:10.22074/ijfs.2015 .4605.

16. "Contraception," CDC.

17. Dane Johnson and Jay I. Sandlow, "Vasectomy: Tips and Tricks," *Translational Andrology and Urology* 6, no. 4 (2017): 704–9, doi:10.21037/tau.2017.07.08.

18. A. Chandra et al., "Fertility, Family Planning, and Reproductive Health of U.S. Women: Data from the 2002 National Survey of Family Growth," *Vital and Health Statistics* no. 25 (2005): 1–160.

19. "How Effective Are Condoms?," Planned Parenthood, https://www.planned parenthood.org/learn/birth-control/condom/how-effective-are-condoms.

20. "How Effective Are Diaphragms?," Planned Parenthood, https://www .plannedparenthood.org/learn/birth-control/diaphragm/how-effective -are-diaphragms.

21. "How Effective Are Cervical Caps?," Planned Parenthood, https://www .plannedparenthood.org/learn/birth-control/cervical-cap/how-effective -are-cervical-caps.

22. "How Effective Is the Sponge?," Planned Parenthood, https://www.planned parenthood.org/learn/birth-control/birth-control-sponge/how-effective -sponge.

23. Katherine A. Liu and Natalie A. Dipietro Mager, "Women's Involvement in Clinical Trials: Historical Perspective and Future Implications," *Pharmacy Practice* 14, no. 1 (Jan.–March 2016): 708, doi:10.18549/PharmPract .2016.01.708.

24. "Technology," Daysy, https://daysy.me/technology/.

25. "How Ava Works," Ava Women, https://www.avawomen.com/how-ava -works/.

INDEX

NOTE: Page numbers in *italics* indicate a figure or chart

food journal, 232
fraternal twins, 8
fructose avoidance, reasons for, 99
fruit, 99–100
FSH. *See* follical stimulating
    hormone
fungal overgrowth in the gut, 149

GABA, 95
gelatin for gut health, 165
genetically modified organisms
    (GMOs), 96, 98, 151
genetics and genetic factors
    overview, 76
    and liver detoxification, 181–82
    and missing periods, 67–68
    and PCOS, 76
    PMS, PMDD, and, 48
    and portal system of the liver, 176
genetic testing, 237
Gersh, Felice, 40
getting grounded (walk barefoot on
    the earth), 204–5
global health crisis, too much sugar
    as, 118–19
glucose. *See entries beginning with*
    "blood sugar"
glucose testing meter, 136–39
glutathione, 181, 185, 187, 242
gluten and gluten sensitivity, 97–98,
    152–4
gluten-free whole grains, 97–99
glycemic index, 99
GMOs (genetically modified organ-
    isms), 96, 98, 151
GnRH (gonadotropin-releasing
    hormone), 6–7
goitrogens, 91–92
gonadotropin-releasing hormone
    (GnRH), 6–7
gonorrhea, 55
Gottfried, Sara, 227
grains, gluten-free whole, 97–99
Grave's disease, 221

Grigg-Spall, Holly, 259–60
gut dysbiosis, 151–52, 155–57, 159
gut-healing supplements, 165
gut health issues
    gluten-related, 98
    gut barrier harm from gluten, 154
    gut-brain axis transmits gut
      inflammation to the brain,
      154–55
    histamine intolerance, 157–58
    PMS, PMDD, and, 48
    from stress, 199
    unhealthy microbiome, 148–49
    vaginal bacteria and gut bacteria
      correlation, 159
    and vaginal infections, 74
    See also leaky gut; Week Three:
      Fix Your Gut
gut microbiome, 148–49, 237

H. pylori in the gut, 149, 237
hangry feelings, 37, 123, 135, 195
Hashimoto's thyroiditis, 198–99,
    221, 224
hCG (human chorionic
    gonadotropin) hormone, 10
heart disease and sugar addiction,
    119
heavy periods (menorrhagia)
    overview, 4, 16–17, 57
    cause of, 57–58
    Jardim's experience with, xvii–xviii
    in perimenopause, 23–24
    with secondary dysmenorrhea, 54
Helicobacter pylori in the gut, 149,
    237
Herxheimer reaction to gut detox,
    165–66
histamine intolerance, 157–58, 165
histamines in fermented foods, 166
hormonal birth control, 21, 67, 72,
    260–62
hormonal cravings and PMS,
    133–35

NFP (natural family planning) birth
control, 263–66
nonhormonal birth control. See
birth control, nonhormonal
No Period. Now What? (Rinaldi), 242
norepinephrine, 134, 191–93, *192*
NSAIDS, 53, 151
nutrients
in leafy greens, 88, 89–90
PMS, PMDD, and deficiencies, 48
in sprouts and microgreens, 93
underexposure to, 169
nutritional therapist or nutrition
consultant, 314
Nutritional Therapy Association, 314
nuts and seeds, 105–6, 107

obesity or excess weight
and addiction to sugar, 119
and anovulatory cycles, 86–87
and aromatase in fat cells, 127, *127*
bisphenol-A exposure related to,
174
estrogen excess due to, 87
oligomenorrhea (erratic menstrual
schedule), 63–65
oligomenorrhea (infrequent or
irregular periods), 4, 22, 31–32,
54, 63–65, 309
oligoovulation (irregular ovulation),
75
omega-3 and omega-6 fatty acids,
102–5, 242
organic pollutants (POPs), 218
organophosphate pesticides, health
problems associated with, 172
ovarian cysts, 55, 128
ovarian follicles, 7
ovaries
inflammation in, 152
insulin receptors on, 125
as source of testosterone, 42
toxic effects of synthetic
xenoestrogens, 174

overweight. *See* obesity or excess
weight
ovulation
overview, 3–4
and basal body temperature, 28–29
birth control pills vs., xxi
cervical fluid during, 28
effect of insulin resistance, 128
estradiol's role in, 40
and infrequent or irregular
periods, 64
irregular ovulation and PCOS, 75
and length of menstrual cycle,
12–13
and likelihood of pregnancy, 8
and melatonin level, 193
melatonin supplements vs., 43–44
mid-cycle or ovulatory pain, 56
ovulatory phase of the menstrual
cycle, 8–9
and PCOS, 74
and peak day, 28
and PMS symptoms, 51
short cycles vs., 62
and thyroid disease, 215
timing of, during menstrual
cycle, 13
ovulatory spotting mid-cycle, 8
oxalic acid (oxalates), 92
oxidized fats, 106
oxytocin, 5

painful bladder syndrome
(interstitial cystitis), 92,
155–57, 160
pancreas as source of insulin, 121–22
Paragard (copper) IUD, 55, 59,
268–69
parasites in the gut, 149, 242
PCBs (polychlorinated biphenyls), 218
PCOS. *See* polycystic ovary
syndrome
peak day, 28
peanuts, 95–96

NICOLE JARDIM is a certified women's health coach, writer, speaker, mentor, and the creator of Fix Your Period, a program that empowers women to reclaim their hormone health using a method that combines evidence-based information with simplicity and sass. Her work has impacted the lives of tens of thousands of women around the world by effectively addressing a wide variety of period problems, including PMS, irregular periods, PCOS, painful and heavy periods, missing periods, and more. Nicole is also a co-host of *The Period Party*, a top-rated podcast on iTunes—be sure to tune in if you want to learn more about how to fix your period.

Her passion for women's health stems from her own health challenges and negative experience with hormonal birth control in her early twenties. After working with an acupuncturist to regain her health, she knew that sharing her experience could benefit many others in the same situation. She became a certified health coach and took further specialised training in women's hormonal health with industry visionaries such as Dr. Sara Gottfried; Dr. Jessica Drummond, founder of the Integrative Women's Health Institute; and Chris Kresser, founder of the Kresser Institute.

Rather than just treating symptoms, Nicole helps women address the root cause of their period problems. She passionately believes that the fundamentals of healing any hormonal imbalance lie in an approach that addresses each woman's unique physiology. This is essential to reclaiming and maintaining optimal health and vitality at any age.